2012
YEAR BOOK OF
ANESTHESIOLOGY AND
PAIN MANAGEMENT™

The 2012 Year Book Series

Year Book of Anesthesiology and Pain Management™: Drs Chestnut, Abram, Black, Gravlee, Lien, Mathru, and Roizen

Year Book of Cardiology®: Drs Gersh, Cheitlin, Elliott, Gold, Graham, and Thourani

Year Book of Critical Care Medicine®: Drs Dries, Zanotti-Cavazzoni, Latenser, Martinez, Rincon, and Zwank

Year Book of Dermatology and Dermatologic Surgery™: Dr Del Rosso

Year Book of Diagnostic Radiology®: Drs Elster, Abbara, Oestreich, Offiah, Rosado de Christenson, Stephens, and Strickland

Year Book of Emergency Medicine®: Drs Hamilton, Bruno, Handly, Minczak, Mullin, Quintana, and Ramoska

Year Book of Endocrinology®: Drs Schott, Apovian, Clarke, Eugster, Ludlam, Meikle, Oetgen, Ovalle, Schteingart, and Toth

Year Book of Gastroenterology™: Drs Talley, DeVault, Harnois, Murray, Pearson, Philcox, Picco, and Smith

Year Book of Hand and Upper Limb Surgery®: Drs Yao, Adams, Isaacs, Lee, and Rizzo

Year Book of Medicine®: Drs Barker, Garrick, Gersh, Khardori, LeRoith, Panush, Talley, and Thigpen

Year Book of Neonatal and Perinatal Medicine®: Drs Fanaroff, Benitz, Donn, Neu, Papile, Polin, and Van Marter

Year Book of Neurology and Neurosurgery®: Drs Klimo, Minagar, Gandhi, House, Liu, Mazia, Panagariya, Ragel, Riesenburger, Robottom, Schwendimann, Shafazand, Uhm, and Yang

Year Book of Obstetrics, Gynecology, and Women's Health®: Drs Dungan and Shulman

Year Book of Oncology®: Drs Arceci, Bauer, Chiorean, Gordon, Lawton, Murphy, Thigpen, and Tsao

Year Book of Ophthalmology®: Drs Rapuano, Cohen, Flanders, Hammersmith, Milman, Myers, Nagra, Nelson, Penne, Pyfer, Sergott, Shields, Talekar, and Vander

Year Book of Orthopedics®: Drs Morrey, Huddleston, Rose, Swiontkowski, and Trigg

Year Book of Otolaryngology-Head and Neck Surgery®: Drs Sindwani, Balough, Franco, Gapany, and Mitchell

Year Book of Pathology and Laboratory Medicine®: Drs Raab and Bissell

Year Book of Pediatrics®: Dr Stockman

Year Book of Plastic and Aesthetic Surgery™: Drs Miller, Gosman, Gurtner, Gutowski, Ruberg, Salisbury, and Smith

Year Book of Psychiatry and Applied Mental Health®: Drs Talbott, Ballenger, Buckley, Frances, Krupnick, and Mack

Year Book of Pulmonary Disease®: Drs Barker, Jones, Maurer, Spradley, Tanoue, and Willsie

Year Book of Sports Medicine®: Drs Shephard, Cantu, Feldman, Galea, Jankowski, Janssen, Lebrun, and Nieman

Year Book of Surgery®: Drs Copeland, Behrns, Daly, Eberlein, Fahey, Huber, Klodell, Mozingo, and Pruett

Year Book of Urology®: Drs Andriole and Coplen

Year Book of Vascular Surgery®: Drs Moneta, Gillespie, Starnes, and Watkins

2012

The Year Book of ANESTHESIOLOGY AND PAIN MANAGEMENT™

Editor-in-Chief
David H. Chestnut, MD

Associate Editors
Stephen E. Abram, MD
Susan Black, MD
Glenn P. Gravlee, MD
Cynthia A. Lien, MD
Mali Mathru, MD, FCCP
Michael F. Roizen, MD

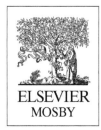

ELSEVIER
MOSBY

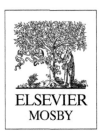

ELSEVIER
MOSBY

Vice President, Continuity: Kimberly Murphy
Developmental Editor: Yonah Korngold
Production Supervisor, Electronic Year Books: Donna M. Skelton
Electronic Article Manager: Mike Sheets
Illustrations and Permissions Coordinator: Dawn A. Vohsen

2012 EDITION

Printed and bound by CPI Group (UK) Ltd, Croydon, CR0 4YY
Transferred to Digital Print 2012

Editorial Office:
Elsevier
1600 John F. Kennedy Boulevard
Suite 1800
Philadelphia, PA 19103-2899

International Standard Serial Number: 1073-5437
International Standard Book Number: 978-0-323-08873-2

Editorial Board

Table of Contents

Journals Represented

Journals represented in this YEAR BOOK are listed below.

Academic Emergency Medicine
Acta Anaesthesiologica Scandinavica
Acta Obstetricia et Gynecologica Scandinavica
AJNR American Journal of Neuroradiology
American Heart Journal
American Journal of Cardiology
American Journal of Clinical Nutrition
American Journal of Emergency Medicine
American Journal of Epidemiology
American Journal of Health Promotion
American Journal of Medicine
American Journal of Obstetrics and Gynecology
American Journal of Pathology
American Journal of Public Health
American Journal of Respiratory and Critical Care Medicine
American Journal of Respiratory Cell and Molecular Biology
Anaesthesia
Anaesthesia and Intensive Care
Anesthesia & Analgesia
Anesthesiology
Annals of Surgical Oncology
Annals of Thoracic Surgery
Archives of Disease in Childhood Fetal and Neonatal Edition
Archives of Internal Medicine
Archives of Neurology
Archives of Ophthalmology
Archives of Otolaryngology Head & Neck Surgery
Australia & New Zealand Journal of Obstetrics & Gynaecology
British Journal of Anaesthesia
British Medical Journal
Canadian Journal of Anaesthesia
Cell
Chest
Circulation
Clinical Journal of Pain Clinical Toxicology
Critical Care Medicine
Diabetes Care
European Journal of Cancer
European Journal of Pain
Gastrointestinal Endoscopy
Intensive Care Medicine
International Journal of Gynaecology & Obstetrics
International Journal of Obstetric Anesthesia
Journal of Applied Physiology
Journal of Bone and Joint Surgery (American)
Journal of Cardiothoracic and Vascular Anesthesia
Journal of Clinical Anesthesia

Journal of Clinical Psychiatry
Journal of Immunology
Journal of Neurosurgery
Journal of Neurosurgery Spine
Journal of Nutrition
Journal of Oral and Maxillofacial Surgery
Journal of Pain
Journal of Pain and Symptom Management
Journal of Pathology
Journal of Surgical Research
Journal of the American College of Cardiology
Journal of the American College of Surgeons
Journal of the American Geriatrics Society
Journal of the American Medical Association
Journal of the American Society of Echocardiography
Journal of Thoracic and Cardiovascular Surgery
Journal of Trauma
Lancet
Laryngoscope
Neurosurgery
New England Journal of Medicine
Obstetrics & Gynecology
Pain
Pediatric Radiology
Pediatrics
Plastic and Reconstructive Surgery
Public Library of Science Medicine
Radiology
Regional Anesthesia and Pain Medicine
Social Science & Medicine
Spine
Spine Journal
Stroke
Surgery
Transfusion
World Neurosurgery

STANDARD ABBREVIATIONS

The following terms are abbreviated in this edition: acquired immunodeficiency syndrome (AIDS), cardiopulmonary resuscitation (CPR), central nervous system (CNS), cerebrospinal fluid (CSF), computed tomography (CT), deoxyribonucleic acid (DNA), electrocardiography (ECG), health maintenance organization (HMO), human immunodeficiency virus (HIV), intensive care unit (ICU), intramuscular (IM), intravenous (IV), magnetic resonance (MR) imaging (MRI), ribonucleic acid (RNA), ultrasound (US), and ultraviolet (UV).

NOTE

The YEAR BOOK OF ANESTHESIOLOGY AND PAIN MANAGEMENT™ is a literature survey service providing abstracts of articles published in the professional literature. Every effort is made to ensure the accuracy of the information presented in these pages.

Neither the editors nor the publisher of the YEAR BOOK OF ANESTHESIOLOGY AND PAIN MANAGEMENT™ can be responsible for errors in the original materials. The editors' comments are their own opinions. Mention of specific products within this publication does not constitute endorsement.

To facilitate the use of the YEAR BOOK OF ANESTHESIOLOGY AND PAIN MANAGEMENT™ as a reference tool, all illustrations and tables included in this publication are now identified as they appear in the original article. This change is meant to help the reader recognize that any illustration or table appearing in the YEAR BOOK OF ANESTHESIOLOGY AND PAIN MANAGEMENT™ may be only one of many in the original article. For this reason, figure and table numbers will often appear to be out of sequence within the YEAR BOOK OF ANESTHESIOLOGY AND PAIN MANAGEMENT™.

1 Studies of Outcomes, Risks, Costs, and Benefits

A meta-analysis shows that docosahexaenoic acid from algal oil reduces serum triglycerides and increases HDL-cholesterol and LDL-cholesterol in persons without coronary heart disease
Bernstein AM, Ding EL, Willett WC, et al (Wellness Inst of the Cleveland Clinic, Lyndhurst, OH; Harvard School of Public Health, Boston, MA)
J Nutr 142:99-104, 2012

Certain algae contain the (n-3) fatty acid DHA, yet the relation between algal oil supplementation and cardiovascular disease risk factors has not been systematically examined. Our objective was to examine the relation between algal oil supplementation and cardiovascular disease risk factors. We conducted a systematic review of randomized controlled trials published between 1996 and 2011 examining the relation between algal oil supplementation and cardiovascular disease risk factors and performed a meta-analysis of the association between algal oil DHA supplementation and changes in the concentrations of TG, LDL-cholesterol (LDL-C), and HDL-cholesterol (HDL-C). We identified 11 randomized controlled trials with 485 healthy participants that evaluated the relation between algal oil DHA supplementation and TG, LDL-C, and HDL-C. The median dose of algal DHA was 1.68 g/d. The pooled estimate for the change in TG concentration was -0.20 mmol/L (95% CI: -0.27 to -0.14), 0.23 mmol/L (95% CI: 0.16$-$0.30) for LDL-C, and 0.07 mmol/L (95% CI: 0.05$-$0.10) for HDL-C. DHA supplementation from algal oil, a marine source of (n-3) fatty acids not extracted from fish, may reduce serum TG and increase HDL-C and LDL-C in persons without coronary heart disease.

▶ There are a lot of reasons to take docosahexaenoic acid (DHA), which really converts back to eicosapentaenoic acid to decrease heart disease. But it is not just the heart that the DHA helps. DHA helps the brain, eyes and joints and decreases inflammation throughout the body. And it seems that it also decreases the lipid risk factors for arterial aging.

M. F. Roizen, MD

1

Accuracy of Stated Energy Contents of Restaurant Foods

Urban LE, McCrory MA, Dallal GE, et al (Tufts Univ, Boston, MA; Purdue Univ, West Lafayette, IN; et al)
JAMA 306:287-293, 2011

Context.—National recommendations for the prevention and treatment of obesity emphasize reducing energy intake. Foods purchased in restaurants provide approximately 35% of the daily energy intake in US individuals but the accuracy of the energy contents listed for these foods is unknown.

Objective.—To examine the accuracy of stated energy contents of foods purchased in restaurants.

Design and Setting.—A validated bomb calorimetry technique was used to measure dietary energy in food from 42 restaurants, comprising 269 total food items and 242 unique foods. The restaurants and foods were randomly selected from quick-serve and sit-down restaurants in Massachusetts, Arkansas, and Indiana between January and June 2010.

Main Outcome Measure.—The difference between restaurant-stated and laboratory-measured energy contents, which were corrected for standard metabolizable energy conversion factors.

Results.—The absolute stated energy contents were not significantly different from the absolute measured energy contents overall (difference of 10 kcal/portion; 95% confidence interval [CI], −15 to 34 kcal/portion; $P=.52$); however, the stated energy contents of individual foods were variable relative to the measured energy contents. Of the 269 food items, 50 (19%) contained measured energy contents of at least 100 kcal/portion more than the stated energy contents. Of the 10% of foods with the highest excess energy in the initial sampling, 13 of 17 were available for a second sampling. In the first analysis, these foods contained average measured energy contents of 289 kcal/portion (95% CI, 186 to 392 kcal/portion) more than the stated energy contents; in the second analysis, these foods contained average measured energy contents of 258 kcal/portion (95% CI, 154 to 361 kcal/portion) more than the stated energy contents ($P<.001$ for each vs 0 kcal/portion difference). In addition, foods with lower stated energy contents contained higher measured energy contents than stated, while foods with higher stated energy contents contained lower measured energy contents ($P<.001$).

Conclusions.—Stated energy contents of restaurant foods were accurate overall. However, there was substantial inaccuracy for some individual foods, with understated energy contents for those with lower energy contents.

▶ This junk food restaurant junking up the calorie counts is disgraceful. Roughly 20% of the tested samples contained at least 100-kcal-per-portion higher than the stated amounts. These are discrepancies in portion size clearly highlighted for desserts, carbohydrate-rich food, and salads—and guess what—the errors were in ways that make the dieter's life more difficult and reduce the job competitiveness of the fast food patron. But even more amazing, collectively, snacks, desserts, and pizza represent 30% of the typical populations' average caloric intake and 40% of that in adolescents from age 14 to 19. We aren't feeding our kids very well. With the passage of the US patient protection and affordable care act, labeling of caloric content is mandated in restaurants and by food needs enhanced by effective public health education to ensure the manufacturers have accurate data on menus...and to penalize them big time if they keep trying to deceive us.

M. F. Roizen, MD

Association of change in daily step count over five years with insulin sensitivity and adiposity: population based cohort study

Dwyer T, Ponsonby A-L, Ukoumunne OC, et al (Royal Children's Hosp, Parkville, Melbourne, Australia; et al)
BMJ 341:c7249, 2010

Objectives.—To investigate the association between change in daily step count and both adiposity and insulin sensitivity and the extent to which the association between change in daily step count and insulin sensitivity may be mediated by adiposity.

Design.—Population based cohort study.

Setting.—Tasmania, Australia.

Participants.—592 adults (men (n=267), mean age 51.4 (SD 12.2) years; women (n=325), mean age 50.3 (12.3) years) who participated in the Tasmanian component of the national AusDiab Study in 2000 and 2005.

Main Outcome Measures.—Body mass index, waist to hip ratio, and HOMA insulin sensitivity at follow-up in 2005.

Results.—Over the five year period, the daily step count decreased for 65% (n=382) of participants. Having a higher daily step count in 2005 than in 2000 was independently associated with lower body mass index (0.08 (95% confidence interval 0.04 to 0.12) lower per 1000 steps), lower waist to hip ratio (0.15 (0.07 to 0.23) lower), and greater insulin sensitivity (1.38 (0.14 to 2.63) HOMA units higher) in 2005. The mean increase in HOMA units fell to 0.34 (−0.79 to 1.47) after adjustment for body mass index in 2005.

Conclusions.—Among community dwelling, middle aged adults, a higher daily step count at five year follow-up than at baseline was associated with better insulin sensitivity. This effect seems to be largely mediated through lower adiposity.

▶ We have known for a long time that for some reason, 10 000 steps is key to preventing type 2 diabetes, but we have never known why. This study helps show that a higher daily step count is associated with better insulin sensitivity. Whether this insulin sensitivity is caused by reduced fat per se or whether this change leads to less fat isn't clear, but what is clear is that all of us should be walking around more in the operating room.

M. F. Roizen, MD

Association of ICU or Hospital Admission With Unintentional Discontinuation of Medications for Chronic Diseases

Bell CM, Brener SS, Gunraj N, et al (Univ of Toronto, Ontario, Canada; Inst for Clinical Evaluative Sciences, Toronto, Ontario, Canada)
JAMA 306:840-847, 2011

Context.—Patients discharged from acute care hospitals may be at risk for unintentional discontinuation of medications prescribed for chronic diseases. The intensive care unit (ICU) may pose an even greater risk because of the focus on acute events and the presence of multiple transitions in care.

Objective.—To evaluate rates of potentially unintentional discontinuation of medications following hospital or ICU admission.

Design, Setting, and Patients.—A population-based cohort study using administrative records from 1997 to 2009 of all hospitalizations and outpatient prescriptions in Ontario, Canada; it included 396 380 patients aged 66 years or older with continuous use of at least 1 of 5 evidence-based medication groups prescribed for long-term use: (1) statins, (2) antiplatelet/anticoagulant agents, (3) levothyroxine, (4) respiratory inhalers, and (5) gastric acid–suppressing drugs. Rates of medication discontinuation were compared across 3 groups: patients admitted to the ICU, patients hospitalized without ICU admission, and nonhospitalized patients (controls). Odds ratios (ORs) were calculated and adjusted for patient demographics, clinical factors, and health services use.

Main Outcome Measures.—The primary outcome was failure to renew the prescription within 90 days after hospital discharge.

Results.—Patients admitted to the hospital (n=187 912) were more likely to experience potentially unintentional discontinuation of medications than controls (n=208 468) across all medication groups examined. The adjusted ORs (AORs) ranged from 1.18 (95% CI, 1.14-1.23) for discontinuing levothyroxine in 12.3% of hospitalized patients (n=6831) vs 11.0% of controls (n=7114) to an AOR of 1.86 (95% CI, 1.77-1.97) for discontinuing antiplatelet/anticoagulant agents in 19.4% of hospitalized patients (n=5564) vs 11.8% of controls (n=2535). With ICU exposure, the AORs ranged from 1.48 (95% CI, 1.39-1.57) for discontinuing statins in 14.6% of ICU patients (n=1484) to an AOR of 2.31 (95% CI, 2.07-2.57) for discontinuing antiplatelet/anticoagulant agents in 22.8% of ICU patients (n=522) vs the control group. Admission to an ICU was associated with an additional risk of medication discontinuation in 4 of 5 medication groups vs hospitalizations without an ICU admission. One-year follow-up of patients who discontinued medications showed an elevated AOR for the secondary composite outcome of death, emergency department visit, or emergent hospitalization of 1.07 (95% CI, 1.03-1.11) in the statins group and of 1.10 (95% CI, 1.03-1.16) in the antiplatelet/anticoagulant agents group.

Conclusions.—Patients prescribed medications for chronic diseases were at risk for potentially unintentional discontinuation after hospital admission.

Admission to the ICU was generally associated with an even higher risk of medication discontinuation.

▶ Geez. I can't believe it. How can medications be discontinued so commonly on admission to an intensive care unit or hospital when you have medication reconciliation lists and all the other devices, instruments, and reminders to try and not have this happen? It is very tough, and clearly the more systems we have that help us, the better we will be.

M. F. Roizen, MD

Conjugated linoleic acid supplementation for 8 weeks does not affect body composition, lipid profile, or safety biomarkers in overweight, hyperlipidemic men

Joseph SV, Jacques H, Plourde M, et al (Laval Univ, Quebec, Canada)
J Nutr 141:1286-1291, 2011

The usefulness of conjugated linoleic acid (CLA) as a nutraceutical remains ambiguous. Our objective was, therefore, to investigate the effect of CLA on body composition, blood lipids, and safety biomarkers in over-weight, hyperlipidemic men. A double-blinded, 3-phase crossover trial was conducted in overweight (BMI $\geq$ 25 kg/m^2), borderline hypercholesterolemic [LDL-cholesterol (C) $\geq$ 2.5 mmol/L] men aged 18-60 y. During three 8-wk phases, each separated by a 4-wk washout period, 27 participants consumed under supervision in random order 3.5 g/d of safflower oil (control), a 50:50 mixture of *trans* 10, *cis* 12 and *cis* 9, *trans* 11 ($c9$, $t11$) CLA:Clarinol G-80, and $c9$, $t11$ isomer:$c9$, $t11$ CLA. At baseline and endpoint of each phase, body weight, body fat mass, and lean body mass were measured by DXA. Blood lipid profiles and safety biomarkers, including insulin sensitivity, blood concentrations of adiponectin, and inflammatory (high sensitive-C-reactive protein, TNFα, and IL-6) and oxidative (oxidized-LDL) molecules, were measured. The effect of CLA consumption on fatty acid oxidation was also assessed. Compared with the control treatment, the CLA treatments did not affect changes in body weight, body composition, or blood lipids. In addition, CLA did not affect the β-oxidation rate of fatty acids or induce significant alterations in the safety markers tested. In conclusion, although no detrimental effects were caused by supplementation, these results do not confirm a role for CLA in either body weight or blood lipid regulation in humans.

▶ This study and the study by Asp et al[1] come to exactly opposite conclusions. They are both randomized, they are both approximately the same length of time, they both seem to be well done, and one was performed in men and the other in women. Are men and women that different in their response to linoleic acid supplementation? This is not clear to me, but what is clear is that whatever the end result, it won't make a huge difference because neither study had large changes in outcome.

M. F. Roizen, MD

Reference

1. Asp ML, Collene AL, Norris LE, et al. Time-dependent effects of safflower oil to improve glycemia, inflammation and blood lipids in obese, post-menopausal women with type 2 diabetes: A randomized, double-masked, crossover study. *Clinical Nutrition.* 2011:1-7.

Diet intervention and cerebrospinal fluid biomarkers in amnestic mild cognitive impairment

Bayer-Carter JL, Green PS, Montine TJ, et al (Veterans Affairs Puget Sound Health Care System, Seattle, WA)
Arch Neurol 68:743-752, 2011

Objective.—To compare the effects of a 4-week high-saturated fat/high-glycemic index (HIGH) diet with a low-saturated fat/low-glycemic index (LOW) diet on insulin and lipid metabolism, cerebrospinal fluid (CSF) markers of Alzheimer disease, and cognition for healthy adults and adults with amnestic mild cognitive impairment (aMCI).

Design.—Randomized controlled trial.

Setting.—Veterans Affairs Medical Center clinical research unit.

Participants.—Forty-nine older adults (20 healthy adults with a mean [SD] age of 69.3 [7.4] years and 29 adults with aMCI with a mean [SD] age of 67.6 [6.8] years).

Intervention.—Participants received the HIGH diet (fat, 45% [saturated fat, > 25%]; carbohydrates, 35%-40% [glycemic index, > 70]; and protein, 15%-20%) or the LOW diet (fat, 25%; [saturated fat, < 7%]; carbohydrates, 55%-60% [glycemic index, < 55]; and protein, 15%-20%) for 4 weeks. Cognitive tests, an oral glucose tolerance test, and lumbar puncture were conducted at baseline and during the fourth week of the diet.

Main Outcome Measures.—The CSF concentrations of β-amyloid (Aβ42 and Aβ40), tau protein, insulin, F2-isoprostanes, and apolipoprotein E, plasma lipids and insulin, and measures of cognition.

Results.—For the aMCI group, the LOW diet increased CSF Aβ42 concentrations, contrary to the pathologic pattern of lowered CSF Aβ42 typically observed in Alzheimer disease. The LOW diet had the opposite effect for healthy adults, ie, decreasing CSF Aβ42, whereas the HIGH diet increased CSF Aβ42. The CSF apolipoprotein E concentration was increased by the LOW diet and decreased by the HIGH diet for both groups. For the aMCI group, the CSF insulin concentration increased with the LOW diet, but the HIGH diet lowered the CSF insulin concentration for healthy adults. The HIGH diet increased and the LOW diet decreased plasma lipids, insulin, and CSF F2-isoprostane concentrations. Delayed visual memory improved for both groups after completion of 4 weeks of the LOW diet.

Conclusion.—Our results suggest that diet may be a powerful environmental factor that modulates Alzheimer disease risk through its effects on central nervous system concentrations of Aβ42, lipoproteins, oxidative stress, and insulin.

▶ The impressive thing with this is that a diet low in saturated fat, high in fruits and vegetables, and low in added sugar rapidly decreases markers of cognitive impairment. The low diet here, I must admit, is exactly what we determined from the literature and published in the *You on a Diet* book as the ideal for healthy living.

M. F. Roizen, MD

Dietary ω-3 fatty acid and fish intake and incident age-related macular degeneration in women
Christen WG, Schaumberg DA, Glynn RJ, et al (Brigham and Women's Hosp and Harvard Med School, Boston, MA)
Arch Ophthalmol 129:921-929, 2011

Objective.—To examine whether intake of ω-3 fatty acids and fish affects incidence of age-related macular degeneration (AMD) in women.

Design.—A detailed food-frequency questionnaire was administered at baseline among 39 876 female health professionals (mean [SD] age: 54.6 [7.0] years). A total of 38 022 women completed the questionnaire and were free of a diagnosis of AMD. The main outcome measure was incident AMD responsible for a reduction in best-corrected visual acuity to 20/30 or worse based on self-report confirmed by medical record review.

Results.—A total of 235 cases of AMD, most characterized by some combination of drusen and retinal pigment epithelial changes, were confirmed during an average of 10 years of follow-up. Women in the highest tertile of intake for docosahexaenoic acid, compared with those in the lowest, had a multivariate-adjusted relative risk of AMD of 0.62 (95% confidence interval, 0.44-0.87). For eicosapentaenoic acid, women in the highest tertile of intake had a relative risk of 0.66 (95% confidence interval, 0.48-0.92). Consistent with the findings for docosahexaenoic acid and eicosapentaenoic acid, women who consumed 1 or more servings of fish per week, compared with those who consumed less than 1 serving per month, had a relative risk of AMD of 0.58 (95% confidence interval, 0.38-0.87).

Conclusion.—These prospective data from a large cohort of female health professionals without a diagnosis of AMD at baseline indicate that regular consumption of docosahexaenoic acid and eicosapentaenoic acid and fish was associated with a significantly decreased risk of incident AMD and may be of benefit in primary prevention of AMD.

▶ This study was part of a women's health study and clearly examined whether omega-3 fatty acid intake was associated with age-related macular degeneration.

These data combine with those on lutein to show that these 2 alone seem to prevent more than 40% of age-related macular degeneration. I guess that means that not only our brains but our eyes, heart, and joints are all beneficiaries of more docosahexaenoic acid (DHA) omega-3. What this means to me is that I will continue to take 900 mg of algal DHA per day. It is clear that 900 mg is good for your brain, but it isn't clear whether you need that much for your eyes.

M. F. Roizen, MD

Differences in health between Americans and Western Europeans: Effects on longevity and public finance
Michaud P-C, Goldman D, Lakdawalla D, et al (Université du Québec à Montréal, Canada; Univ of Southern California and RAND Corporation, CA; et al)
Soc Sci Med 73:254-263, 2011

In 1975, 50 year-old Americans could expect to live slightly longer than most of their Western European counterparts. By 2005, American life expectancy had fallen behind that of most Western European countries. We find that this growing longevity gap is primarily due to real declines in the health of near-elderly Americans, relative to their Western European peers. We use a microsimulation approach to project what US longevity would look like, if US health trends approximated those in Western Europe. The model implies that differences in health can explain most of the growing gap in remaining life expectancy. In addition, we quantify the public finance consequences of this deterioration in health. The model predicts that gradually moving American cohorts to the health status enjoyed by Western Europeans could save up to $1.1 trillion in discounted total health expenditures from 2004 to 2050.

▶ This article goes to the heart of the matter of job noncompetitiveness in the United States. Not only are we living less long than Western Europeans, but we pay considerably more in total medical costs for illness care. That leads to job discompetitiveness as well as a $1.1 trillion extra expenditure. If we took control of the 5 major factors in health—tobacco use, physical activity, food choices and portion size, stress, and sleep, we could reduce costs for illness care related to chronic disease to such a degree as to cut our budget deficit by more than 75% per year. And we actually could be much more competitive for jobs. This article strikes at the heart of what we need to do in America if we are to be job competitive with the rest of the world. Without this we will have much higher illness care costs that will eventually lead to rationing or loss of freedom. But this article shows that we/you are in control.

M. F. Roizen, MD

Effect of a dietary portfolio of cholesterol-lowering foods given at 2 levels of intensity of dietary advice on serum lipids in hyperlipidemia: a randomized controlled trial

Jenkins DJ, Jones PJ, Lamarche B, et al (St Michael's Hosp, Toronto, Ontario, Canada; Univ of Toronto, Ontario, Canada; Laval Univ, Quebec City, Canada; et al)

JAMA 306:831-839, 2011

Context.—Combining foods with recognized cholesterol-lowering properties (dietary portfolio) has proven highly effective in lowering serum cholesterol under metabolically controlled conditions.

Objective.—To assess the effect of a dietary portfolio administered at 2 levels of intensity on percentage change in low-density lipoprotein cholesterol (LDL-C) among participants following self-selected diets.

Design, Setting, and Participants.—A parallel-design study of 351 participants with hyperlipidemia from 4 participating academic centers across Canada (Quebec City, Toronto, Winnipeg, and Vancouver) randomized between June 25, 2007, and February 19, 2009, to 1 of 3 treatments lasting 6 months.

Intervention.—Participants received dietary advice for 6 months on either a low–saturated fat therapeutic diet (control) or a dietary portfolio, for which counseling was delivered at different frequencies, that emphasized dietary incorporation of plant sterols, soy protein, viscous fibers, and nuts. Routine dietary portfolio involved 2 clinic visits over 6 months and intensive dietary portfolio involved 7 clinic visits over 6 months.

Main Outcome Measures.—Percentage change in serum LDL-C.

Results.—In the modified intention-to-treat analysis of 345 participants, the overall attrition rate was not significantly different between treatments (18% for intensive dietary portfolio, 23% for routine dietary portfolio, and 26% for control; Fisher exact test, $P = .33$). The LDL-C reductions from an overall mean of 171 mg/dL (95% confidence interval [CI], 168–174 mg/dL) were −13.8% (95% CI, −17.2% to −10.3%; $P < .001$) or −26 mg/dL (95% CI, −31 to −21 mg/dL; $P < .001$) for the intensive dietary portfolio; −13.1% (95% CI, −16.7% to −9.5%; $P < .001$) or −24 mg/dL (95% CI, −30 to −19 mg/dL; $P < .001$) for the routine dietary portfolio; and −3.0% (95% CI, −6.1% to 0.1%; $P = .06$) or −8 mg/dL (95% CI, −13 to −3 mg/dL; $P = .002$) for the control diet. Percentage LDL-C reductions for each dietary portfolio were significantly more than the control diet ($P < .001$, respectively). The 2 dietary portfolio interventions did not differ significantly ($P = .66$). Among participants randomized to one of the dietary portfolio interventions, percentage reduction in LDL-C on the dietary portfolio was associated with dietary adherence (r = −0.34, n = 157, $P < .001$).

Conclusion.—Use of a dietary portfolio compared with the low-saturated fat dietary advice resulted in greater LDL-C lowering during 6 months of follow-up.

Trial Registration.—clinicaltrials.gov Identifier: NCT00438425.

▶ Nuts, viscous fiber, soy protein, plant sterols, and the avoidance of saturated fat seem to be lifestyle changes that result in significant and major reductions in low-density lipoprotein cholesterol. Is it possible to have this and enjoy food and eating? Absolutely. I do it every day.

M. F. Roizen, MD

Effects of prenatal fish-oil and 5-methyltetrahydrofolate supplementation on cognitive development of children at 6.5 y of age
Campoy C, Escolano-Margarit MV, Ramos R, et al (Univ of Granada, Spain; Clinical Univ Hosp San Cecilio, Granada, Spain; et al)
Am J Clin Nutr 94:1880S-1888S, 2011

Background.—The influence of prenatal long-chain polyunsaturated fatty acids (LC-PUFAs) and folate on neurologic development remains controversial.

Objective.—The objective was to assess the long-term effects of n−3 (omega-3) LC-PUFA supplementation, 5-methyltetrahydrofolate (5-MTHF) supplementation, or both in pregnant women on cognitive development of offspring at 6.5 y of age.

Design.—This was a follow-up study of the NUHEAL (Nutraceuticals for a Healthier Life) cohort. Healthy pregnant women in 3 European centers were randomly assigned to 4 intervention groups. From the 20th week of pregnancy until delivery, they received a daily supplement of 500 mg docosahexaenoic acid (DHA) + 150 mg eicosapentaenoic acid [fish oil (FO)], 400 µg 5-MTHF, or both or a placebo. Infants received formula containing 0.5% DHA and 0.4% arachidonic acid (AA) if they were born to mothers receiving FO supplements or were virtually free of DHA and AA until the age of 6 mo if they belonged to the groups that were not supplemented with FO. Fatty acids and folate concentrations were determined in maternal blood at weeks 20 and 30 of pregnancy, at delivery, and in cord blood. Cognitive function was assessed at 6.5 y of age with the Kaufman Assessment Battery for Children (K-ABC).

Results.—We observed no significant differences in K-ABC scores between intervention groups. Higher DHA in maternal erythrocytes at delivery was associated with a Mental Processing Composite Score higher than the 50th percentile in the offspring.

Conclusion.—We observed no significant effect of supplementation on the cognitive function of children, but maternal DHA status may be related to later cognitive function in children. This trial was registered at clinicaltrials.gov as NCT01180933.

▶ Higher docosahexaenoic acid (DHA) levels—that is, the active omega-3 brain component in fish oil—have been related to better childhood development. This study showed no benefit of DHA therapy and 5-methyltetrahydrofolate supplementation in the prenatal period. Although this was true, higher DHA in maternal erythrocytes at delivery was associated with an improvement in mental processing scores. Does this mean we should or shouldn't give DHA prenatally? Know that current therapy (ie, to give DHA prenatally because of higher IQ tests in kids from other studies) still represents the preponderance of evidence, but these data probably make it less mandatory or less clear that this is absolutely necessary for normal childhood development.

M. F. Roizen, MD

Fibroblast Growth Factor 23 and Risks of Mortality and End-Stage Renal Disease in Patients With Chronic Kidney Disease

Isakova T, for the Chronic Renal Insufficiency Cohort (CRIC) Study Group (Univ of Miami Miller School of Medicine, FL; et al)
JAMA 305:2432-2439, 2011

Context.—A high level of the phosphate-regulating hormone fibroblast growth factor 23 (FGF-23) is associated with mortality in patients with end-stage renal disease, but little is known about its relationship with adverse outcomes in the much larger population of patients with earlier stages of chronic kidney disease.

Objective.—To evaluate FGF-23 as a risk factor for adverse outcomes in patients with chronic kidney disease.

Design, Setting, and Participants.—A prospective study of 3879 participants with chronic kidney disease stages 2 through 4 who enrolled in the Chronic Renal Insufficiency Cohort between June 2003 and September 2008.

Main Outcome Measures.—All-cause mortality and end-stage renal disease.

Results.—At study enrollment, the mean (SD) estimated glomerular filtration rate (GFR) was 42.8 (13.5) mL/min/1.73 m^2, and the median FGF-23 level was 145.5 RU/mL (interquartile range [IQR], 96-239 reference unit [RU]/mL). During a median follow-up of 3.5 years (IQR, 2.5-4.4 years), 266 participants died (20.3/1000 person-years) and 410 reached end-stage renal disease (33.0/1000 person-years). In adjusted analyses, higher levels of FGF-23 were independently associated with a greater risk of death (hazard ratio [HR], per SD of natural log-transformed FGF-23, 1.5; 95% confidence interval [CI], 1.3-1.7). Mortality risk increased by quartile of FGF-23: the HR was 1.3 (95% CI, 0.8-2.2) for the second quartile, 2.0 (95% CI, 1.2-3.3) for the third quartile, and 3.0 (95% CI, 1.8-5.1) for the fourth quartile. Elevated fibroblast growth factor 23 was independently associated with significantly higher risk of end stage renal disease among participants with an estimated GFR between 30 and 44 mL/min/1.73 m^2 (HR, 1.3 per SD of FGF-23 natural log-transformed FGF-23; 95% CI, 1.04-1.6) and 45 mL/min/1.73 m^2 or higher (HR, 1.7; 95% CI, 1.1-2.4), but not less than 30 mL/min/1.73 m^2.

Conclusion.—Elevated FGF-23 is an independent risk factor for end-stage renal disease in patients with relatively preserved kidney function and for mortality across the spectrum of chronic kidney disease.

▶ I had never heard of fibroblast growth factor 23 before reading this article but clearly will hear more of it because it is an independent risk factor for end-stage renal disease in patients across the spectrum of chronic kidney disease, including diabetics. What will we do differently? Well, I suppose we do the same thing we do differently for patients with known chronic kidney disease—that is, make sure that their hydration is such that we may sacrifice other things to ensure appropriate kidney output and kidney perfusion during the operation and perioperative periods.

M. F. Roizen, MD

Forecasting the Future of Cardiovascular Disease in the United States: A Policy Statement From the American Heart Association
Heidenreich PA, on behalf of the American Heart Association Advocacy Coordinating Committee, Stroke Council, Council on Cardiovascular Radiology and Intervention, Council on Clinical Cardiology, Council on Epidemiology and Prevention, Council on Arteriosclerosis, Thrombosis and Vascular Biology, Council on Cardiopulmonary, Critical Care, Perioperative and Resuscitation, Council on Cardiovascular Nursing, Council on the Kidney in Cardiovascular Disease, Council on Cardiovascular Surgery and Anesthesia, and Interdisciplinary Council on Quality of Care and Outcomes Research
Circulation 123:933-944, 2011

Background.—Cardiovascular disease (CVD) is the leading cause of death in the United States and is responsible for 17% of national health expenditures. As the population ages, these costs are expected to increase substantially.

Methods and Results.—To prepare for future cardiovascular care needs, the American Heart Association developed methodology to project future costs of care for hypertension, coronary heart disease, heart failure, stroke, and all other CVD from 2010 to 2030. This methodology avoided double counting of costs for patients with multiple cardiovascular conditions. By 2030, 40.5% of the US population is projected to have some form of CVD. Between 2010 and 2030, real (2008$) total direct medical costs of CVD are projected to triple, from $273 billion to $818 billion. Real indirect costs (due to lost productivity) for all CVD are estimated to increase from $172 billion in 2010 to $276 billion in 2030, an increase of 61%.

Conclusions.—These findings indicate CVD prevalence and costs are projected to increase substantially. Effective prevention strategies are needed if we are to limit the growing burden of CVD.

▶ This article is striking in that it is from the American Heart Association and looks at how much cardiovascular disease we will have in the future and how hazardous it is to our security and well-being as a country. It is amazing that this comes from the American Heart Association, and, worse, it is amazing how much control we could have of our future health and well-being if we wanted and frightening how little we as a profession and the government, with its reimbursement system, have done to encourage health.

M. F. Roizen, MD

Hallmarks of Cancer: The Next Generation
Hanahan D, Weinberg RA (The Swiss Inst for Experimental Cancer Res (ISREC), Lausanne, Switzerland; Whitehead Inst for Biomedical Res, Cambridge, MA)
Cell 144:646-674, 2011

The hallmarks of cancer comprise six biological capabilities acquired during the multistep development of human tumors. The hallmarks constitute an organizing principle for rationalizing the complexities of neoplastic disease. They include sustaining proliferative signaling, evading growth suppressors, resisting cell death, enabling replicative immortality, inducing angiogenesis, and activating invasion and metastasis. Underlying these hallmarks are genome instability, which generates the genetic diversity that expedites their acquisition, and inflammation, which fosters multiple hallmark functions. Conceptual progress in the last decade has added two emerging hallmarks of potential generality to this list—reprogramming of energy metabolism and evading immune destruction. In addition to cancer cells, tumors exhibit another dimension of complexity: they contain a repertoire of recruited, ostensibly normal cells that contribute to the acquisition of hallmark traits by creating the "tumor microenvironment." Recognition of the widespread applicability of these concepts will increasingly affect the development of new means to treat human cancer.

▶ This is an important article for any of us interested in learning about cancer. It talks about why cancers grow and what we can do to prevent them. It is clear from this review and from other studies that extra sugar and maybe extra saturated fat are clearly risk factors for cancer. Is there a way to avoid immune dysfunction as well? Like all good data, I think this article brings up more questions and more stimulation than it provides answers.

M. F. Roizen, MD

Low-Risk Lifestyle Behaviors and All-Cause Mortality: Findings From the National Health and Nutrition Examination Survey III Mortality Study
Ford ES, Zhao G, Tsai J, et al (Ctrs for Disease Control and Prevention, Atlanta, GA)
Am J Public Health 101:1922-1929, 2011

Objectives.—We examined the relationship between 4 low-risk behaviors—never smoked, healthy diet, adequate physical activity, and moderate alcohol consumption—and mortality in a representative sample of people in the United States.

Methods.—We used data from 16958 participants aged 17 years and older in the National Health and Nutrition Examination Survey III Mortality Study from 1988 to 2006.

Results.—The number of low-risk behaviors was inversely related to the risk for mortality. Compared with participants who had no low-risk behaviors, those who had all 4 experienced reduced all-cause mortality (adjusted hazard ratio [AHR]=0.37; 95% confidence interval [CI]=0.28, 0.49), mortality from malignant neoplasms (AHR=0.34; 95% CI=0.20, 0.56), major cardiovascular disease (AHR=0.35; 95% CI=0.24, 0.50), and other causes (AHR=0.43; 95% CI=0.25, 0.74). The rate advancement periods, representing the equivalent risk from a certain number of years of chronological age, for participants who had all 4 high-risk behaviors compared with those who had none were 11.1 years for all-cause mortality, 14.4 years for malignant neoplasms, 9.9 years for major cardiovascular disease, and 10.6 years for other causes.

Conclusions.—Low-risk lifestyle factors exert a powerful and beneficial effect on mortality.

▶ Avoiding smoking, having a diet filled with vegetables, doing adequate physical activity, and moderate alcohol consumption resulted in a more than 60% reduction in all-cause mortality. This meant that Real Ages (in my terms) were more than 20 years younger if you include reduction in disabilities, and you would live more than 10 years longer just from these 4 behaviors.

M. F. Roizen, MD

Milk Intake in Early Life and Risk of Advanced Prostate Cancer

Torfadottir JE, Steingrimsdottir L, Mucci L, et al (Univ of Iceland, Reykjavik; Univ of Iceland and Landspitali Univ Hosp, Reykjavik; Harvard School of Public Health, Boston, MA; et al)
Am J Epidemiol 175:144-153, 2012

The authors investigated whether early-life residency in certain areas of Iceland marked by distinct differences in milk intake was associated with risk of prostate cancer in a population-based cohort of 8,894 men born between 1907 and 1935. Through linkage to cancer and mortality registers, the men were followed for prostate cancer diagnosis and mortality from study entry (in waves from 1967 to 1987) through 2009. In 2002–2006, a subgroup of 2,268 participants reported their milk intake in early, mid-, and current life. During a mean follow-up period of 24.3 years, 1,123 men were diagnosed with prostate cancer, including 371 with advanced disease (stage 3 or higher or prostate cancer death). Compared with early-life residency in the capital area, rural residency in the first 20 years of life was marginally associated with increased risk of advanced prostate cancer (hazard ratio = 1.29, 95% confidence interval (CI): 0.97, 1.73), particularly among men born before 1920 (hazard ratio = 1.64, 95% CI: 1.06, 2.56). Daily milk consumption in adolescence (vs. less than daily), but not in midlife or currently, was associated with a 3.2-fold risk of advanced prostate cancer (95% CI: 1.25, 8.28). These data suggest that frequent milk intake in adolescence increases risk of advanced prostate cancer.

▶ Wow—does the white mustache promote prostate and breast cancer? This study confirms some of the data from T. Colin Campbell's work in the China study and Dr Esselstyn's (Essy) op-ed commented on elsewhere in this YEAR BOOK. Essy may be right for both heart disease and cancer—do not eat anything with a face or a mother, including milk. In this study, older Icelandic men who remember chugging a lot of milk in their teens are 3 times as likely to be diagnosed with advanced prostate cancer as more moderate milk drinkers, researchers have found.

The data suggest that a "sensitive period" occurs during adolescence during which the prostate may be more susceptible to cancer. However, the 2 studies on prostate cancer and milk intake in adolescents have come to mixed conclusions—one found milk lovers seemed to be somewhat protected against the disease, while the other found no link at all. The study included men that had been part of a medical study started in the 1960s and, in the early 2000s, had answered questions about their diet in early and midlife as part of another study. Among 463 men who recalled drinking milk less than once a day in their teens, 1% developed advanced prostate cancer or died of the disease over a quarter century of follow-up. That figure was 3% among the more than 1800 men who said they drank milk at least daily in adolescence. How much milk men drank had no connection to their risk of early-stage tumors, however. And intake in midlife—the age group most other studies have focused on—didn't seem to matter either. All results and mechanisms are speculative at this point, and further investigation needs to be done.

M. F. Roizen, MD

Orthopaedic surgeons: as strong as an ox and almost twice as clever? Multicentre prospective comparative study

Subramanian P, Kantharuban S, Subramanian V, et al (Whipps Cross Hosp, Leytonstone, London, UK; Milton Keynes Hosp, Eaglestone, UK; Southport General Hosp, UK; et al)
BMJ 343:d7506, 2011

Objective.—To compare the intelligence and grip strength of orthopaedic surgeons and anaesthetists.

Design.—Multicentre prospective comparative study.

Setting.—Three UK district general hospitals in 2011.

Participants.—36 male orthopaedic surgeons and 40 male anaesthetists at consultant or specialist registrar grade.

Main Outcome Measures.—Intelligence test score and dominant hand grip strength.

Results.—Orthopaedic surgeons had a statistically significantly greater mean grip strength (47.25 (SD 6.95) kg) than anaesthetists (43.83 (7.57) kg). The mean intelligence test score of orthopaedic surgeons was also statistically significantly greater at 105.19 (10.85) compared with 98.38 (14.45) for anaesthetists.

Conclusions.—Male orthopaedic surgeons have greater intelligence and grip strength than their male anaesthetic colleagues, who should find new ways to make fun of their orthopaedic friends.

▶ Well, we all know that orthopedic surgeons are stronger than anesthesiologists, but smarter? I refuse to accept this conclusion. The non-London anesthesiologist in this study must have been outcast, drugged, or given too much alcohol before the intelligence test.

M. F. Roizen, MD

Participation in fitness-related activities of an incentive-based health promotion program and hospital costs: a retrospective longitudinal study
Patel D, Lambert EV, da Silva R, et al (Univ of Cape Town, Cape Town South Africa)
Am J Health Promot 25:341-348, 2011

Purpose.—A retrospective, longitudinal study examined changes in participation in fitness-related activities and hospital claims over 5 years amongst members of an incentivized health promotion program offered by a private health insurer.

Design.—A 3-year retrospective observational analysis measuring gym visits and participation in documented fitness-related activities, probability of hospital admission, and associated costs of admission.

Setting.—A South African private health plan, Discovery Health and the Vitality health promotion program.

Participants.—304,054 adult members of the Discovery medical plan, 192,467 of whom registered for the health promotion program and 111,587 members who were not on the program.

Intervention.—Members were incentivised for fitness-related activities on the basis of the frequency of gym visits.

Measures.—Changes in electronically documented gym visits and registered participation in fitness-related activities over 3 years and measures of association between changes in participation (years 1-3) and subsequent probability and costs of hospital admission (years 4-5). Hospital admissions and associated costs are based on claims extracted from the health insurer database.

Analysis.—The probability of a claim modeled by using linear logistic regression and costs of claims examined by using general linear models.

Propensity scores were estimated and included age, gender, registration for chronic disease benefits, plan type, and the presence of a claim during the transition period, and these were used as covariates in the final model.

Results.—There was a significant decrease in the prevalence of inactive members (76% to 68%) over 5 years. Members who remained highly active (years 1-3) had a lower probability ($p < .05$) of hospital admission in years 4 to 5 (20.7%) compared with those who remained inactive (22.2%). The odds of admission were 13% lower for two additional gym visits per week (odds ratio, .87; 95% confidence interval [CI], .801-.949).

Conclusion.—We observed an increase in fitness-related activities over time amongst members of this incentive-based health promotion program, which was associated with a lower probability of hospital admission and lower hospital costs in the subsequent 2 years.

▶ This is one of the few times I've seen a study with incentives that are not large increases in physical activity that are sustained for at least 8% of the population. And for those in whom it is sustained, it is associated with a decrease in hospitalization and decreased medical costs.

M. F. Roizen, MD

Public health importance of triggers of myocardial infarction: a comparative risk assessment
Nawrot TS, Perez L, Künzli N, et al (Hasselt Univ, Diepenbeek, Belgium; Univ of Basel, Switzerland)
Lancet 377:732-740, 2011

Background.—Acute myocardial infarction is triggered by various factors, such as physical exertion, stressful events, heavy meals, or increases in air pollution. However, the importance and relevance of each trigger are uncertain. We compared triggers of myocardial infarction at an individual and population level.

Methods.—We searched PubMed and the Web of Science citation databases to identify studies of triggers of non-fatal myocardial infarction to calculate population attributable fractions (PAF). When feasible, we did a meta-regression analysis for studies of the same trigger.

Findings.—Of the epidemiologic studies reviewed, 36 provided sufficient details to be considered. In the studied populations, the exposure prevalence for triggers in the relevant control time window ranged from $0·04\%$ for cocaine use to 100% for air pollution. The reported odds ratios (OR) ranged from $1·05$ to $23·7$. Ranking triggers from the highest to the lowest OR resulted in the following order: use of cocaine, heavy meal, smoking of marijuana, negative emotions, physical exertion, positive emotions, anger, sexual activity, traffic exposure, respiratory infections, coffee consumption, air pollution (based on a difference of 30 µg/m^3 in particulate matter with a diameter <10 µm [PM_{10}]). Taking into account the OR and the prevalences of exposure, the highest PAF was estimated for traffic exposure (7·4%), followed by physical exertion (6·2%), alcohol (5·0%), coffee (5·0%), a difference of 30 μg/m³ in PM_{10} (4·8%), negative emotions (3·9%), anger (3·1%), heavy meal (2·7%), positive emotions (2·4%), sexual activity (2·2%), cocaine use (0·9%), marijuana smoking (0·8%) and respiratory infections (0·6%).

Interpretation.—In view of both the magnitude of the risk and the prevalence in the population, air pollution is an important trigger of myocardial infarction, it is of similar magnitude (PAF 5−7%) as other well accepted triggers such as physical exertion, alcohol, and coffee. Our work shows that ever-present small risks might have considerable public health relevance.

▶ Everyone knows air pollution is a problem; all you have to do is look at Google and see the pictures from Beijing or Shanghai in the afternoon. It's hard to believe that air pollution is this great a trigger of acute myocardial infarction, but there is no doubt it is probably the result of the inflammation it causes.

M. F. Roizen, MD

Rapid Response Team in an Academic Institution: Does It Make a Difference?
Shah SK, Cardenas VJ Jr, Kuo Y-F, et al (Univ of Texas Med Branch, Galveston)
Chest 139:1361-1367, 2011

Background.—Although data remain contradictory, rapid response systems are implemented across US hospitals. We aimed to determine whether implementation of a rapid response team (RRT) in a tertiary academic hospital improved outcomes.

Methods.—Our hospital is a tertiary academic medical center with 24-h in-house resident coverage. We conducted a retrospective cohort study comparing 27 months after implementation of the RRT (April 1, 2006, to June 31, 2008) and 9 months before (January 1, 2005, to September 31, 2005). Outcomes included incidence of codes (cardiac and/or respiratory arrests), outcome of the codes, and overall hospital mortality.

Results.—We analyzed 16,244 nonobstetrics hospital admissions and 70,208 patient days in the control period and 45,145 nonobstetrics hospital admissions and 161,097 patient days after the RRT was implemented. The RRT was activated 1,206 times (7.7 calls per 1,000 patient days). There was no difference in the code rate (0.83 vs 0.98 per 1,000 patient days, $P = .3$). There was a modest but nonsustained improvement in nonobstetrics hospital mortality during the study period (2.40% vs 2.15%; $P = .05$), which could not be explained by the RRT effect on code rates. The mortality was 2.40% in the control group and 2.06%, 1.94%, and 2.46%, respectively, during the next three consecutive 9-month intervals.

Conclusions.—In our single-institution study involving an academic hospital with 24-h in-house coverage, we found that RRT implementation did not reduce code rates in the 27 months after intervention. Although there was a decrease in overall hospital mortality, this decrease was small, nonsustained, and not explained by the RRT effect on code rates.

▶ Enthusiasm abounds for the rapid response team (RRT) concept, yet the literature about outcomes is mixed. The authors found a negative result in a tertiary care center, which may be attributable to other factors nicely described in their discussion: tertiary care centers have readily available house officers 24/7, nursing thresholds for activation of RRTs may vary, inpatient disease acuity outside the intensive care unit (ICU) varies substantially even among tertiary referral centers, and the definition of the "denominator" in previous studies varies (per 1000 admissions vs per 1000 inpatient non-ICU days, the latter being favored). In addition, this article contained a historical control group, which admittedly is difficult to avoid in a study of this type. Hospitals seem to be jumping on the RRT bandwagon, but the cost effectiveness, perhaps as compared with more intense or scientifically driven nurse-to-patient ratios, requires substantial further investigation.

G. P. Gravlee, MD

Red meat consumption and risk of type 2 diabetes: 3 cohorts of US adults and an updated meta-analysis

Pan A, Sun Q, Bernstein AM, et al (Harvard School of Public Health, Boston, MA; et al)
Am J Clin Nutr 94:1088-1096, 2011

Background.—The relation between consumption of different types of red meats and risk of type 2 diabetes (T2D) remains uncertain.

Objective.—We evaluated the association between unprocessed and processed red meat consumption and incident T2D in US adults.

Design.—We followed 37,083 men in the Health Professionals Follow-Up Study (1986–2006), 79,570 women in the Nurses' Health Study I (1980–2008), and 87,504 women in the Nurses' Health Study II (1991–2005). Diet was assessed by validated food-frequency questionnaires, and data were updated every 4 y. Incident T2D was confirmed by a validated supplementary questionnaire.

Results.—During 4,033,322 person-years of follow-up, we documented 13,759 incident T2D cases. After adjustment for age, BMI, and other lifestyle and dietary risk factors, both unprocessed and processed red meat intakes were positively associated with T2D risk in each cohort (all P-trend <0.001). The pooled HRs (95% CIs) for a one serving/d increase in unprocessed, processed, and total red meat consumption were 1.12 (1.08, 1.16), 1.32 (1.25, 1.40), and 1.14 (1.10, 1.18), respectively. The results were confirmed by a meta-analysis (442,101 participants and 28,228 diabetes cases): the RRs (95% CIs) were 1.19 (1.04, 1.37) and 1.51 (1.25, 1.83) for 100 g unprocessed red meat/d and for 50 g processed red meat/d, respectively. We estimated that substitutions of one serving of nuts, low-fat dairy, and whole grains per day for one serving of red meat per day were associated with a 16—35% lower risk of T2D.

Conclusion.—Our results suggest that red meat consumption, particularly processed red meat, is associated with an increased risk of T2D.

▶ This is scary stuff. Red meat is clearly related to the cause of type 2 diabetes, based on this cohort study, adding to its known risks as shown by Micha et al[1] in the systemic review in meta-analysis, where it is associated with coronary heart disease. While we don't know the effects or why red meat causes the risk of type 2 diabetes (and this is in health professionals, so all of us have to pay attention), it is clear that red meat is probably a cause of type 2 diabetes as well as coronary heart disease and stroke. Another nail Essy can put in the coffin of saturated fat.

M. F. Roizen, MD

Reference

1. Micha R, Wallace SK, Mozaffarian D. Red and processed meat consumption and risk of incident coronary heart disease, stroke, and diabetes mellitus: a systematic review and meta-analysis. *Circulation.* 2010;121:2271-2283.

Reduced Lung-Cancer Mortality with Low-Dose Computed Tomographic Screening

The National Lung Screening Trial Research Team (Univ of California at Los Angeles; Brown Univ, Providence, RI; Natl Cancer Inst, Bethesda, MD; et al)
N Engl J Med 365:395-409, 2011

Background.—The aggressive and heterogeneous nature of lung cancer has thwarted efforts to reduce mortality from this cancer through the use of screening. The advent of lowdose helical computed tomography (CT) altered the landscape of lung-cancer screening, with studies indicating that low-dose CT detects many tumors at early stages. The National Lung Screening Trial (NLST) was conducted to determine whether screening with low-dose CT could reduce mortality from lung cancer.

Methods.—From August 2002 through April 2004, we enrolled 53,454 persons at high risk for lung cancer at 33 U.S. medical centers. Participants were randomly assigned to undergo three annual screenings with either low-dose CT (26,722 participants) or single-view posteroanterior chest radiography (26,732). Data were collected on cases of lung cancer and deaths from lung cancer that occurred through December 31, 2009.

Results.—The rate of adherence to screening was more than 90%. The rate of positive screening tests was 24.2% with low-dose CT and 6.9% with radiography over all three rounds. A total of 96.4% of the positive screening results in the low-dose CT group and 94.5% in the radiography group were false positive results. The incidence of lung cancer was 645 cases per 100,000 person-years (1060 cancers) in the low-dose CT group, as compared with 572 cases per 100,000 person-years (941 cancers) in the radiography group (rate ratio, 1.13; 95% confidence interval [CI], 1.03 to 1.23). There were 247 deaths from lung cancer per 100,000 person-years in the low-dose CT group and 309 deaths per 100,000 person-years in the radiography group, representing a relative reduction in mortality from lung cancer with low-dose CT screening of 20.0% (95% CI, 6.8 to 26.7; $P = 0.004$). The rate of death from any cause was reduced in the low-dose CT group, as compared with the radiography group, by 6.7% (95% CI, 1.2 to 13.6; $P = 0.02$).

Conclusions.—Screening with the use of low-dose CT reduces mortality from lung cancer. (Funded by the National Cancer Institute; National Lung Screening Trial ClinicalTrials.gov number, NCT00047385.)

▶ This is validation of prior studies showing that routine (easy to obtain) low-dose CT screening in persons who have quit smoking but consequently are at high risk of lung cancer saves lives by resulting in early detection. Fig 1 in the original article in this article clearly shows the improvement in detection, and Table 7 in the original article shows the roughly 7% reduction in death rate by low-dose CT screening.

M. F. Roizen, MD

Sugar-Sweetened Beverages and Risk of Metabolic Syndrome and Type 2 Diabetes: A meta-analysis

Malik VS, Popkin BM, Bray GA, et al (Harvard School of Public Health, Boston, MA; Univ of North Carolina, Chapel Hill; Pennington Biomedical Res Ctr, Baton Rouge, LA; et al)
Diabetes Care 33:2477-2483, 2010

Objective.—Consumption of sugar-sweetened beverages (SSBs), which include soft drinks, fruit drinks, iced tea, and energy and vitamin water drinks has risen across the globe. Regular consumption of SSBs has been associated with weight gain and risk of overweight and obesity, but the role of SSBs in the development of related chronic metabolic diseases, such as metabolic syndrome and type 2 diabetes, has not been quantitatively reviewed.

Research Design and Methods.—We searched the MEDLINE database up to May 2010 for prospective cohort studies of SSB intake and risk of metabolic syndrome and type 2 diabetes. We identified 11 studies (three for metabolic syndrome and eight for type 2 diabetes) for inclusion in a random-effects meta-analysis comparing SSB intake in the highest to lowest quantiles in relation to risk of metabolic syndrome and type 2 diabetes.

Results.—Based on data from these studies, including 310,819 participants and 15,043 cases of type 2 diabetes, individuals in the highest quantile of SSB intake (most often 1—2 servings/day) had a 26% greater risk of developing type 2 diabetes than those in the lowest quantile (none or <1 serving/month) (relative risk [RR] 1.26 [95% CI 1.12–1.41]). Among studies evaluating metabolic syndrome, including 19,431 participants and 5,803 cases, the pooled RR was 1.20 [1.02–1.42].

Conclusions.—In addition to weight gain, higher consumption of SSBs is associated with development of metabolic syndrome and type 2 diabetes. These data provide empirical evidence that intake of SSBs should be limited to reduce obesity-related risk of chronic metabolic diseases.

▶ This study of soft drinks, fruit drinks, iced tea, and energy and vitamin water drinks that are sugar sweetened is a little scary. The fact that it was conducted in more than 300 000 participants with 15 000 cases of type 2 diabetes means that these data are much more likely to be found true in the long run. But the fact that it was only a 20% to 25% increase in type 2 diabetes means that there is still some doubt. While red meat clearly is associated with type 2 diabetes initiation, as is obesity, we don't know if sugar-sweetened beverages really do the trick or are the cause of this in humans.

M. F. Roizen, MD

Suicide Deaths of Active-Duty US Military and Omega-3 Fatty-Acid Status: A Case-Control Comparison

Lewis MD, Hibbeln JR, Johnson JE, et al (Uniformed Services Univ of the Health Sciences, Bethesda, MD; Natl Insts of Health (NIH), Bethesda, MD)
J Clin Psychiatry 72:1585-1590, 2011

Background.—The recent escalation of US military suicide deaths to record numbers has been a sentinel for impaired force efficacy and has accelerated the search for reversible risk factors.

Objective.—To determine whether deficiencies of neuroactive, highly unsaturated omega-3 essential fatty acids (n-3 HUFAs), in particular docosahexaenoic acid (DHA), are associated with increased risk of suicide death among a large random sample of active-duty US military.

Method.—In this retrospective case-control study, serum fatty acids were quantified as a percentage of total fatty acids among US military suicide deaths (n = 800) and controls (n = 800) matched for age, date of collection of sera, sex, rank, and year of incident. Participants were active-duty US military personnel (2002–2008). For cases, age at death ranged from 17–59 years (mean = 27.3 years, SD = 7.3 years). Outcome measures included death by suicide, postdeployment health assessment questionnaire (Department of Defense Form 2796), and ICD-9 mental health diagnosis data.

Results.—Risk of suicide death was 14% higher per SD of lower DHA percentage (OR = 1.14; 95% CI, 1.02–1.27; *P* < .03) in adjusted logistic regressions. Among men, risk of suicide death was 62% greater with low serum DHA status (adjusted OR = 1.62; 95% CI, 1.12–2.34; *P* < .01, comparing DHA below 1.75% [n = 1,389] to DHA of 1.75% and above [n = 141]). Risk of suicide death was 52% greater in those who reported having seen wounded, dead, or killed coalition personnel (OR = 1.52; 95% CI, 1.11–2.09; $P < .01$).

Conclusion.—This US military population had a very low and narrow range of n-3 HUFA status. Although these data suggest that low serum DHA may be a risk factor for suicide, well-designed intervention trials are needed to evaluate causality.

▶ A large series of epidemiological data suggest that getting the right amount of omega-3 fatty-acids decreases mental illness. In this study, the risk of suicide was slightly higher in those with a low docosahexaenoic acid (DHA). Because there is little risk from DHA, it is available in algal capsules (ie, capsules from algae where the fish get their DHA) and it decreases age-related macular degeneration, cognitive dysfunction as well as heart disease risk and probably joint disease, we should probably all be taking DHA omega-3 fatty-acids. However, whether it decreases mortality rates or just improves quality of life is not clear to me.

M. F. Roizen, MD

Survival Among High-Risk Patients After Bariatric Surgery
Maciejewski ML, Livingston EH, Smith VA, et al (Durham VA Med Ctr, NC; Univ of Texas, Arlington; et al)
JAMA 305:2419-2426, 2011

Context.—Existing evidence of the survival associated with bariatric surgery is based on cohort studies of predominantly younger women with a low inherent obesity-related mortality risk. The association of survival and bariatric surgery for older men is less clear.

Objective.—To determine whether bariatric surgery is associated with reduced mortality in a multisite cohort of predominantly older male patients who have a high baseline mortality rate.

Design, Setting, and Participants.—Retrospective cohort study of bariatric surgery programs in Veterans Affairs medical centers. Mortality was examined for 850 veterans who had bariatric surgery in January 2000 to December 2006 (mean age 49.5 years; SD 8.3; mean body mass index [BMI] 47.4; SD 7.8) and 41 244 nonsurgical controls (mean age 54.7 years, SD 10.2; mean BMI 42.0, SD 5.0) from the same 12 Veteran Integrated Service Networks; the mean follow-up was 6.7 years. Four Cox proportional hazards models were assessed: unadjusted and controlled for baseline covariates on unmatched and propensity-matched cohorts.

Main Outcome Measure.—All-cause mortality through December 2008.

Results.—Among patients who had bariatric surgery, the 1-, 2-, and 6-year crude mortality rates were, respectively, 1.5%, 2.2%, and 6.8% compared with 2.2%, 4.6%, and 15.2% for nonsurgical controls. In unadjusted Cox regression, bariatric surgery was associated with reduced mortality (hazard ratio [HR], 0.64; 95% confidence interval [CI], 0.51-0.80). After covariate adjustment, bariatric surgery remained associated with reduced mortality (HR, 0.80; 95% CI, 0.63-0.995). In analysis of 1694 propensity-matched patients, bariatric surgery was no longer significantly associated with reduced mortality in unadjusted (HR, 0.83; 95% CI, 0.61-1.14) and time-adjusted (HR, 0.94; 95% CI, 0.64-1.39) Cox regressions.

Conclusion.—In propensity score—adjusted analyses of older severely obese patients with high baseline mortality in Veterans Affairs medical centers, the use of bariatric surgery compared with usual care was not associated with decreased mortality during a mean 6.7 years of follow-up.

▶ Bariatric surgery would not be necessary if people weren't obese and gaining weight by eating enlarged portions. But bariatric surgery is needed. What was disappointing to me from this study was not that bariatric patients did as well as high-risk patients who were treated medically but that these older, severely obese patients didn't do better after bariatric surgery compared with usual care. We should have better outcomes than usual low-cost care if we are going to have high-cost procedures.

M. F. Roizen, MD

The Effect of Chromosome 9p21 Variants on Cardiovascular Disease May Be Modified by Dietary Intake: Evidence from a Case/Control and a Prospective Study
Do R, on behalf of the INTERHEART investigators (McGill Univ, Montré al, Quebec, Canada; et al)
PLoS Med 8:e1001106, 2011

Background.—One of the most robust genetic associations for cardiovascular disease (CVD) is the Chromosome 9p21 region. However, the interaction of this locus with environmental factors has not been extensively explored. We investigated the association of 9p21 with myocardial infarction (MI) in individuals of different ethnicities, and tested for an interaction with environmental factors.

Methods and Findings.—We genotyped four 9p21 SNPs in 8,114 individuals from the global INTERHEART study. All four variants were associated with MI, with odds ratios (ORs) of 1.18 to 1.20 ($1.85 \times 10^{-8} \leq p \leq 5.21 \times 10^{-7}$). A significant interaction ($p = 4.0 \times 10^{-4}$) was observed between rs2383206 and a factor-analysis-derived "prudent" diet pattern score, for which a major component was raw vegetables. An effect of 9p21 on MI was observed in the group with a low prudent diet score (OR = 1.32, $p = 6.82 \times 10^{-7}$), but the effect was diminished in a step-wise fashion in the medium (OR = 1.17, $p = 4.9 \times 10^{-3}$) and high prudent diet scoring groups (OR = 1.02, $p = 0.68$) ($p = 0.014$ for difference). We also analyzed data from 19,129 individuals (including 1,014 incident cases of CVD) from the prospective FINRISK study, which used a closely related dietary variable. In this analysis, the 9p21 risk allele demonstrated a larger effect on CVD risk in the groups with diets low or average for fresh vegetables, fruits, and berries (hazard ratio [HR] = 1.22, $p = 3.0 \times 10^{-4}$, and HR = 1.35, $p = 4.1 \times 10^{-3}$, respectively) compared to the group with high consumption of these foods (HR = 0.96, $p = 0.73$) ($p = 0.0011$ for difference). The combination of the least prudent diet and two copies of the risk allele was associated with a 2-fold increase in risk for MI (OR = 1.98, $p = 2.11 \times 10^{-9}$) in the INTERHEART study and a 1.66-fold increase in risk for CVD in the FINRISK study (HR = 1.66, $p = 0.0026$).

Conclusions.—The risk of MI and CVD conferred by Chromosome 9p21 SNPs appears to be modified by a prudent diet high in raw vegetables and fruits.

▶ You might guess from the abstract that this says it all: raw vegetables and high "prudent" diet, as in what Dr. Esselstyn recommends in another study in this YEAR BOOK, change gene function. This change in gene function by diet decreases the effect of chromosome variants that increase heart disease; it turned these genes off. That is, to be clear, raw veggies decrease heart disease by changing gene function.

M. F. Roizen, MD

2 Anesthesia-Related Pharmacology and Toxicology

Comparison of Succinylcholine and Rocuronium for First-attempt Intubation Success in the Emergency Department
Patanwala AE, Stahle SA, Sakles JC, et al (Univ of Arizona, Tucson)
Acad Emerg Med 18:11-14, 2011

Objectives.—The objective was to determine the effect of paralytic type and dose on first-attempt rapid sequence intubation (RSI) success in the emergency department (ED).

Methods.—This was a retrospective evaluation of information collected prospectively in a quality improvement database between July 1, 2007, and October 31, 2008. Information regarding all intubations performed in a tertiary care ED was recorded in this database. All RSI performed using succinylcholine or rocuronium were included. Logistic regression was used to analyze the effect of paralytic type and dosing, as well as age, sex, body mass index, physician experience, device type, and presence of difficult airway predictors on first attempt RSI success.

Results.—A total of 327 RSI were included in the final analyses. All patients received etomidate as the induction sedative and were successfully intubated. Of these, 113 and 214 intubations were performed using succinylcholine and rocuronium, respectively. The rate of first-attempt intubation success was similar between the succinylcholine and rocuronium groups (72.6% vs. 72.9%, $p = 0.95$). Median doses used for succinylcholine and rocuronium were 1.65 mg/kg (interquartile range [IQR] = 1.26–1.95 mg/kg) and 1.19 mg/kg (IQR = 1–1.45 mg/kg), respectively. In the univariate logistic regression analyses, variables predictive of first-attempt intubation success were laryngeal view (more success if Grade 1 or 2 compared to Grade 3 or 4 of the Cormack-Lehane classification, odds ratio [OR] = 55.18, 95% confidence interval [CI] = 18.87 to 161.39), intubation device (less success if direct laryngoscopy, OR = 0.57, 95% CI = 0.34 to 0.96), and presence of a difficult airway predictor (OR = 0.55, 95% CI = 0.31 to 0.99). In the multivariate analysis, the only variable predictive of first-attempt intubation success was laryngeal view.

Conclusions.—Succinylcholine and rocuronium are equivalent with regard to first-attempt intubation success in the ED when dosed according to the ranges used in this study.

▶ The results of this study, that success of intubation with first laryngoscopy is the same regardless of whether succinylcholine (median dose, 1.65 mg/kg) or rocuronium (median dose, 1.19 mg/kg) is used, corroborate the findings of an earlier study comparing onset of neuromuscular blockade with succinylcholine and increasing doses of rocuronium.[1]

Because data were collected prospectively, it is surprising that some of the data (drug doses, patient height, and weight) had to be collected retrospectively. This information is important in data analysis, as an adequate dose of induction agents has been found to allow intubating conditions that were similar to those with succinylcholine.[2] In the study being reviewed, the authors found no impact of medication dose on the success of intubation with first laryngoscopy. Yet, the specifics of that data are not presented. One would have expected, based on earlier trials, that intubation would have been more difficult with smaller doses of rocuronium.[3]

Also of note is the manner in which the authors grouped physicians in terms of their experience. Physicians were grouped in 1 of 3 ways: (1) first-year resident, (2) second-year resident, or (3) third-year resident or attending physician. Creating a separate fourth group for faculty would seem reasonable given the faculty's greater degree of experience than that of residents in training. Additionally, because the data were collected over 15 months (July through October), residents in any given year of training would have had much less experience in months 1 through 6 of the study and months 13 through 15 than those intubating patients in the emergency department during months 7 through 12. The success of first-year residents in intubating patients is not indicated in Table 2 in the original article, and one has to wonder whether their participation was predictive of first attempt success.

In a clinical setting such as the emergency department, controlling for the myriad of factors that will influence the ease of intubation in a study is extremely difficult. As observed in this study, many questions are likely to remain unanswered in the clinical setting.

C. Lien, MD

References

1. Magorian T, Flannery KB, Miller RD. Comparison of rocuronium, succinylcholine, and vecuronium for rapid-sequence induction of anesthesia in adult patients. *Anesthesiology.* 1993;79:913-918.
2. Scheller MS, Zornow MH, Saidman LJ. Tracheal intubation without the use of muscle relaxants: a technique using propofol and varying doses of alfentanil. *Anesth Analg.* 1992;75:788-793.
3. Mallon WK, Keim SM, Shoenberger JM, Walls RM. Rocuronium vs. succinylcholine in the emergency department: a critical appraisal. *J Emerg Med.* 2009;37:183-188.

ED procedural sedation of elderly patients: is it safe?

Weaver CS, Terrell KM, Bassett R, et al (Indiana Univ School of Medicine, Indianapolis)
Am J Emerg Med 29:541-544, 2011

Objective.—Emergency physicians routinely perform emergency department procedural sedation (EDPS), and its safety is well established. We are unaware of any published reports directly evaluating the safety of EDPS in older patients (≥65 years old). Many EDPS experts consider seniors to be at higher risk. The objective was to evaluate the complication rate of EDPS in elderly adults.

Methods.—This was a prospective, observational study of EDPS patients at least 65 years old, as compared with patients aged 18 to 49 and 50 to 64 years. Physicians were blind to the objectives of this research. The study protocol required an ED nurse trained in data collection to be present to record vital signs and assess for any prospectively defined complications. We used American Society of Anesthesiologists (ASA) physical status classification for systemic disease to evaluate and account for the comorbidities of patients. We used the Fisher exact test for the difference in proportions across age groups and analysis of variance for the differences in dosing across age and ASA categories.

Results.—During the 4-year study, we enrolled 50 patients at least 65 years old, 149 patients aged 50 to 64 years, and 665 patients aged 18 to 49 years. Adverse event rates were 8%, 5.4%, and 5.2%, respectively ($P = .563$). The at least 65 years age group represented a greater percentage of those with higher ASA scores ($P < .001$). The average total sedative dose in the at least 65 years group was significantly lower than the comparisons ($P < .001$).

Conclusions.—This study demonstrated no statistically significant difference in complication rate for patients 65 years or older. There was a significant decrease in mean sedation dosing with increased age and ASA score.

▶ This is an observational study conducted over the course of 4 years in a single emergency department. During this period of time, more than 850 patients were enrolled into the study. Unfortunately, only 50 of them (5.8%) were elderly as defined by age 65 years or greater. For an emergency room with more than 100 000 visits per year, this is a relatively small number of visits by elderly patients who may require sedation. Whether enrollment was due to patient agreement to participate, the nature of the treatment required, or the demographics of the population, presenting to the emergency room is not clear.

Because no power analysis was performed to determine the number of patients needed in each of the 3 study groups, ages 18 to 49, 50 to 64, and 65 and older, the validity of the lack of significance found in the frequency of adverse events in the oldest group of patients is unclear. In 2 of the 3 adverse events reported, hypotension and unsuccessful treatment, there was an increased frequency of events in the oldest patient group. The frequency of hypotension, as noted by the authors, increased 3-fold in the elderly. They did not note the degree of decrease in blood pressure, considering hypotension to a systolic blood pressure less than 90 mmHg. Whether the elderly had more pronounced hypotension would have been useful information. Elderly patients did not decrease their oxygen saturation to less than 90% any more frequently than young adults. How the airways of these patients were managed compared with the young adults is not described, and whether they received oxygen supplementation more frequently would have been useful information in determining the applicability of the results to practice in other emergency departments.

Interestingly, the authors described studying the incidence of apnea, bradycardia, and aspiration. How frequently they occurred, however, is not presented. Given the changes in physiology that accompany aging, it is not surprising that elderly patients received less medication. From this article, it is not clear whether the dosing was guided by level of sedation or concern about adverse events with overdosing of medication. Information regarding level of sedation in the different patient groups would have been useful in this regard.

From the data presented, sedation can be safely provided to elderly patients in this one emergency department. Without greater details regarding the specifics of care for the elderly by these physicians, however, these data cannot be generalized to other emergency rooms.

C. Lien, MD

Effect of an intravenous infusion of lidocaine on cisatracurium-induced neuromuscular block duration: a randomized-controlled trial
Hans GA, Defresne A, Ki B, et al (Univ of Liège, Belgium; et al)
Acta Anaesthesiol Scand 54:1192-1196, 2010

Background.—Intravenous lidocaine can be used intraoperatively for its analgesic and antihyperalgesic properties but local anaesthetics may also prolong the duration of action of neuromuscular blocking agents. We hypothesized that intravenous lidocaine would prolong the time to recovery of neuromuscular function after cisatracurium.

Methods.—Forty-two patients were enrolled in this randomized, double-blind, placebo-controlled study. Before induction, patients were administered either a 1.5 mg/kg bolus of intravenous lidocaine followed by a 2 mg/kg/h infusion or an equal volume of saline. Anaesthesia was induced and maintained using propofol and remifentanil infusions. After loss of consciousness, a 0.15 mg/kg bolus of cisatracurium was administered. No additional cisatracurium injection was allowed. Neuromuscular function was assessed every 20 s using kinemyography. The primary endpoint was the time to spontaneous recovery of a train-of-four (TOF) ratio ≥ 0.9.

Results.—The time to spontaneous recovery of a TOF ratio ≥ 0.9 was 94 ± 15 min in the control group and 98 ± 16 min in the lidocaine group ($P = 0.27$).

Conclusions.—No significant prolongation of spontaneous recovery of a TOF ratio ≥ 0.9 after cisatracurium was found in patients receiving intravenous lidocaine.

▶ Lidocaine potentially impacts neuromuscular transmission through more than 1 mechanism. As noted by the authors of this study, it has been found in vitro to block open junctional nicotinic acetylcholine receptors.[1-3] Through its effect on voltage-gated sodium channels, it may also inhibit the propogation of an electrical impulse through the perijunctional muscle membrane.[4] It also has prejunctional effects.[5] There are many ways that lidocaine can interfere in neuromuscular transmission. Therefore, in research involving neuromuscular blockade, administration of lidocaine is not allowed as any part of an anesthetic. Bolus administration of lidocaine, 0.5 to 1.0 mg/kg, during a stable or recovering block will potentiate the depth of block for a period of several minutes. Administration of lidocaine has also been found to speed onset of neuromuscular block.[6]

Why the authors of this study found no prolongation of recovery is unclear. Dosing of lidocaine used in the study is what would commonly be administered. Perhaps the dosing of cisatracurium was such that changes in pharmacodynamics could not be identified. Ideally, studies of the impact of comorbidities or medications on potency and recovery from neuromuscular blockade involve the administration of doses of neuromuscular blocking agents that do not cause 100% neuromuscular block. This is the way that the impact of age on vecuronium-induced neuromuscular block was determined.[7]

While an infusion of lidocaine as a supplement to general anesthetics was used more commonly in the past, its current use in this fashion is not as common. Similarly, it may have previously been used as an infusion in a patient with a recent history of ventricular fibrillation. Now, however, other antiarrhythmics, such as amiodarone, are preferred and have shown improved patient outcomes.[8] Because of changing clinical practices, the clinical applicability of the results of this study is limited.

C. Lien, MD

References

1. Steinbach AB. Alteration by xylocaine (lidocaine) and its derivatives of the time course of the end plate potential. *J Gen Physiol.* 1968;52:144-161.
2. Neher E, Steinbach JH. Local anaesthetics transiently block currents through single acetylcholine-receptor channels. *J Physiol.* 1978;277:153-176.
3. Ruff RL. The kinetics of local anesthetic blockade of end-plate channels. *Biophys J.* 1982;37:625-631.
4. Usubiaga JE, Standaert F. The effects of local anesthetics on motor nerve terminals. *J Pharmacol Exp Ther.* 1968;159:353-361.
5. Kordas M. The effect of procaine on neuromuscular transmission. *J Physiol.* 1970;209:689-699.
6. Nonaka A, Sugawara T, Suzuki S, Masamune T, Kumazawa T. Pretreatment with lidocaine accelerates onset of vecuronium-induced neuromuscular blockade. *Masui.* 2002;51:880-883.
7. Koscielniak-Nielsen ZJ, Bevan JC, Popovic V, Baxter MR, Donati F, Bevan DR. Onset of maximum neuromuscular block following succinylcholine or vecuronium in four age groups. *Anesthesiology.* 1993;79:229-234.

8. Dorian P, Cass D, Schwartz B, Cooper R, Gelaznikas R, Barr A. Amiodarone as compared with lidocaine for shock-resistant ventricular fibrillation. *N Engl J Med.* 2002;346:884-890.

Effect of phenylephrine and ephedrine bolus treatment on cerebral oxygenation in anaesthetized patients

Meng L, Cannesson M, Alexander BS, et al (Univ of California, Orange; et al)
Br J Anaesth 107:209-217, 2011

Background.—How phenylephrine and ephedrine treatments affect global and regional haemodynamics is of major clinical relevance. Cerebral tissue oxygen saturation (Sct_{o_2})-guided management may improve postoperative outcome. The physiological variables responsible for Sct_{o_2} changes induced by phenylephrine and ephedrine bolus treatment in anaesthetized patients need to be defined.

Methods.—A randomized two-treatment cross-over trial was conducted: one bolus dose of phenylephrine (100–200 µg) and one bolus dose of ephedrine (5–20 mg) were given to 29 ASA I–III patients anaesthetized with propofol and remifentanil. Sct_{o_2}, mean arterial pressure (MAP), cardiac output (CO), and other physiological variables were recorded before and after treatments. The associations of changes were analysed using linear-mixed models.

Results.—The CO decreased significantly after phenylephrine treatment [$\Delta CO = -2.1$ (1.4) litre min^{-1}, $P<0.001$], but was preserved after ephedrine treatment [$\Delta CO = 0.5$ (1.4) litre min^{-1}, $P>0.05$]. The Sct_{o_2} was significantly decreased after phenylephrine treatment [$\Delta Sct_{o_2} = -3.2$ (3.0)%, $P<0.01$] but preserved after ephedrine treatment [$\Delta Sct_{o_2} = 0.04$ (1.9)%, $P>0.05$]. CO was identified to have the most significant association with Sct_{o_2} ($P<0.001$). After taking CO into consideration, the other physiological variables, including MAP, were not significantly associated with Sct_{o_2} ($P>0.05$).

Conclusions.—Associated with changes in CO, Sct_{o_2} decreased after phenylephrine treatment, but remained unchanged after ephedrine treatment. The significant correlation between CO and Sct_{o_2} implies a cause–effect relationship between global and regional haemodynamics (Table 1).

▶ The ideal bolus pharmacologic treatment of anesthesia-related hypotension remains unclear, but in my local practice, phenylephrine dominates over ephedrine. The apparent rationale is fear of ephedrine-induced tachycardia. In this study, ephedrine did induce a small increase in heart rate, but phenylephrine induced a substantial decrease that likely accounts for much of its observed decrease in cardiac output (Table 1). The surprising finding is a reduction in cerebral tissue O_2 saturation after phenylephrine, despite an increase in MAP. Theoretically, cerebral autoregulation as well as cerebrovascular resistance to the direct effects of circulating catecholamines should prevent this from occurring. Debate continues about the importance of catecholamine effects on conductance and resistance cerebral arteries. Of potential concern is the authors' use of excessively deep anesthesia using the cerebral vasoconstrictor propofol.

TABLE 1.—Summarized Physiological Measurements Before (Pre) and After (Post) Treatments (Tx). Data are Presented as Means (SD). Δ = Post−Pre; Sct_{O_2}, Cerebral Tissue Oxygen Saturation; MAP, Mean Arterial Pressure; CO, Cardiac Output; HR, Heart Rate (Beats min^{-1}); SV, Stroke Volume; E'_{CO_2}, End-Tidal CO_2; Sp_{O_2}, Oxygen Saturation Per Pulse Oximetry; BIS, Bispectral Index

	Phenylephrine First Tx (n=13)			Phenylephrine Second Tx (n=16)			Ephedrine First Tx (n=16)			Ephedrine Second Tx (n=13)		
	Pre	Post	Δ	Pre	Post	Δ	Pre	Post	Δ	Pre	Post	Δ
Sct_{O_2} (%)	68.8 (8.8)	63.9 (10.4)	−4.9 (2.8)*	66.4 (6.7)	64.5 (6.7)	−1.8 (2.4)†	67.4 (6.3)	67.1 (6.0)	−0.4 (2.3)	65.7 (8.5)	66.2 (8.9)	0.5 (1.1)
MAP (mm Hg)	60.8 (12.1)	90.3 (14.5)	29.5 (9.3)*	58.8 (9.3)	101.3 (14.7)	42.6 (15.7)*	48.1 (8.9)	72.3 (10.7)	24.1 (13.5)*	62.4 (5.3)	90.7 (13.7)	28.3 (13.3)*
CO (litre min^{-1})	5.3 (1.1)	3.6 (0.7)	−1.7 (1.0)*	6.8 (1.7)	4.5 (2.2)	−2.3 (1.7)*	6.0 (1.8)	6.5 (1.8)	0.5 (1.7)	5.0 (0.9)	5.4 (1.0)	0.4 (0.9)
HR (beats min^{-1})	71.2 (15.2)	53.9 (8.6)	−17.3 (11.4)*	64.7 (12.1)	48.0 (6.6)	−16.7 (12.1)*	65.3 (14.1)	67.6 (12.6)	2.3 (5.8)†	59.5 (9.6)	67.0 (11.3)	7.5 (7.8)
SV (ml)	77.2 (16.7)	68.7 (14.4)	−8.5 (9.2)†	105.8 (31.0)	90.7 (39.5)	−15.2 (22.3)‡	92.2 (30.4)	97.4 (29.7)	5.3 (21.6)	85.5 (17.9)	83.1 (18.0)	−2.4 (11.9)
E'_{CO_2} (kPa)	5.1 (0.7)	4.9 (0.6)	−0.2 (0.3)‡	4.7 (0.4)	4.6 (0.5)	−0.1 (0.3)	4.7 (0.4)	4.7 (0.4)	0.04 (0.3)	4.9 (0.7)	5.0 (0.6)	0.2 (0.3)
Sp_{O_2} (%)	99.5 (0.7)	99.9 (0.3)	0.4 (0.7)	99.1 (1.4)	99.5 (1.2)	0.4 (0.7)	99.3 (1.4)	99 (2.7)	−0.3 (1.8)	99.1 (1.9)	99.4 (0.9)	0.3 (1.2)
BIS	25.5 (11.9)	27.8 (11.4)	2.3 (5.2)	34.9 (7.8)	30.5 (11.0)	−4.3 (8.4)	25.7 (12.5)	26.5 (8.5)	0.7 (6.0)	29.8 (12.9)	29.0 (11.2)	−0.9 (3.3)

*$P<0.001$.
†$P<0.01$.
‡$P<0.05$ (post *vs* pre, paired Student's *t*-test).

Nevertheless, this study suggests that ephedrine may be a more appropriate first-line bolus vasopressor during general anesthesia than phenylephrine.

G. P. Gravlee, MD

Neostigmine/Glycopyrrolate Administered after Recovery from Neuromuscular Block Increases Upper Airway Collapsibility by Decreasing Genioglossus Muscle Activity in Response to Negative Pharyngeal Pressure
Herbstreit F, Zigrahn D, Ochterbeck C, et al (Universitätsklinikum Essen, Germany; Universität Duisburg-Essen, Germany)
Anesthesiology 113:1280-1288, 2010

Background.—Reversal of residual neuromuscular blockade by acetylcholinesterase inhibitors (e.g., neostigmine) improves respiratory function. However, neostigmine may also impair muscle strength. We hypothesized that neostigmine administered after recovery of the train-of-four (TOF) ratio impairs upper airway integrity and genioglossus muscle function.

Methods.—We measured, in 10 healthy male volunteers, epiglottic and nasal mask pressures, genioglossus electromyogram, air flow, respiratory timing, and changes in lung volume before, during (TOF ratio: 0.5), and after recovery of the TOF ratio to unity, and after administration of neostigmine 0.03 mg/kg IV (with glycopyrrolate 0.0075 mg/kg). Upper airway critical closing pressure (Pcrit) was calculated from flow-limited breaths during random pharyngeal negative pressure challenges.

Results.—Pcrit increased significantly after administration of neostigmine/glycopyrrolate compared with both TOF recovery (mean ± SD, by 27 ± 21%; $P = 0.02$) and baseline (by 38 ± 17%; $P = 0.002$). In parallel, phasic genioglossus activity evoked by negative pharyngeal pressure decreased (by 37 ± 29%, $P = 0.005$) compared with recovery, almost to a level observed at a TOF ratio of 0.5. Lung volume, respiratory timing, tidal volume, and minute ventilation remained unchanged after neostigmine/glycopyrrolate injection.

Conclusion.—Neostigmine/glycopyrrolate, when administered after recovery from neuromuscular block, increases upper airway collapsibility and impairs genioglossus muscle activation in response to negative pharyngeal pressure. Reversal with acetylcholinesterase inhibitors may be undesirable in the absence of neuromuscular blockade.

▶ Whether to administer an anticholinesterase to anyone who has received a neuromuscular blocking agent is a decision the clinician frequently makes. Neostigmine and glycopyrrolate have several dose-related adverse effects that include arrhythmias, nausea and vomiting, bronchospasm, and tension on intestinal anastomoses. However, not infrequently patients are admitted to the pediatric acute care unit with postoperative residual paralysis even when they received only a single intubating dose of vecuronium, rocuronium, or atracurium.[1] Subtle degrees of residual neuromuscular block may be difficult to detect, yet they are associated with adverse consequences.[2-4] Although not administering an anticholinesterase to everyone increases the likelihood of inadequate recovery of neuromuscular function,[5] not all patients require it, and administering it to patients who have spontaneously recovery from neuromuscular block may cause weakness.[6,7] The increase in weakness may be due to the excessive amount of acetylcholine at the neuromuscular junction.[8]

These authors have previously reported that unnecessary administration of anticholinesterases can impair genioglossus and diaphragm function.[7] The genioglossus is a dilator of the upper airway, and weakness of this muscle can lead to upper airway collapse. In the current volunteer trial, healthy men receiving rocuronium to establish a train-of-4 ratio (TOFR) of 0.5 were allowed to recover spontaneously to a TOFR of 1 and then received neostigmine and glycopyrrolate. Importantly, the dose of neostigmine that was administered was small (30 mcg/kg). Even following administration of this small dose of neostigmine, the upper airway critical closing pressure increased after administration of neostigmine, and the genioglossus activity generated with negative pharyngeal pressure, rather than increasing as it does in the absence of neuromuscular blockade, decreased to values observed during partial paralysis (TOFR = 0.5).

The results of this study speak to the inadequacy of our monitors of neuromuscular blockade. If a clinician can document that a patient has complete recovery of muscle strength, no anticholinesterase will be administered. Our monitors of neuromuscular blockade, however, do not allow us to do this,[9] and the decision as to whether to administer anticholinesterase is based on clinical judgment. Previously, administration of small doses (10, 20, or 30 mcg/kg) of neostigmine was recommended when no fade was palpable in the train-of-4[10] so as to not cause weakness. However, on the basis of the results of the current study, 30 mcg/kg may be too much to administer when muscle strength has recovered to a TOFR = 1.

C. Lien, MD

References

1. Debaene B, Plaud B, Dilly MP, Donati F. Residual paralysis in the PACU after a single intubating dose of nondepolarizing muscle relaxant with an intermediate duration of action. *Anesthesiology.* 2003;98:1042-1048.
2. Murphy GS, Szokol JW, Marymont JH, Greenberg SB, Avram MJ, Vender JS. Residual neuromuscular blockade and critical respiratory events in the postanesthesia care unit. *Anesth Analg.* 2008;107:130-137.
3. Sundman E, Witt H, Olsson R, Ekberg O, Kuylenstierna R, Eriksson LI. The incidence and mechanisms of pharyngeal and upper esophageal dysfunction in partially paralyzed humans: pharyngeal videoradiography and simultaneous manometry after atracurium. *Anesthesiology.* 2000;92:977-984.
4. Eriksson LI, Sato M, Severinghaus JW. Effect of a vecuronium-induced partial neuromuscular block on hypoxic ventilatory response. *Anesthesiology.* 1993; 78:693-699.
5. Tramèr MR, Fuchs-Buder T. Omitting antagonism of neuromuscular block: effect on postoperative nausea and vomiting and risk of residual paralysis. A systematic review. *Br J Anaesth.* 1999;82:379-386.
6. Caldwell JE. Reversal of residual neuromuscular block with neostigmine at one to four hours after a single intubating dose of vecuronium. *Anesth Analg.* 1995;80:1168-1174.

7. Eikermann M, Fassbender P, Malhotra A, et al. Unwarranted administration of acetylcholinesterase inhibitors can impair genioglossus and diaphragm muscle function. *Anesthesiology.* 2007;107:621-629.
8. Bevan DR, Donati F, Kopman AF. Reversal of neuromuscular blockade. *Anesthesiology.* 1992;77:785-805.
9. Viby-Mogensen J, Jensen NH, Engbaek J, Ording H, Skovgaard LT, Chraemmer-Jørgensen B. Tactile and visual evaluation of the response to train-of-four nerve stimulation. *Anesthesiology.* 1985;63:440-443.
10. Fuchs-Buder T, Meistelman C, Alla F, Grandjean A, Wuthrich Y, Donati F. Antagonism of low degrees of atracurium-induced neuromuscular blockade: dose-effect relationship for neostigmine. *Anesthesiology.* 2010;112:34-40.

Onset time and haemodynamic response after thiopental vs. propofol in the elderly: a randomized trial

Sørensen MK, Dolven TL, Rasmussen LS (Copenhagen Univ Hosp, Denmark)
Acta Anaesthesiol Scand 55:429-434, 2011

Background.—The induction dose of hypnotic agents should be reduced in the elderly, but it is not well studied whether thiopental or propofol should be preferred in this group of patients. The aim of this study was to compare onset time, hypnosis level and the haemodynamic response after thiopental vs. propofol for induction of anaesthesia. Our primary hypothesis was that in the elderly, thiopental had a shorter onset time than propofol, defined as time to bispectral index (BIS) <50.

Methods.—In this randomized and double-blinded study, we included 78 patients. Patients were eligible, if they were scheduled for elective surgery with general anaesthesia and aged 60 or older. Patients received alfentanil 10 μg/kg and either thiopental 2.5 mg/kg or propofol 1.0 mg/kg, and depth of anaesthesia was determined with BIS the following 120 s along with clinical assessment of anaesthetic depth. The primary endpoint was the time from start of injection of the hypnotic to a BIS value below 50.

Results.—Time to BIS <50 was significantly shorter in patients receiving thiopental, where onset time was 52 s (median value) compared with 65 s in the propofol group ($P = 0.01$). Mean arterial pressure decreased 25.6 mmHg in the propofol group and 15.6 mmHg in the thiopental group ($P = 0.003$) within 120 s. Heart rate decreased 9.1 b.p.m. within 120 s in the patients receiving propofol compared with a decrease of 5.1 b.p.m. in patients receiving thiopental ($P = 0.04$).

Conclusion.—Thiopental was found to have a faster onset than propofol in elderly surgical patients.

▶ Unfortunately, thiopental is no longer available for use in the United States. There are potentially a number of reasons that its use would be preferred over that of propofol in the geriatric patient population. Although commonly used in all patients, propofol does have significant cardiovascular effects. Blood pressure decreases of up to 40% occur following administration of induction doses in patients who do not have cardiac disease,[1] and there is a decrease in cardiac output.[2] Hypotension due to the administration of propofol is not accompanied by tachycardia.[3] One of the predictors of severe hypotension within 10 minutes of induction of anesthesia with propofol and fentanyl is an age of 50 years or older.[4]

Clinical onset of the doses of each drug studied for this work were essentially indistinguishable. A bispectral index value is of little consequence in an unresponsive patient and sets an artificial end point as a primary marker of onset.

The difference in hemodynamic effects was large. To interpret the potential significance of these data, information regarding comorbidities such as hypertension and cardiac disease, medications, and baseline blood pressure values would have been useful.

What this study nicely documents is that geriatric patients do not require large doses of sedative hypnotics to induce unconsciousness. Patients enrolled in this study received 1 mg/kg propofol or 2.5 mg/kg thiopental for induction of anesthesia. These doses are far lower than those recommended for induction in young, healthy individuals. Had larger doses been administered to the elderly patients in this study, greater hemodynamic effects may have been observed.

C. Lien, MD

References

1. Larsen R, Rathgeber J, Bagdahn A, Lange H, Rieke H. Effects of propofol on cardiovascular dynamics and coronary blood flow in geriatric patients: a comparison with etomidate. *Anaesthesia.* 1988;43:25-31.
2. Van Aken H, Meinshausen E, Prien T, Brüssel T, Heinećke A, Lawin P. The influence of fentanyl and tracheal intubation on the hemodynamic effects of anesthesia induction with propofol/N2O in humans. *Anesthesiology.* 1988;58:157-163.
3. Ebert TJ, Muzi M, Berens R, Goff D, Kampine JP. Sympathetic responses to induction of anesthesia in humans with propofol or etomidate. *Anesthesiology.* 1992;76:725-733.
4. Reich DL, Hossain S, Krol M, et al. Predictors of hypotension after induction of general anesthesia. *Anesth Analg.* 2005;101:622-628.

Pharmacodynamics and Cardiopulmonary Side Effects of CW002, a Cysteine-reversible Neuromuscular Blocking Drug in Dogs
Heerdt PM, Malhotra JK, Pan BY, et al (Weill Med College of Cornell Univ, NY)
Anesthesiology 112:910-916, 2010

Background.—CW002 is a novel neuromuscular blocking drug with a duration dependent on the rate of cysteine adduction to the molecule. The current study characterized the pharmacodynamics and cardiopulmonary side effects of CW002 in dogs.

Methods.—In eight beagles, the dose required to produce 95% neuromuscular blockade (ED_{95}) for CW002 was first determined and cysteine reversibility was confirmed. Five to 7 days later, incrementally larger doses were injected starting with $6.25 \times ED_{95}$ and doubling the dose every 15 min. Before and after injection, blood was obtained for histamine analysis. Systemic and pulmonary arterial pressures, cardiac output, and left ventricular pressure and volume were recorded along with inspiratory pressure and pulmonary compliance. Ventricular contractility and lusi-tropy were indexed from pressure and volume data.

Results.—The ED_{95} for CW002 from pooled data was 0.009 mg/kg. At $3 \times ED_{95}$, onset time was 2.6 ± 0.9 min and duration was 47 ± 9 min. The duration was shortened to 3.7 ± 0.6 min by 50 mg/kg L-cysteine injected 1 min after CW002. At $25 \times ED_{95}$, CW002 reduced mean arterial pressure with concomitant decreases in systemic vascular resistance, mean pulmonary artery pressure, cardiac output, contractility, and lusitropy, beginning at $50 \times ED_{95}$. However, even at a dose of $100 \times ED_{95}$, the average change in any variable was less than 20%. There were no changes in pulmonary vascular resistance or ventilation mechanics at any dose, and histamine release occurred in only two of eight animals.

Conclusions.—CW002 is a potent neuromuscular blocking drug that at doses up to $100 \times ED_{95}$ produces modest hemodynamic effects that are not associated with bronchoconstriction or consistent histamine release.

▶ CW002 is a nonhalogenated, benzylisoquinolinium fumarate diester that, in animals, has a rapid onset of effect and an intermediate duration of action. As part of its preclinical evaluation, it has undergone evaluation of its hemodynamic safety. This is a report of the results of these trails in dogs. A dose of 25 times the ED_{95} (the dose that, on average, will cause 95% suppression of neuromuscular response to stimulation) caused an average decrease in mean arterial pressure of 4 mm Hg. Administration of 50 and then 100 times the ED_{95} resulted in more substantial changes of, on average, a 20% decrease in mean arterial pressure. Other hemodynamic changes, such as decreased cardiac output, pulmonary artery pressure, and systemic vascular resistance, also occurred. Histamine release is likely to cause the hemodynamic changes. Other changes observed with histamine release, such as increases in peak inspiratory pressure and decreases in pulmonary compliance, were not observed—even at the highest doses of CW002.

What is interesting is that mean arterial pressure changes were related to the dose of CW002 administered. The greatest decreases in mean arterial pressure, however, occurred in those animals that did not release histamines. An interesting figure that the authors did not include would have been the maximal change in mean arterial pressure versus the maximal change in heart rate for each animal at each dose. With histamine release, decreases in mean arterial pressure are accompanied by a transient decrease in blood pressure and an increase in heart rate. Study design, as noted by the authors, was not optimal for identifying histamine release. To do this, the authors would have needed to study each dose of CW002 in a different animal.

Because of the difference in potency of CW002 in beagles and nonhuman primates, prediction of how this compound will behave in humans is difficult. Phase 1 trials that will begin later this year will help to define the hemodynamic safety of this neuromuscular blocking agent in humans.

C. Lien, MD

Postoperative nausea and vomiting in patients after craniotomy: incidence and risk factors

Latz B, Mordhorst C, Kerz T, et al (Universitätsmedizin der Johannes Gutenberg—Universität Mainz, Germany)
J Neurosurg 114:491-496, 2011

Object.—The purpose of this study was to assess the incidence and risk factors of postoperative nausea and vomiting (PONV) after craniotomy because most available data about PONV in neurosurgical patients are retrospective in nature or derive from small prospective studies.

Methods.—Postoperative nausea and vomiting was prospectively assessed within 24 hours after surgery in 229 patients requiring supratentorial or infratentorial craniotomy. To rule out the relevance of the neurosurgical procedure itself to the development of PONV, the observed incidence of vomiting was compared with the rate of vomiting predicted with a surgery-independent risk score (Apfel postoperative vomiting score).

Results.—The overall incidence of PONV after craniotomy was 47%. Logistic regression identified female sex as a risk factor for postoperative nausea (OR 4.25, 95% CI 2.3−7.8) and vomiting (OR 2.62, 95% CI 1.4−4.9). Both the incidence of nausea (OR 3.76, 95% CI 2.06−6.88) and vomiting (OR 4.48, 95% CI 2.4−8.37) were increased in patients not receiving steroids. Postoperative nausea and vomiting occurred after infratentorial as well as after supratentorial procedures. The observed incidence of vomiting within 24 hours after surgery was higher (49%) than would be predicted with the Apfel surgery-independent risk score (31%; p = 0.0004).

Conclusions.—The overall incidence of PONV within 24 hours after craniotomy was approximately 50%. One possible reason is that intracranial surgeries pose an additional and independent risk factor for vomiting, especially in female patients. Patients undergoing craniotomy should be identified as high-risk patients for PONV.

▶ Because the risks associated with postoperative nausea and vomiting in patients who have had craniotomies are so great, knowing whether the surgery itself is associated with an increased incidence of postoperative nausea and vomiting is important in determining whether routine prophylaxis is indicated. Based on the results of this work, it is. Craniotomies can be added to the list of procedures associated with an increased risk of postoperative nausea and vomiting. Because of their study design, the incidence may be even higher than found by the authors. Because the type of anesthesia was left to the anesthesiologist's discretion, patients with a history of postoperative nausea and vomiting received total intravenous anesthesia with propofol. Because propofol has antiemetic properties, the frequency of postoperative nausea and vomiting (PONV) in this subset of patients may have been lower than it would have been had they received a balanced anesthetic.

The question is, how can the incidence of PONV that is almost 50% be lowered? The administration of dexamethasone intraoperatively lowered the incidence of PONV. While perioperative administration of steroids has been found to increase risk of postoperative infection,[1] it does decrease intracranial pressure as well as, as found in this study, the incidence of both nausea and vomiting. Intraoperative prophylaxis with the 5-HT3 antagonist, granisetron, however, did not appreciably decrease the incidence of PONV in this patient population. As the authors note, this may have been caused by its being administered to patients with a history of PONV. Additional studies of the best means of reducing the incidence of PONV in patients undergoing craniotomy seem warranted.

C. Lien, MD

Reference

1. Percival VG, Riddell J, Corcoran TB. Singe dose dexamethasone for postoperative nausea and vomiting—a matched case-control study of postoperative infection risk. *Anaesth Intensive Care.* 2010;38:661-666.

Reversibility of rocuronium-induced profound neuromuscular block with sugammadex in younger and older patients
Suzuki T, Kitajima O, Ueda K, et al (Nihon Univ School of Medicine, Tokyo, Japan)
Br J Anaesth 106:823-826, 2011

Background.—This study compared the reversibility of rocuronium-induced profound neuromuscular block with sugammadex in younger and older patients.

Methods.—Fifteen younger (20—50 yr) and 15 older ($\geq$70 yr) patients were sequentially enrolled in this study. After induction of anaesthesia and laryngeal mask insertion, contraction of the adductor pollicis muscle in response to ulnar nerve stimulation was quantified using acceleromyography during 1.0—1.5% end-tidal sevoflurane and remifentanil anaesthesia. All patients initially received rocuronium 1 mg kg^{-1}, followed by 0.02 mg kg^{-1} when a post-tetanic count (PTC) of 1 or 2 was observed. After completion of surgery, at reappearance of 1—2 PTC, the time required for a single bolus dose of 4 mg kg^{-1} sugammadex to produce recovery to a train-of-four (TOF) ratio of 0.9 was recorded.

Results.—There were no differences in the total dose of rocuronium administered between the younger [mean (SD): 93.4 (17.5) mg] and the older [97.5 (32.2) mg] groups. In all patients, adequate recovery of the TOF ratio to 0.9 was achieved after administration of sugammadex, although it was significantly slower in the older [3.6 (0.7) min, $P < 0.0001$] than in the younger group [1.3 (0.3) min]. There were no clinical events attributable to recurarization.

Conclusions.—Sugammadex can adequately restore neuromuscular function in older patients, although a longer time is required to recover from profound rocuronium-induced neuromuscular block than in younger patients.

▶ This is another study of the efficacy of sugammadex in reversing profound rocuronium-induced neuromuscular block. What makes this study different is that it studied the efficacy of sugammadex in geriatric patients. Although effective in the elderly, patients of advanced age required more time than young adults for recovery of neuromuscular function. As noted by the authors, this finding may have been due to physiologic changes associated with aging.

Studies comparing pharmacodynamics in the elderly and the young are difficult to design because there are many differences between the 2 patient populations, such as decreases in renal function, changes in cardiac function, greater comorbidities in and more medications taken by the elderly, and decreases in anesthetic requirements with advanced age.

Information not provided in the description of this study and its results that would have aided in interpreting the outcomes include subjects' comorbidities, the medications the subjects were taking, and the amount of sevoflurane administered, because any of these could have affected the pharmacodynamics of either rocuronium or sugammadex. Other information that would have been useful from the aspect of data gathered during the study includes the intervals between the maintenance doses of rocuronium in each of the study groups. Additionally, the interval between the last dose of rocuronium and the administration of sugammadex would have helped to put in perspective the 2.3-minute increase in time for recovery of neuromuscular function in the elderly. Based on the data provided, in which geriatric patients had longer anesthetics and received the same dose of rocuronium as their younger counterparts, it is likely that the dosing intervals were greater in the elderly. Not delivering sevoflurane in age-adjusted multiples of minimum alveolar concentration would likely not, as the authors noted, have affected the efficacy of sugammadex. However, it may have potentiated neuromuscular block in the elderly more than it did in the young.

Without these details, it is difficult to determine the overall applicability of the slight increase in time required for complete recovery of neuromuscular function in the elderly from profound rocuronium-induced neuromuscular block.

C. Lien, MD

The Duration of Residual Neuromuscular Block After Administration of Neostigmine or Sugammadex at Two Visible Twitches During Train-of-Four Monitoring

Illman HL, Laurila P, Antila H, et al (Turku Univ Hosp and Univ of Turku, Finland; Oulu Univ Hosp, Oulu, Finland; et al)
Anesth Analg 112:63-68, 2011

Background.—Adequate recovery from neuromuscular block (NMB) is imperative for the patient to have full control of pharyngeal and respiratory muscles. The train-of-4 (TOF) ratio should return to at least 0.90

to exclude potentially clinically significant postoperative residual block. Fade cannot be detected reliably with a peripheral nerve stimulator (PNS) at a TOF ratio >0.4. The time gap between loss of visual fade by using a PNS until objective TOF ratio has returned to >0.90 can be considered "the potentially unsafe period of recovery." According to our hypothesis the duration of this period would be significantly shorter with sugammadex than with neostigmine.

Methods.—Fifty patients received volatile anesthetics, opioids, and a rocuronium-induced NMB. TOF-Watch® without a preload was used, but the anesthesiologist relied on visual evaluation of the TOF responses only. At end of operation, patients were randomized to receive either neostigmine 50 μg/kg or sugammadex 2 mg/kg, when 2 twitch responses were detected after the last dose of rocuronium. Timing of tracheal extubation was based on PNS and clinical data. Duration of the potentially unsafe period of recovery after reversal by either neostigmine or sugammadex was analyzed. Mann–Whitney *U* test and Pearson χ^2 test were used for statistical analysis.

Results.—The times [mean ± SD (range)] from loss of visual fade to TOF ratio >0.90 were 10.3 ± 5.5 (1.3 to 26.0) minutes and 0.3 ± 0.3 (0.0 to 1.0) minutes in the neostigmine and sugammadex groups, respectively ($P < 0.001$). The times from reversal by neostigmine or sugammadex to TOF ratio >0.90 were 13.3 ± 5.7 (3.5 to 28.9) and 1.7 ± 0.7 (0.7 to 3.5) minutes, respectively ($P < 0.001$). The values of TOF ratios at the time of loss of visual fade were 0.34 ± 0.14 (0.00 to 0.56) in patients given neostigmine and 0.86 ± 0.11 (0.64 to 1.04) in patients given sugammadex ($P < 0.001$).

Conclusions.—There is a significant time gap between visual loss of fade and return of TOF ratio >0.90 after reversal of a rocuronium block by neostigmine. Sugammadex in comparison with neostigmine allows a safer reversal of a moderate NMB when relying on visual evaluation of the TOF response.

▶ The results of this study are not surprising given the number of studies that have shown more rapid recovery of neuromuscular function after the administration of sugammadex than neostigmine.[1-4] The specific hypothesis the authors chose to study, however, is both interesting and unique. They attempted to define the period at which patients would be most at risk for complications of residual neuromuscular block. When patients are extubated with inadequate recovery of neuromuscular strength, they are at greatest risk for aspiration[5,6] and critical respiratory events.[7] Based on early studies of the inadequacies of qualitative monitors of neuromuscular function and the overall lack of adequate recovery at time of extubation,[8] the authors hypothesized that this period of increased risk would occur over the time that it takes a patient to recover from a train-of-four ratio (TOFR) of 0.4, when fade is not reliably detectable in the TOFR, to a TOFR of 0.9.

In this study, the authors found that the average TOFR at which fade is no longer detectable is lower than had been previously described.[8] It was 0.34

and ranged from 0.0 to 0.56. Based on the authors' observations of times to recovery to a TOFR of 0.9, the at-risk period ranged from 0 to 1 minute in the sugammadex group and 1.3 to 26.0 minutes in the neostigmine group. Interestingly, in this study, clinicians did not extubate the trachea of their patients until a greater degree of neuromuscular function, than reported in previous trials, had occurred. On average, patients had recovered to a TOFR of 0.82 in the neostigmine group (range 0.44-1.00) and 0.99 in the sugammadex group (range 0.93-1.04), decreasing the at-risk period to 2.4 minutes in the neostigmine group and 0 minutes in the sugammadex group. The later extubation in the sugammadex group may have been because of rapid recovery following sugammadex administration at return of 2 responses to TOF stimulation.

The authors did not report on the frequency of critical respiratory events in each study group, and based on an earlier trial,[7] their study would have had to be much larger to do so. With recovery being so great in the sugammadex group, however, one would have expected the incidence of critical respiratory events caused by residual neuromuscular blockade to be nil in patients receiving this selective relaxant binding agent.

Although quantitative monitors of depth of neuromuscular block are not routinely used when nondepolarizing neuromuscular blocking agents are administered,[9] they are available. Sugammadex, in contrast, is not available for use in the United States. Therefore, encouraging routine use of these monitors would currently seem to be the most reliable way to decrease the incidence of postoperative residual neuromuscular block.[10]

C. Lien, MD

References

1. Lemmens HJ, El-Orbany MI, Berry J, Morte JB Jr, Martin G. Reversal of profound vecuronium-induced neuromuscular block under sevoflurane anesthesia: sugammadex versus neostigmine. *BMC Anesthesiol.* 2010;10:15.
2. Blobner M, Eriksson LI, Scholz J, Motsch J, Della Rocca G, Prins ME. Reversal of rocuronium-induced neuromuscular blockade with sugammadex compared with neostigmine during sevoflurane anaesthesia: results of a randomised, controlled trial. *Eur J Anaesthesiol.* 2010;27:874-881.
3. Khuenl-Brady KS, Wattwil M, Vanacker BF, Lora-Tamayo JI, Rietbergen H, Alvarez-Gómez JA. Sugammadex provides faster reversal of vecuronium-induced neuromuscular blockade compared with neostigmine: a multicenter, randomized, controlled trial. *Anesth Analg.* 2010;110:64-73.
4. Jones RK, Caldwell JE, Brull SJ, Soto RG. Reversal of profound rocuronium-induced blockade with sugammadex: a randomized comparison with neostigmine. *Anesthesiology.* 2008;109:816-824.
5. Eriksson LI, Sundman E, Olsson R, et al. Functional assessment of the pharynx at rest and during swallowing in partially paralyzed humans: simultaneous videomanometry and mechanomyography of awake human volunteers. *Anesthesiology.* 1997;87:1035-1043.
6. Berg H, Roed J, Viby-Mogensen J, et al. Residual neuromuscular block is a risk factor for postoperative pulmonary complications. A prospective, randomised, and blinded study of postoperative pulmonary complications after atracurium, vecuronium and pancuronium. *Acta Anaesthesiol Scand.* 1997;41:1095-1103.
7. Murphy GS, Szokol JW, Marymont JH, Greenberg SB, Avram MJ, Vender JS. Residual neuromuscular blockade and critical respiratory events in the postanesthesia care unit. *Anesth Analg.* 2008;107:130-137.

8. Viby-Mogensen J, Jensen NH, Engbaek J, Ording H, Skovgaard LT, Chraemmer-Jørgensen B. Tactile and visual evaluation of the response to train-of-four nerve stimulation. *Anesthesiology.* 1985;63:440-443.
9. Naguib M, Kopman AF, Lien CA, Hunter JM, Lopez A, Brull SJ. A survey of current management of neuromuscular block in the United States and Europe. *Anesth Analg.* 2010;111:110-119.
10. Murphy GS, Szokol JW, Marymont JH, et al. Intraoperative acceleromyographic monitoring reduces the risk of residual neuromuscular blockade and adverse respiratory events in the postanesthesia care unit. *Anesthesiology.* 2008;109:389-398.

The Effect of Antihypertensive Class on Intraoperative Pressor Requirements During Carotid Endarterectomy

Anastasian ZH, Gaudet JG, Connolly ES Jr, et al (Columbia Univ, NY)
Anesth Analg 112:1452-1460, 2011

Background.—Certain classes of antihypertensive drugs have been associated with intraoperative hypotension, and frequently, patients are receiving multiple classes of antihypertensive medications. We sought to determine whether one class of antihypertensive medication either alone, or in combination with other classes of antihypertensive medications, increased the probability of intraoperative hypotension, determined by the amount of vasopressor required during carotid endarterectomy (CEA) performed under general anesthesia with specific arterial blood pressure management.

Methods.—This is a post hoc analysis of 252 patients scheduled for elective CEA under general anesthesia, all of whom participated in a prospective evaluation of cognitive dysfunction. Patients were characterized by class and number of preoperative antihypertensive medications taken. A predetermined anesthetic regimen was administered to all patients, with a phenylephrine infusion titrated to maintain mean arterial blood pressure at baseline before clamping the carotid artery, and approximately 20% above baseline during clamping. Computerized anesthesia records were used to record hemodynamics and to quantify medication administered intraoperatively.

Results.—Patients taking diuretics as part of their antihypertensive regimen required significantly more (1.6 times) total intraoperative phenylephrine than those not taking diuretics, independently of the number of other antihypertensive medications. This difference in the phenylephrine requirement occurs only during the preclamp period, i.e., from induction to application of carotid artery clamping for the maintenance of preoperative blood pressure. However, in contrast to this result, there is no difference in pressor requirement comparing classes of antihypertensive medications to increase the mean arterial blood pressure 20% above baseline during the period when the carotid artery is clamped.

Conclusion.—Diuretics are associated with increased vasopressor requirements in patients having a CEA under general anesthesia in the pre-clamp period, which is likely true for any patient having a general anesthetic.

▶ Perioperative hypotension has been associated with significant perioperative morbidity. Identifying patients most at risk for this is important because it may influence choices made for perianesthetic management and anesthetic medications. Adult patients presenting for surgery frequently take antihypertensive medications. Based on the results of this retrospective trial, we can expect that patients taking multiple antihypertensive medications and those taking diuretics will require more phenylephrine than those taking fewer medications or non-diuretic-type medications for hypertension.

Perhaps because the data were not collected prospectively, details of the various groups studied are not provided. One of the interesting things about the design of this study is that the anesthetic had been standardized for the study in which patients were initially enrolled. How this affected the findings is not evident. Administration of volatile anesthetics, a minimum of 0.3% isoflurane, to all patients, may have contributed to the incidence and severity of hypotension. Of note, despite standardization of the anesthetic, doses of individual anesthetic agents varied widely. Unfortunately, the amount of each agent administered to the different study groups is not quantified. In contrast, details regarding intravenous fluid administration were provided and, surprisingly, all groups received, on average, the same volume of intravenous fluid, regardless of whether they had been taking diuretics.

This post hoc analysis was done on a very specific set of patients receiving a particular anesthetic type. All took their antihypertensive medications the morning of surgery. Whether this information is applicable to patients presenting for different surgeries will, as noted by the authors, have to be studied. However, based on the results of this study, greater intraoperative hypotension can be anticipated in patients taking diuretics than in patients taking other classes of antihypertensive agents.

C. Lien, MD

The effects of low-dose ephedrine on intubating conditions following low-dose priming with cisatracurium
Leykin Y, Dalsasso M, Setti T, et al (Santa Maria degli Angeli Hosp, Pordenone, Italy)
J Clin Anesth 22:425-431, 2010

Study Objective.—To determine whether low-dose ephedrine plus priming with low-dose cisatracurium improves intubating conditions.
Design.—Prospective, randomized, double-blinded study.
Setting.—Operating room.
Patients.—124 ASA physical status I and II patients scheduled for elective surgery.

Interventions.—Patients were randomly assigned to 4 groups (n = 31): Group PE (priming + ephedrine), Group P (priming), Group E (ephedrine), and Group NPE (no priming, no ephedrine). All patients were induced with propofol two mg/kg and sulfentanil 0.15 μg/kg. In the priming groups, 0.005 mg/kg (10% ED95) cisatracurium was given, followed three minutes later by 0.145 mg/kg of cisatracurium. In Groups E and NPE, a single dose of 0.15 mg/kg cisatracurium was given. Intravenous ephedrine 70 μg/kg was given in Groups PE and E. Tracheal intubation was attempted 60 seconds after the intubating dose of cisatracurium and was considered successful only if performed within 20 seconds.

Measurements.—Intubating conditions were graded. Heart rate and non-invasive blood pressure, at one-minute intervals, were recorded during and 5 minutes after induction.

Main Results.—The tracheas of all patients in Group PE were success-fully intubated within 20 seconds versus 74% in Group P, 77% in Group E, and 64% in Group NPE ($P < 0.001$ vs. Group PE). Intubating conditions were graded good to excellent in all PE patients, but in only 52% of Groups P and E, and 48% of NPE patients ($P < 0.001$). Hemody-namic variables were comparable among groups ($P = $ ns).

Conclusions.—Low-dose ephedrine plus priming with low-dose cisatra-curium before an intubating dose, significantly improved clinical intubat-ing conditions at 60 seconds.

▶ This is yet another study of ways to speed onset of neuromuscular block and improve intubating conditions at 60 seconds. Increasing cardiac output with ephedrine and priming does, based on the results of this trial and others,[1] allow for early intubation with acceptable intubating conditions.

The authors are to be commended for using an appropriate priming dose (one-tenth of an ED95 dose). Frequently, clinicians prime with a fraction of an intubating dose, which can range from 1 to 4 times the ED95.

In priming with cisatracurium, the slow onset of the effect of the compound should be considered. The priming interval allowed in this study was 3 minutes, yet the maximal effect of cisatracurium occurs more than 4 minutes after admin-istration of a dose.[2] Had a greater time interval been allowed between priming and administration of the intubating dose, perhaps a greater percentage of patients would have had excellent intubating conditions.

There are a number of reasons to not prime. Studies have demonstrated that neuromuscular block develops even with small doses of neuromuscular block-ing agents. Accompanying this loss of muscle strength are symptoms ranging from visual changes to difficulty swallowing and breathing.[3,4] When one considers which patients require intubation in 60 seconds, their health is compromised and they are at increased risk of aspiration. Although the authors of this study did not find that any patients complained of feeling weak, they did not monitor depth of neuromuscular block. Additionally, the patients enrolled in this study were adults 65 years and younger and generally healthy (ASA phys-ical status 1 or 2). Elderly patients develop greater muscle weakness and decreases in oxygen saturation and respiratory function following precurarizing doses of neuromuscular blocking agents.[5] The practice of priming may render those patients who are most at risk for aspiration more susceptible to it.[6]

Similarly, the healthy patients enrolled in this study were not hemodynamically compromised by the administration of 70 µg/kg ephedrine; however, administration of this same dose to patients with cardiovascular disease may have different results.

Given the availability of other neuromuscular blocking agents with pharmacodynamic properties that would be more suitable for a rapid sequence induction and intubation, the similar duration of action of equivalent doses of rocuronium. Other means of facilitating rapid-sequence induction and intubation, such as the administration of lidocaine to potentiate existing neuromuscular block, should be considered prior to priming and administration of ephedrine.

C. Lien, MD

References

1. Leykin Y, Pellis T, Lucca M, Gullo A. Effects of ephedrine on intubating conditions following priming with rocuronium. *Acta Anaesthesiol Scand*. 2005;49:792-797.
2. Belmont MR, Lien CA, Quessy S, et al. The clinical neuromuscular pharmacology of 51W89 in patients receiving nitrous oxide/opioid/barbiturate anesthesia. *Anesthesiology*. 1995;82:1139-1145.
3. Engbaek J, Howardy-Hansen P, Ording H, Viby-Mogensen J. Precurarization with vecuronium and pancuronium in awake, healthy volunteers: the influence on neuromuscular transmission and pulmonary function. *Acta Anaesthesiol Scand*. 1985;29:117-120.
4. Howardy-Hansen P, Møller J, Hansen B. Pretreatment with atracurium: the influence on neuromuscular transmission and pulmonary function. *Acta Anaesthesiol Scand*. 1987;31:642-644.
5. Aziz L, Jahangir SM, Choudhury SN, Rahman K, Ohta Y, Hirakawa M. The effect of priming with vecuronium and rocuronium on young and elderly patients. *Anesth Analg*. 1997;85:663-666.
6. Shorten GD, Braude BM. Pulmonary aspiration of gastric contents after a priming dose of vecuronium. *Paediatr Anaesth*. 1997;7:167-169.

The use of rocuronium in a patient with cystic fibrosis and end-stage lung disease made safe by sugammadex reversal
Porter MV, Paleologos MS (Royal Prince Alfred Hosp, New South Wales, Australia)
Anaesth Intensive Care 39:299-302, 2011

While the pharmacology of sugammadex has been extensively reviewed, there is limited literature regarding its use in specific clinical settings. Several case reports describe its use in patients with the potential for postoperative respiratory dysfunction; in the settings of myasthenia gravis, Duchenne muscular dystrophy and myotonic dystrophy. We describe the use of sugammadex in a patient with severe bronchiectasis related to cystic fibrosis who required neuromuscular block for percutaneous endoscopic gastrostomy insertion. The use of rocuronium for neuromuscular block was preferred in order to avoid the potential complications associated with the use of suxamethonium. However, we wished to ensure complete neuromuscular block reversal for this short duration procedure in this high-risk patient and also to avoid the side-effects of traditional reversal agents. We therefore planned in advance to use sugammadex for neuromuscular block reversal, and this approach proved successful. Overall, the combination of rocuronium and sugammadex improved perioperative surgical and anaesthetic management in this patient.

▶ Postoperative residual neuromuscular block results in decreased hypoxic drive,[1] increased incidence of postoperative pulmonary complications,[2,3] and decreased coordination of the musculature involved in swallowing.[4] While estimates are that postoperative residual neuromuscular block occurs in 10% to 40% of patients receiving a general anesthetic with neuromuscular blockade, it is generally not appreciated in the clinical setting.[5] There is, however, a subset of patients that will tolerate this compromise of muscle strength more poorly than the general population. The authors of this case report mention some of these, including patients with myasthenia gravis and patients with compromised pulmonary function, especially those needing to have a short surgical procedure where complete recovery from neuromuscular blockade (even after the administration of an anticholinesterase) is unlikely.

These authors describe the successful use of the combination of rocuronium and sugammadex, the selective-relaxant binding agent, in a patient with cystic fibrosis requiring placement of a percutaneous endoscopic gastrostomy to allow for improvement of her nutritional status. She received approximately 0.75 mg/kg rocuronium for a rapid sequence induction of anesthesia and appropriately, with the return of 2 twitches in response to train-of-four stimulation, 5 mg/kg sugammadex for reversal of residual neuromuscular block. The patient's trachea was extubated, and her postoperative course uneventful.

Sugammadex binds to rocuronium so that the neuromuscular blocking agent is unable to bind to the acetylcholine receptor of the neuromuscular junction. The rocuronium-sugammadex complex is eliminated in the urine.[6] Because of its mechanism of action, sugammadex will cause more rapid recovery of neuromuscular function than an anticholinesterase administered at the same point in spontaneous recovery.[7] Because complete recovery of neuromuscular function (a train-of-four ratio > 0.9) is increasingly recognized as adequate recovery, this type of rapid and complete recovery profile will become increasingly necessary. In addition to decreasing the incidence of postoperative pulmonary complications, complete recovery of neuromuscular function after the administration of sugammadex results in shorter postanesthesia care unit stays and shorter times to discharge from the hospital. Whether the savings in medical care costs will be enough to off set the acquisition cost of sugammadex will have to be determined. Because sugammadex is not available for use in the United States, clinicians practicing here will have to continue to optimize care using agents that are available.

C. Lien, MD

References

1. Jonsson M, Wyon N, Lindahl SG, Fredholm BB, Eriksson LI. Neuromuscular blocking agents block carotid body neuronal nicotinic acetylcholine receptors. *Eur J Pharmacol.* 2004;497:173-180.
2. Berg H, Roed J, Viby-Mogensen J, et al. Residual neuromuscular block is a risk factor for postoperative pulmonary complications. A prospective, randomised, and blinded study of postoperative pulmonary complications after atracurium, vecuronium and pancuronium. *Acta Anaesthesiol Scand.* 1997;41:1095-1103.
3. Murphy GS, Szokol JW, Marymont JH, Greenberg SB, Avram MJ, Vender JS. Residual neuromuscular blockade and critical respiratory events in the postanesthesia care unit. *Anesth Analg.* 2008;107:130-137.
4. Hårdemark Cedborg AI, Sundman E, Bodén K, et al. Co-ordination of spontaneous swallowing with respiratory airflow and diaphragmatic and abdominal muscle activity in healthy adult humans. *Exp Physiol.* 2009;94:459-468.
5. Naguib M, Kopman AF, Lien CA, Hunter JM, Lopez A, Brull SJ. A survey of current management of neuromuscular block in the United States and Europe. *Anesth Analg.* 2010;111:110-119.
6. Epemolu O, Mayer I, Hope F, Scullion P, Desmond P. Liquid chromatography/mass spectrometric bioanalysis of a modified gamma-cyclodextrin (Org 25969) and Rocuronium bromide (Org 9426) in guinea pig plasma and urine: its application to determine the plasma pharmacokinetics of Org 25969. *Rapid Commun Mass Spectrom.* 2002;16:1946-1952.
7. Blobner M, Eriksson LI, Scholz J, Motsch J, Della Rocca G, Prins ME. Reversal of rocuronium-induced neuromuscular blockade with sugammadex compared with neostigmine during sevoflurane anaesthesia: results of a randomised, controlled trial. *Eur J Anaesthesiol.* 2010;27:874-881.

3　Anesthesia Techniques and Monitors

Acceleromyographic monitoring of neuromuscular block over the orbicularis oris muscle in anesthetized patients receiving vecuronium
Saitoh Y, Oshima T, Nakata Y (Tsujinaka Hosp Kashiwanoha, Chiba, Japan;
The Cancer Inst Hosp of Japanese Foundation for Cancer Res, Tokyo, Japan;
Teikyo Univ School of Medicine, Tokyo, Japan)
J Clin Anesth 22:318-323, 2010

Study Objective.—To evaluate the level of neuromuscular block acceleromyographically over the orbicularis oris muscle.

Design.—Prospective, randomized, controlled study.

Setting.—Operating room of a university-affiliated hospital.

Patients.—36 adult, ASA physical status I and II women scheduled for mastectomy with air-oxygen-isoflurane-fentanyl anesthesia.

Interventions.—Patients were randomized to two groups. In the orbicularis oris group (n=18), the facial nerve was stimulated and movement of the orbicularis oris muscle was measured acceleromyographically. In the control group (n=18), adduction of the thumb was quantified mechanically.

Measurements.—Onset and recovery of neuromuscular block caused by vecuronium 0.1 mg/kg were compared between the groups.

Main Results.—Time to onset of neuromuscular block in the orbicularis oris group was significantly shorter than in the control group (176 ± 52 vs. 220 ± 34 sec, mean ± SD; $P = 0.004$). Times to return of the first, second, third, or fourth (T1, T2, T3, or T4) response of train-of four (TOF), and recovery of T1/control were comparable between the groups. Train-of-four ratio (T4/T1) in the orbicularis oris group was significantly higher than in the control group 50 to 120 minutes after vecuronium administration ($P < 0.05$).

Conclusion.—Depth of neuromuscular block can be assessed acceleromyographically over the orbicularis oris muscle. Onset of neuromuscular block is quicker and recovery of TOF ratio is faster over the orbicularis oris muscle than at the thumb in patients receiving vecuronium.

▶ When providing anesthesia for patients undergoing surgical or diagnostic procedures, the patients' arms are likely to be tucked tightly by their sides, making monitoring at the adductor pollicis impossible. These authors confirm that monitoring at the orbicularis oris of the face provides clinicians with the ability to have a sense of how profound neuromuscular block is in their patients.

As found in other studies, the onset of neuromuscular block occurs more quickly and recovery more slowly in the muscles of the face than in the muscles of the arm.[1] In the current study, the use of different monitoring modalities, acceleromyography and electromyography, makes comparison of the results obtained in the face and at the arm difficult. That being said, it is interesting that the first, second, third, and fourth twitches in the train-of-4 response to stimulation reappeared at the same time intervals in both locations. This is important because dosing recommendations for anticholinesterases, when the train-of-4 count is less than 4, have been made based on the number of responses that are present to stimulation.[2] If these results are confirmed in other trials, neuromuscular block can be monitored at the orbicularis oris, and neuromuscular blocking agents can be dosed on the basis of monitoring results. Importantly, anticholinesterase could also be appropriately dosed on the basis of these results without access to the adductor pollicis. Clinicians should always remember when determining adequacy of recovery of neuromuscular function, however, that the train-of-4 ratio will be less at the arm than any location on the face.

C. Lien, MD

References

1. Donati F, Meistelman C, Plaud B. Vecuronium neuromuscular blockade at the adductor muscles of the larynx and adductor pollicis. *Anesthesiology.* 1991;74: 833-837.
2. Kopman AF, Eikermann M. Antagonism of non-depolarising neuromuscular block: current practice. *Anaesthesia.* 2009;64:22-30.

Automated Cuff Pressure Modulation: A Novel Device to Reduce Endotracheal Tube Injury
Chadha NK, Gordin A, Luginbuehl I, et al (Hosp for Sick Children, Toronto, Ontario, Canada)
Arch Otolaryngol Head Neck Surg 137:30-34, 2011

Objective.—To assess whether dynamically modulating endotracheal tube (ETT) cuff pressure, by decreasing it during each ventilatory cycle instead of maintaining a constant level, would reduce the extent of intubationrelated laryngotracheal injury.

Design.—Single-blind, randomized controlled animal study using a previously validated live porcine model of accelerated intubation-related tracheal injury.

Setting.—Animal research facility.

Patients.—Ten piglets (weight, 16-20 kg each) were anesthetized and underwent intubation using a cuffed ETT.

Interventions.—The animals were randomized into the following 2 groups: 5 pigs had a novel device to modulate their cuff pressure from 25 cm H_2O during inspiration to 7 cm H_2O during expiration, and 5 pigs had a constant cuff pressure of 25 cm H_2O. Both groups underwent ventilation under hypoxic conditions for 4 hours.

Main Outcome Measure.—Laryngotracheal mucosal injury after blinded histopathological assessment.

Results.—The modulated-pressure group showed significantly less overall laryngotracheal damage than the constant-pressure group (mean grades, 1.2 vs 2.1; $P < .001$). Subglottic damage and tracheal damage were significantly less severe in the modulated-pressure group (mean grades, 1.0 vs 2.2; $P < .001$, and 1.9 vs 3.2; $P < .001$, respectively). There was no significant difference in glottic or supraglottic damage between the groups ($P = .06$ and .27, respectively).

Conclusions.—This novel device reduces the risk of subglottic and tracheal injury by modulating ETT cuff pressure in synchronization with the ventilatory cycle. This finding could have far-reaching implications for reducing the risk of airway injury in patients undergoing long-term intubation. Further clinical study of this device is warranted.

▶ This is an interesting study of a device designed to regulate the pressure in the cuff of an endotracheal tube. The device does more than ensure that pressure does not increase too much. It varies cuff pressure with respiration, increasing the pressure during inspiration, to allow delivery of a positive pressure breath and then decreasing it during exhalation. The authors studied the efficacy of the device using a hypoxic animal model that they had previously described.[1] They determined cuff-induced damage to the tracheal mucosa over the course of 4 hours of mechanical ventilation with a hypoxic gas mixture. Although interesting, how relevant the model is to current intraoperative patient care and patient management in the intensive care unit is of concern.

If these same results are found in a clinical setting of prolonged ventilation with a gas mixture that was not hypoxic, incorporating this type of device into routine clinical practice could improve the care of patients requiring intubation and mechanical ventilation. Of note, the authors were looking for the presence of subglottic damage caused by cuff pressure. The frequency of laryngeal edema resulting from intubation was not documented. The impact of the device on the incidence of subglottic mucosal damage would be difficult to determine, as clinical practice varies, and the frequency of subglottic tracheal damage ranges from 20% to 100%.[2-4]

One piece of information not provided by the authors that would have been interesting was the volume of gas removed from the cuff of the endotracheal tubes over the 4-hour course of the experiment in control animals. Nitrous oxide is used less frequently in clinical practice now than it was prior to the addition of propofol and desflurane to the list of available anesthetics. In anesthetized or sedated patients, therefore, who are not straining on the endotracheal tube and not receiving nitrous oxide, one would expect little variation in cuff pressure over the course of an anesthetic.

Simple maintenance of a constant cuff pressure at or below a reasonable pressure may represent an improvement in clinical practice, where hyperinflation of the cuff is common.[4,5] Use of a device such as the one described in this article may further reduce the morbidity associated with endotracheal intubation, as it is not feasible for a clinician to vary the cuff pressure of the endotracheal tube with the respiratory cycle.

C. Lien, MD

References

1. Gordin A, Chadha NK, Campisi P, Luginbuehl I, Taylor G, Forte V. Effect of a novel anatomically shaped endotracheal tube on intubation-related injury. *Arch Otolaryngol Head Neck Surg.* 2010;136:54-59.
2. Wittekamp BH, van Mook WN, Tjan DH, Zwaveling JH, Bergmans DC. Clinical review: post-extubation laryngeal edema and extubation failure in critically ill adult patients. *Crit Care.* 2009;13:233.
3. Wain JC Jr. Postintubation tracheal stenosis. *Semin Thorac Cardiovasc Surg.* 2009; 21:284-289.
4. Combes X, Schauvliege F, Peyrouset O, et al. Intracuff pressure and tracheal morbidity: influence of filling with saline during nitrous oxide anesthesia. *Anesthesiology.* 2001;95:1120-1124.
5. Nseir S, Brisson H, Marquette CH, et al. Variations in endotracheal cuff pressure in intubated critically ill patients: prevalence and risk factors. *Eur J Anaesthesiol.* 2009;26:229-234.

Capnography enhances surveillance of respiratory events during procedural sedation: a meta-analysis

Waugh JB, Epps CA, Khodneva YA (Univ of Alabama at Birmingham)
J Clin Anesth 23:189-196, 2011

Study Objective.—To determine if capnography, in addition to standard monitoring, identified more respiratory complications than standard monitoring alone.

Design.—Meta-analysis.

Setting.—University medical center.

Measurements.—The electronic databases PubMed, CINAHL, and Cochrane Library (Cochrane Reviews, CENTRAL) were searched for studies published between 1995-2009 reporting adverse respiratory events during procedural sedation and analgesia (PSA) with clearly defined end-tidal carbon dioxide threshold, adult population, clear study design, P-value calculation, similar outcome and predictor variable definitions, and binary independent and dependent variable raw data. Five such studies were evaluated independently. A meta-analysis of these studies was performed.

Main Results.—During PSA, cases of respiratory depression were 17.6 times more likely to be detected if monitored by capnography than cases not monitored by capnography (95% CI, 2.5-122.1; $P < 0.004$).

Conclusion.—End-tidal carbon dioxide monitoring is an important addition in detecting respiratory depression during PSA.

▶ The results of this meta-analysis—that capnography improves detection of respiratory events during sedation—is not surprising. The pulse oximeter reacts slowly to changes in oxygenation saturation. After a period of apnea and desaturation, oxygen saturation continues to fall despite adequate ventilation and can be alarming. Anyone who works with these monitors anticipates the worsening SpO_2 value, knowing that it is only a period of time before the oximeter will begin to reflect the patient's improving oxygen saturation.

Capnography, on the other hand, monitors the concentration of carbon dioxide in the inspired and expired gases and provides a waveform indicative of the amount of carbon dioxide measure with each breath. Therefore, a period of apnea or any airway obstruction can be immediately detected with this monitor, as can the restoration of respiration. These monitors are not without problems when used during sedation. Not infrequently, the sampling port will be displaced so that it cannot sample properly, and the patient will appear as if he or she is not breathing. Additionally, because the gas the system is sampling contains room air in addition to what the patient is exhaling, the measured value of carbon dioxide may be more a reflection of relative changes in respiration rather than an indication of the absolute value of exhaled carbon dioxide. Nevertheless, the monitors are required during the administration of general anesthesia and are frequently used in the operating room when providing sedation.

What is surprising about this study is that the authors were able to identify only 5 studies meeting their inclusion criteria published over a 14-year span. As suggested by this meta-analysis, as more procedures requiring sedation are being done outside of the operating room, more prospective trials documenting the utility of end-tidal capnography as a monitor for these procedures will need to be done.

C. Lien, MD

Endobronchial intubation detected by insertion depth of endotracheal tube, bilateral auscultation, or observation of chest movements: randomised trial
Sitzwohl C, Langheinrich A, Schober A, et al (Med Univ of Vienna General Hosp, Austria; et al)
BMJ 341:c5943, 2010

Objective.—To determine which bedside method of detecting inadvertent endobronchial intubation in adults has the highest sensitivity and specificity.

Design.—Prospective randomised blinded study.

Setting.—Department of anaesthesia in tertiary academic hospital.

Participants.—160 consecutive patients (American Society of Anesthesiologists category I or II) aged 19-75 scheduled for elective gynaecological or urological surgery.

Interventions.—Patients were randomly assigned to eight study groups. In four groups, an endotracheal tube was fibreoptically positioned 2.5-4.0 cm above the carina, whereas in the other four groups the tube was positioned in the right mainstem bronchus. The four groups differed in the bedside test used to verify the position of the endotracheal tube. To determine whether the tube was properly positioned in the trachea, in each patient first year residents and experienced anaesthetists were randomly assigned to independently perform bilateral auscultation of the chest (auscultation); observation and palpation of symmetrical chest movements (observation); estimation of the position of the tube by the insertion depth (tube depth); or a combination of all three (all three).

Main Outcome Measures.—Correct and incorrect judgments of endotracheal tube position.

Results.—160 patients underwent 320 observations by experienced and inexperienced anaesthetists. First year residents missed endobronchial intubation by auscultation in 55% of cases and performed significantly worse than experienced anaesthetists with this bedside test (odds ratio 10.0, 95% confidence interval 1.4 to 434). With a sensitivity of 88% (95% confidence interval 75% to 100%) and 100%, respectively, tube depth and the three tests combined were significantly more sensitive for detecting endobronchial intubation than auscultation (65%, 49% to 81%) or observation(43%, 25% to 60%) (P<0.001). The four tested methods had the same specificity for ruling out endobronchial intubation (that is, confirming correct tracheal intubation). The average correct tube insertion depth was 21 cm in women and 23 cm in men. By inserting the tube to these distances, however, the distal tip of the tube was less than 2.5 cm away from the carina (the recommended safety distance, to prevent inadvertent endobronchial intubation with changes in the position of the head in intubated patients) in 20% (24/118) of women and 18% (7/42) of men. Therefore optimal tube insertion depth was considered to be 20 cm in women and 22 cm in men.

Conclusion.—Less experienced clinicians should rely more on tube insertion depth than on auscultation to detect inadvertent endobronchial intubation. But even experienced physicians will benefit from inserting tubes to 20-21 cm in women and 22-23 cm in men, especially when high ambient noise precludes accurate auscultation (such as in emergency situations or helicopter transport). The highest sensitivity and specificity for ruling out endobronchial intubation, however, is achieved by combining tube depth, auscultation of the lungs, and observation of symmetrical chest movements.

Trial Registration.—NCT01232166.

▶ This is a straightforward study that validates some of the things that we do on a daily basis to confirm that each endotracheal tube is positioned properly. In the clinical setting, where we are also concerned that the endotracheal tube (ETT) is in the trachea and not the esophagus, we look for condensation in the ETT and the presence of end-tidal to carbon dioxide on our monitors, in addition to auscultating the chest, observing chest movement, and looking at the depth of the endotracheal tube.

In terms of accurately detecting endobronchial placement of the endotracheal tube, it is not surprising that, regardless of the method of assessment (observation, auscultation, or tube depth), experienced clinicians more reliably noted actual location of the endotracheal tube. These differences were less marked when the ETT was correctly positioned in the trachea.

As with any monitor in the operating room, no single piece of information should be used in isolation to diagnose a clinical situation. Rather, a constellation of findings should be used to determine the cause of any clinical issue. To ensure that an ETT has not been advanced into the bronchus, clinicians should observe chest movement, auscultate the lungs, and look at the depth of the ETT. If, for any reason, all 3 cannot be done, based on the results of this study, confirming that the ETT is at the proper depth—20 cm in women and 22 cm in men—allows for the most reliable confirmation of a tracheal, rather than endobronchial, intubation.

As noted by the authors, 20 cm may not be the correct depth of the ETT in female patients. In women of short stature, a depth of 19 cm may be more appropriate. To determine other means of identifying the proper depth of the endotracheal tube, the utility of other bedside tests, such as palpation of the cuff of the ETT in the suprasternal notch, should be investigated in a prospective randomized fashion.

C. Lien, MD

Learning curves of novice anesthesiology residents performing simulated fibreoptic upper airway endoscopy

Dalal PG, Dalal GB, Pott L, et al (Penn State Milton S Hershey Med Ctr, PA)
Can J Anesth 58:802-809, 2011

Background.—In various medical and surgical specialties, it is essential to acquire fibreoptic upper airway endoscopy skills for successful endotracheal intubation, especially when faced with a difficult airway. The aim of our study was to evaluate the learning curves of residents performing fibreoptic upper airway endoscopy in the simulation environment.

Methods.—Following a standardized video and practice session, 16 residents newly enrolled in the anesthesiology program performed nasal fibreoptic endoscopy of the upper airway (endpoint being the carina) on a high fidelity simulator. Weekly 20-min sessions continued for a period of one month. Each attempt was designated as either a "success" or a "failure" based on the study participant's ability or inability to visualize the carina in ≤60 sec and with ≤five collisions with the simulated mucosal wall. Proficiency was attained when the downward graphical trend of the cumulative sum (CUSUM) analysis crossed two adjacent boundary lines, i.e., an acceptable failure rate was reached.

Results.—The residents' mean number of attempts at fibreoptic airway endoscopy was 47 (9) with a range of 32–64. Time to visualization of the carina was 51 (36) sec. Three classical patterns of CUSUM trends were observed: proficient ($n = 7$); not proficient with a downward (improvement) trend ($n = 3$); and not proficient with an upward (worsening) trend ($n = 6$). The number of attempts at which proficiency was achieved varied from 27 to 58.

Conclusion.—There is a large variation in the learning curves of residents performing fibreoptic upper airway endoscopy. The training for fibreoptic airway endoscopy should be tailored to the needs of each individual.

▶ This is an interesting study that looks at establishing criteria for successful performance of a fiberoptic bronchoscopy and then the number of attempts over a period of time for novices in that task to become proficient.

Of note, more than half of the 16 residents participating in the trial did not become proficient with 58 attempts at fiberoptic intubation. For those students whose skills improved with repeated exposure, improvements occurred over varying amounts of time.

Initial instruction included video clips and 15-minute practice sessions. The study participants then spent 20 minutes each week attempting nasal fiberoptic bronchoscopy with feedback provided after each session.

The study demonstrates that use of the simulator alone will not make everyone proficient, and for those not following the anticipated course toward success, additional active instruction may be necessary. One of the appeals of the simulator as an educational tool is that it allows for individualized instruction over a longer period of time than could be tolerated when learning in the clinical setting. Practice in a simulated scenario requires constant feedback so that correct habits are learned and ineffective practices are not repeated.

An interesting aspect of this study was that it set a measurable goal applicable to clinical practice in determining the proficiency of students. Keeping in mind that skill increases over the course of a residency and once training is completed, where the standard should be for a resident new to a technique is not immediately apparent. As more of these studies are done with an increasing number of students and students at different levels of training, how to define adequate performance may become clearer.

C. Lien, MD

Learning Endotracheal Intubation Using a Novel Videolaryngoscope Improves Intubation Skills of Medical Students

Herbstreit F, Fassbender P, Haberl H, et al (Univ Hosp Essen, Germany)
Anesth Analg 113:586-590, 2011

Introduction.—Teaching endotracheal intubation to medical students is a task provided by many academic anesthesia departments. We tested the hypothesis that teaching with a novel videolaryngoscope improves students' intubation skills.

Methods.—We prospectively assessed in medical students (2nd clinical year) intubation skills acquired by intubation attempts in adult anesthetized patients during a 60-hour clinical course using, in a randomized fashion, either a conventional Macintosh blade laryngoscope or a videolaryngoscope (C-MAC®). The latter permits direct laryngoscopy with a Macintosh blade and provides a color image on a video screen. Skills were measured before and after the course in a standardized fashion (METI Emergency Care

Simulator) using a conventional laryngoscope. All 1-semester medical students ($n = 93$) were enrolled.

Results.—The students' performance did not significantly differ between groups before the course. After the course, students trained with the video-laryngoscope had an intubation success rate on a manikin 19% higher (95% CI 1.1%−35.3%; $P < 0.001$) and intubated 11 seconds faster (95% CI 4−18) when compared with those trained using a conventional laryngo-scope. The incidence of "difficult (manikin) laryngoscopy" was less frequent in the group trained with the videolaryngoscope (8% vs 34%; $P = 0.005$).

Conclusion.—Education using a video system mounted into a traditional Macintosh blade improves intubation skills in medical students.

▶ This article provides evidence that traditional methods of teaching can be improved upon. It is not unexpected that learning is improved when both instructor and student can see what is being visualized during a laryngoscopy. If the instructor is looking at what the student sees in real time, directions as to how to specifically maneuver the laryngoscope to improve visualization of the larynx can be given. The student will understand what the instructor wants him/her to see because both are looking at the same image and he/she can perse-vere with each laryngoscopy until both he/she and the instructor have an ideal view of the larynx. When teaching in the more traditional method, the student inserts the laryngoscope with instruction, finds the larynx, and then allows the instructor to confirm that his/her view is adequate. In doing this, the view that the student had may be lost.

Because C-MACs are not available throughout most operating room suites, it is reassuring that the skills learned with videolaryngoscopy were retained when using a traditional Macintosh blade. These results were somewhat surprising, because with direct laryngoscopy, the clinician looks directly at the larynx. And with the C-MAC, the clinician is looking at a video screen. In determining how these results would apply to other teaching settings, it would have been useful to know what experience each student had in addition to that obtained in the simulation setting and whether experiences were comparable amongst students. One aspect of teaching intubation skills with a C-MAC that was not addressed in this study was how long skills were retained after instruction. This type of data would be important as educators plan courses of study over a 4-year residency.

C. Lien, MD

Local Is Better Than General Anesthesia During Endovascular Acute Stroke Interventions
Gupta R (Grady Memorial Hosp, Atlanta, GA)
Stroke 41:2718-2719, 2010

Background.—Patients suffering acute ischemic stroke often undergo endovascular reperfusion techniques to improve clinical outcome. Acute stroke protocols are usually designed for emergency departments and stroke units, but procedures done in the endovascular suite may not adhere to standard protocols such as close monitoring of all medical parameters. General anesthesia (GA) is typically used in endovascular suites, but the safety of GA compared to conscious sedation (CS) has not been closely analyzed.

Safety Analysis.—The criteria used to assess the safety of GA versus CS focus on the rate of intracranial hemorrhages that occur, which is a surrogate for wire perforations, and the number of patients who require emergency intubation who were initially given CS. Recent publications demonstrate no difference in hemorrhage statistics between the two approaches, so procedures can be safely performed under CS. The conversion rate from CS to GA is only 2.7%. In addition, patients treated under GA have had higher rates of pneumonia, longer stays in the intensive care unit (ICU), and larger infarct volumes.

Advantage Analysis.—GA is favored for endovascular reperfusion because it provides patient immobility, allows tight control of hemodynamics, may protect the brain, and addresses compromised airway concerns, a common problem in acute stroke. However, evidence does not support a need for patient immobility. Awake patients can participate in neurological assessments that help the operator to determine their neurological status. This real-time determination can impact neurological outcome, especially with aggressive attempts to achieve an angiographic result.

Patients with acute stroke often have other problems such as coronary artery disease, pulmonary disease, cardiac dysrhythmias, renal disease, and valve disease. These increase the possibility that semielective or planned surgical procedures will be done under GA. Comorbidities may be incompletely characterized in the acute stroke situation. Emergency intubation may also increase the risk of airway injury and pulmonary aspiration, especially when rapid sequence intubation is not done.

Protection for cerebral structures from inhaled gases is based on an as-yet-unproved hypothesis. Maintaining cerebral autoregulation with arterial occlusion is needed so cerebral perfusion pressure remains sufficient to the target penumbra where therapy is being delivered. Anesthetic induction often causes hypotension, which is managed with vasopressors that can breach the upper limits of autoregulation. Clinical outcomes of acute stroke are worse with wide fluctuations in blood pressure.

When patients are intubated for acute stroke interventions, they are often brought to the ICU before being extubated. Although there is understandable reluctance to extubate patients with moderate to severe strokes, each day the tube remains in place raises the risk of nosocomial infections, delays rehabilitation, and complicates discharge planning. Care withdrawal is more likely when the family sees loved ones on "life support" and having a profound neurological deficit.

Conclusions.—CS appears to be as safe as GA for endovascular acute stroke situations. The use of GA may not improve clinical outcomes.

Further clinical trials are needed to justify the use of GA and explore the possible advantages of CS for acute stroke.

▶ In this editorial, Dr Gupta raises the possibility that use of conscious sedation, rather than general anesthesia, during endovascular interventions for acute stroke management may allow for better outcomes. Certainly, for select patients, sedation may be the better anesthetic choice. However, as the author notes, patients who have had a stroke often have significant comorbidities, and their assessment is essential before the choice of the most appropriate anesthetic is made. Sedation is not optimal for all patients. A patient with significant pulmonary disease who is hypoxemic may not be an ideal candidate for sedation. Those with expressive aphasia because of their central nervous system (CNS) injury will not be able to express their concerns to their physicians in the radiology suite. Those with receptive aphasia will be unable to understand and follow simple instructions, possibly making the procedure more difficult.

There are risks associated with general anesthesia. However, with careful choice and dosing of induction agents, the risk of hypotension can be minimized. Elective endotracheal intubation for endovascular stroke management is not an emergent process. If chosen as part of an anesthetic, it will be done after establishment of appropriate intravenous access, application of monitors, and preoxygenation. With a quick airway assessment, potential difficulty with intubation can be anticipated and airway adjuvants made available.

As with general anesthesia, there are risks associated with sedation. Perhaps most important among these risks is hypoventilation. Sedative hypnotics are all respiratory depressants, as are the opioids that may be used as part of a sedative technique. One agent that may be used for sedation, dexmedetomidine, is not associated with respiratory depression. It, however, is not frequently used as the sole sedative agent. Neither hypoxia nor hypercapnea will be tolerated well in a brain that has a fresh ischemic insult. Additional swelling because of these induced physiologic derangements could lead to decreased cerebral perfusion and greater injury.

As endovascular treatment of acute strokes is becoming increasingly common, studies of how to best treat these patients are required. They will be difficult to design, though, because of the variability in presentation of the patient regarding the extent and type of CNS injury, the initial time of onset of symptoms, and the many different comorbidities that they may have.

C. Lien, MD

Meta-analysis of desflurane and propofol average times and variability in times to extubation and following commands
Wachtel RE, Dexter F, Epstein RH, et al (Univ of Iowa; Jefferson Med College, Philadelphia, PA)
Can J Anaesth 58:714-724, 2011

Purpose.—We performed a meta-analysis to compare the operating room recovery time of desflurane with that of propofol.

Methods.—Studies were included in which a) humans were assigned randomly to propofol or desflurane groups without other differences between groups (e.g., induction drugs) and b) mean and standard deviation were reported for extubation time and/or time to follow commands. Since there was heterogeneity of variance between treatment groups in the log-scale (i.e., unequal coefficients of variation of observations in the time scale), generalized pivotal methods for the lognormal distribution were used as inputs of the random effects meta-analyses.

Results.—Desflurane reduced the variability (i.e., standard deviation) in time to extubation by 26% relative to propofol (95% confidence interval [CI], 6% to 42%; $P = 0.006$) and reduced the variability in time to follow commands by 39% (95% CI, 25% to 51%; $P < 0.001$). Desflurane reduced the mean time to extubation by 21% (95% CI, 9% to 32%; $P = 0.001$) and reduced the mean time to follow commands by 23% (95% CI, 16% to 30%; $P < 0.001$).

Conclusions.—The mean reduction in operating room recovery time for desflurane relative to propofol was comparable with that shown previously for desflurane relative to sevoflurane. The reduction in variability exceeded that of sevoflurane. Facilities can use the percentage differences when making evidence-based pharmacoeconomic decisions.

▶ This type of study is extremely important in characterizing the dynamic behavior of an anesthetic. Application of the results to clinical practice, however, is not as easily accomplished. Generally, however, general anesthetics consist of combinations of different medications titrated to the desired effect. Typically, benzodiazepines and analgesics are administered in addition to desflurane and may cause a delay in emergence from anesthesia. If administration of one anesthetic reliably provided, in addition to more rapid emergence from general anesthesia and more rapid operating room turnover and greater patient satisfaction, more anesthesiologists would be practicing in that fashion. Solutions to slow patient throughput, however, are not that simple. Other factors are likely more important in causing delays than the time required to set up a propofol infusion. Some that warrant consideration include the nature of the surgery, the duration of the surgery, availability of space in the postanesthesia care unit, and the experience of the anesthesia care provider. Most anesthetics can be titrated to surgical requirement and, even with complex and prolonged anesthetics, medications titrated so that patients emerge from anesthesia as the surgical dressing is being applied. That desflurane allows for a reduction in operating room time relative to propofol is one specific factor to consider when determining how to decrease patient costs and increase operating room throughput. Other factors are also likely to be significant.

C. Lien, MD

Patient safety incidents involving neuromuscular blockade: analysis of the UK National Reporting and Learning System data from 2006 to 2008
Arnot-Smith J, Smith AF (Royal Bolton Hosp Foundation Trust, Bolton, UK; Royal Lancaster Infirmary, UK)
Anaesthesia 65:1106-1113, 2010

Neuromuscular blockade is a powerful anaesthetic tool that has the potential for significant adverse outcomes. We sought to explore the national picture by analysing incidents relating to neuromuscular blockade in anaesthesia from the National Reporting and Learning System from England and Wales between 2006 and 2008. We searched the database of incidents using SNOMED CT® search terms and reading the free text of relevant incidents. There were 231 incidents arising from the use or reversal of neuromuscular blocking agents. The main themes identified were: non-availability of drugs (45 incidents, 19%), possible unintentional awareness under general anaesthesia (42 incidents, 18%), potential allergic reaction (31 incidents, 13%), problems with reversal of blockade (13 incidents, 6%), storage (13 incidents, 6%) and prolonged apnoea (11 incidents, 5%). We make recommendations to reduce human error in the use of neuromuscular blocking agents and on future incident reporting in anaesthesia.

▶ Databases are most useful when the data in them can be reviewed by practitioners to look at their practice as it compares with others and to determine what benchmarks there are for adverse incidents. The study found a total of 231 incidents related to neuromuscular blocking agents of almost 200 000 reported incidents, giving an incidence of just over 0.1%. Adverse incidents were further examined to determine the degree of harm resulting from the incident and where the adverse incidents occurred. From the text entered with each reported incident, common themes were developed. These included lack of availability of drugs, reversal problems, prolonged apnea, drug ineffective, no neuromuscular blockade monitor available, and drugs stored incorrectly. Based on this scheme, the most frequent adverse event was lack of availability of drug (19.5%), followed by possible awareness (18.2%). Incidents related to residual neuromuscular block, such as reversal problems and prolonged apnea, were reported far less frequently (10.4% of incidents). Interestingly, the search terms did not include words such as reintubation, airway obstruction, weakness, or hypoxia. Because of this, complications related to postoperative residual neuromuscular block may have been missed.

How to interpret the frequency reported in this study is not clear. Reporting of incidents to the National Reporting and Learning System over the course of the 3 years included in this article increased markedly in 2008, the last year reviewed. Unless this number of reportable incidents actually increased, reporting during at least the first 2 years of review was incomplete. Whether or not what was reported each year was representative of actual incidents is not known. Reexamination of the database for adverse incidents should be undertaken after several years of robust reporting to begin to understand how frequently they happen.

Expansion of the searched terms may allow for identification of more adverse events related to the use of neuromuscular blocking agents.

C. Lien, MD

Residual Neuromuscular Block: Lessons Unlearned. Part I: Definitions, Incidence, and Adverse Physiologic Effects of Residual Neuromuscular Block
Murphy GS, Brull SJ (Univ of Chicago, Evanston, IL; Mayo Clinic College of Medicine, Jacksonville, FL)
Anesth Analg 111:120-128, 2010

In this review, we summarize the clinical implications of residual neuromuscular block. Data suggest that residual neuromuscular block is a common complication in the postanesthesia care unit, with approximately 40% of patients exhibiting a train-of-four ratio <0.9. Volunteer studies have demonstrated that small degrees of residual paralysis (train-of-four ratios 0.7—0.9) are associated with impaired pharyngeal function and increased risk of aspiration, weakness of upper airway muscles and airway obstruction, attenuation of the hypoxic ventilatory response (approximately 30%), and unpleasant symptoms of muscle weakness. Clinical studies have also identified adverse postoperative events associated with intraoperative neuromuscular management. Large databased investigations have identified intraoperative use of muscle relaxants and residual neuromuscular block as important risk factors in anesthetic-related morbidity and mortality. Furthermore, observational and randomized clinical trials have demonstrated that incomplete neuromuscular recovery during the early postoperative period may result in acute respiratory events (hypoxemia and airway obstruction), unpleasant symptoms of muscle weakness, longer postanesthesia care unit stays, delays in tracheal extubation, and an increased risk of postoperative pulmonary complications. These recent data suggest that residual neuromuscular block is an important patient safety issue and that neuromuscular management affects postoperative outcomes.

▶ This article details the findings of studies done over the past 10 years that involved identification of postoperative residual neuromuscular block. Although not all studies found a high incidence of postoperative residual neuromuscular block (defined as a train-of-4 ratio less than 70%, 80%, or 90%), a few patterns were apparent. The frequency of unacceptable levels of paralysis increased as the minimally acceptable train-of-4 ratio increased to 90%. Although use of the long-acting compound, pancuronium, was associated with more patients having inadequate recovery of neuromuscular function, the use of the short-acting neuromuscular blocking agent, mivacurium, offered no advantage over the intermediate-acting agent, rocuronium.

Residual neuromuscular block has been found to be associated with increases in anesthetic mortality, difficulty speaking, swallowing, seeing, sitting up without assistance, hypoxemia, airway obstruction and pneumonia. Of note, although some patients with a train-of-4 ratio less than 90% will develop adverse postoperative respiratory events, most patients with residual neuromuscular block seem to tolerate it without sequelae. As noted by the authors, adverse events attributable to residual neuromuscular block may be difficult to distinguish from those attributable to the prolonged effects of anesthetic medications; however, reducing the incidence of residual neuromuscular block may decrease the incidence of these complications.

C. Lien, MD

Residual Neuromuscular Block: Lessons Unlearned. Part II: Methods to Reduce the Risk of Residual Weakness
Brull SJ, Murphy GS (Mayo Clinic College of Medicine, Jacksonville, FL; Univ of Chicago, Evanston, IL)
Anesth Analg 111:129-140, 2010

The aim of the second part of this review is to examine optimal neuromuscular management strategies that can be used by clinicians to reduce the risk of residual paralysis in the early postoperative period. Current evidence has demonstrated that frequently used clinical tests of neuromuscular function (such as head lift or hand grip) cannot reliably exclude the presence of residual paralysis. When qualitative (visual or tactile) neuromuscular monitoring is used (train-of-four [TOF], double-burst, or tetanic stimulation patterns), clinicians often are unable to detect fade when TOF ratios are between 0.6 and 1.0. Furthermore, the effect of qualitative monitoring on postoperative residual paralysis remains controversial. In contrast, there is strong evidence that acceleromyography (quantitative) monitoring improves detection of small degrees (TOF ratios >0.6) of residual blockade. The use of intermediate-acting neuromuscular blocking drugs (NMBDs) can reduce, but do not eliminate, the risk of residual paralysis when compared with long-acting NMBDs. In addition, complete recovery of neuromuscular function is more likely when anticholinesterases are administered early (>15−20 minutes before tracheal extubation) and at a shallower depth of block (TOF count of 4). Finally, the recent development of rapid-onset, short-acting NMBDs and selective neuromuscular reversal drugs that can effectively antagonize deep levels of blockade may provide clinicians with novel pharmacologic approaches for the prevention of postoperative residual weakness and its associated complications.

▶ This review is a continuation of the author's other review article in the same journal.[1] While the other review article focused on defining residual neuromuscular block and its adverse effects and determining the incidence of unacceptable levels of recovery of neuromuscular strength at the end of a surgical procedure, this review describes some of the ways that the risk of residual neuromuscular block can be reduced. The author's task was relatively complex in that few studies actually define how to decrease the incidence of residual neuromuscular block. Most studies have described it, defined its incidence, or looked at adverse events associated with it, but, with the exception of studies of quantitative monitors of the depth of neuromuscular block, essentially none have prospectively identified ways to reduce the risk of residual neuromuscular block.

That being said, the authors, in summarizing available data, develop suggestions to decrease the risk of residual neuromuscular block. These include not using long-acting neuromuscular blocking agents, such as pancuronium, approaching appropriate monitoring as a tool (the results on which additional dosing of neuromuscular blocking agents or anticholinesterases will be predicated), understanding that clinical tests are limited in the information that they can provide and that none is adequately sensitive or specific to routinely identify the presence of residual neuromuscular block, and appropriately dosing anticholinesterases.

Without quantitative monitoring of depth of neuromuscular block, it is impossible to know whether a patient has or has not fully recovered from neuromuscular block. Use of shorter-acting neuromuscular blocking agents or compounds that are more reliable and quickly speed up recovery of neuromuscular function may reduce the incidence of residual neuromuscular block.

C. Lien, MD

Reference

1. Brull SJ, Murphy GS. Residual neuromuscular block: lessons unlearned. Part 1: definitions, incidence and adverse physiologic effects of residual neuromuscular block. *Anesth Analg.* 2010;111:120-128.

The effect of neuromuscular blockade on mask ventilation
Warters RD, Szabo TA, Spinale FG, et al (Med Univ of South Carolina, Charleston)
Anaesthesia 66:163-167, 2011

We wished to test the hypothesis that neuromuscular blockade facilitates mask ventilation. In order reliably and reproducibly to assess the efficiency of mask ventilation, we developed a novel grading scale (Warters scale), based on attempts to generate a standardised tidal volume. Following induction of general anaesthesia, a blinded anaesthesia provider assessed mask ventilation in 90 patients using our novel grading scale. The non-blinded anaesthesiologist then randomly administered rocuronium or normal saline. After 2 min, mask ventilation was reassessed by the blinded practitioner. Rocuronium significantly improved ventilation scores on the Warters scale (mean (SD) 2.3 (1.6) vs 1.2 (0.9), $p < 0.001$). In a subgroup of patients with a baseline Warters scale value of > 3 (i.e. difficult to mask ventilate; $n = 14$), the ventilation scores also showed significant improvement (4.2 (1.2) vs 1.9 (1.0), $p = 0.0002$). Saline administration had no effect on ventilation scores. Our data indicate that neuromuscular blockade facilitates mask ventilation. We discuss the implications of this finding for unexpected difficult airway management and for the practice of confirming adequate mask ventilation before the administration of neuro-muscular blockade (Fig 1).

▶ This article demonstrates that ventilation will most likely become easier after administration of a neuromuscular blocking agent. It also describes a system in which ease of ventilation can be quantified and compares the system with one described by Han in 2004.[1] The system described by Han assigns a score of 1 through 4 to the ease of ventilation, based on whether patients could be venti-lated by mask (score of 1) or were impossible to ventilate (score of 4). The grading scale proposed in this article considers factors such as use of an oral airway, peak inspiratory pressures required to ventilate a patient, the number of anesthesia providers required to ventilate the patient, and the tidal volume gener-ated with mask ventilation. The goal of ventilation is delivery of a 5 mL/kg tidal volume. It is not apparent from the article how points are assigned. One can easily imagine a clinical situation in which a peak inspiratory pressure of more than 30 cmH2O is required to generate a tidal volume of 2 mL/kg. Would this patient warrant a score of 2 or 3? Similarly, what score is assigned to the individual easily ventilated with 5 mL/kg and a peak inspiratory pressure less than 20 cmH2O?

As shown in the histograms in Fig 1,[2] none of the patients enrolled were, based on the Han scale, impossible to ventilate. Distribution of the ventilation scores based on the Warters scale is not presented. The only data presented from grading on this scale are that average scores in the saline and rocuronium groups were 1.9 and 2.3, respectively. Therefore, it is not possible to determine

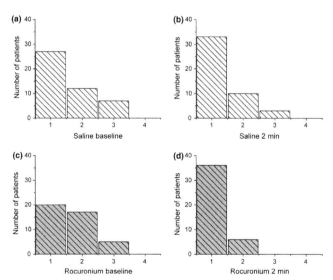

FIGURE 1.—Histograms presenting raw data and estimated distribution of ventilation scores for the Han scale at baseline and 2 min after saline (a, b) or rocuronium (c, d) administration. (Reprinted from Warters RD, Szabo TA, Spinale FG, et al. The effect of neuromuscular blockade on mask ventilation. *Anaesthesia.* 2011;66:163-167, with permission from The Association of Anaesthetists of Great Britain and Ireland.)

the clinical utility of this alternative scale or how it actually compares with one that is currently used in practice.

Regardless of the applicability of the Warters scale, the results of this study, that ventilation became, on average, easier following administration of the neuromuscular blocking agent, support not checking ease of ventilation before administering a neuromuscular blocking agent.[3] Had any patients in the saline and rocuronium study groups been impossible to ventilate following induction of anesthesia, the argument to administer the neuromuscular blocking agent without checking for ease of ventilation would have been strengthened.

C. Lien, MD

References

1. Han R, Tremper KK, Kheterpal S, O'Reilly M. Grading scale for mask ventilation. *Anesthesiology.* 2004;101:267.
2. Warters RD, Szabo TA, Spinale FG, DeSantis SM, Reves JG. The effect of neuro-muscular blockade on mask ventilation. *Anaesthesia.* 2011;66:163-167.
3. Broomhead RH, Marks RJ, Ayton P. Confirmation of the ability to ventilate by facemask before administration of neuromuscular blocker: a non-instrumental piece of information. *Br J Anaesth.* 2010;104:313-317.

Train-of-four ratio recovery often precedes twitch recovery when neuromuscular block is reversed by sugammadex

Staals LM, Driessen JJ, van Egmond J, et al (Erasmus Univ Med Centre, Rotterdam, The Netherlands; Radboud Univ Nijmegen Med Centre, The Netherlands; et al)
Acta Anaesthesiol Scand 55:700-707, 2011

Background.—Sugammadex reverses rocuronium-induced neuromuscular block (NMB). In all published studies investigating sugammadex, the primary outcome parameter was a train-of-four (TOF) ratio of 0.9. The recovery time of T1 was not described. This retrospective investigation describes the recovery of T1 vs. TOF ratio after the reversal of NMB with sugammadex.

Methods.—Two studies were analyzed. In study A, a phase II dose-finding study, ASA I–II patients received an intravenous (IV) dose of rocuronium 1.2 mg/kg, followed by an IV dose of sugammadex (2.0, 4.0, 8.0, 12.0 or 16.0 mg/kg) or placebo (0.9% saline) after 5 min. In study B, a phase III trial comparing patients with renal failure and healthy controls, rocuronium 0.6 mg/kg was used to induce NMB; sugammadex 2.0 mg/kg was administered at reappearance of T2. Neuromuscular monitoring was performed by acceleromyography and TOF nerve stimulation. The primary efficacy variable was time from the administration of sugammadex to recovery of the TOF ratio to 0.9. Retrospectively, the time to recovery of T1 to 90% was calculated.

Results.—After the reversal of rocuronium-induced NMB with an optimal dose of sugammadex [16 mg/kg (A) or 2 mg/kg (B)], the TOF ratio recovered to 0.9 significantly faster than T1 recovered to 90%. Clinical signs of residual paralysis were not observed.

Conclusion.—After the reversal of NMB by sugammadex, full recovery of the TOF ratio is possible when T1 is still depressed. The TOF ratio as the only measurement for the adequate reversal of NMB by sugammadex may not always be reliable. Further investigations for clinical implications are needed.

▶ While the results of this post-hoc analysis of 2 studies[1,2] are interesting, their significance is not clear. The results from re-examination of the data are conflicting. As described by the authors, results from the first study[1] indicate that as long as a dose of sugammadex that is ≤4 mg/kg is administered to antagonize profound neuromuscular block, recovery of neuromuscular function occurs as would be expected. That is, twitch height (the first response to train-of-four stimulation) occurs first and recovery of the train-of-four response follows. Following administration of 8-16 mg/kg sugammadex, though, the train-of-four response (TOFR) is completely recovered before the first twitch in the train-of-four has recovered to baseline. Recovery of the TOFR occurs on average 1 to 2 minutes more quickly than recovery of T1 (the first twitch in the train-of-four). Based on these findings, it would seem prudent to use smaller doses of sugammadex to antagonize residual neuromuscular block.

In the second study,[2] however, smaller doses of sugammadex (2 mg/kg) were used to facilitate recovery from less-profound depths of neuromuscular block. Sugammadex was administered once the second twitch reappeared in response to train-of-four stimulation. In this study, administration of sugammadex resulted in recovery of the TOFR an average of 1.2 minutes before T1 had returned to baseline. The recovery of T1 was even slower in patients with renal failure (2.6 minutes after recovery of the TOFR). Perhaps it is the dose of sugammadex relative to the depth of neuromuscular block that is important in determining whether T1 or the train-of-four recovers first. This relationship will need to be determined in properly designed, prospective trials.

Adequacy of recovery is defined in terms of the response to train-of-four stimulation. A TOFR where the fourth response is 90% of the first response is considered adequate recovery for extubation of a patient's trachea. The significance of a train-of-four ratio of 0.9 and T1 less than baseline has not yet been determined. The authors of the 2 studies in this report did not comment on any patient exhibiting signs of residual neuromuscular block. More recently, a train-of-four ratio obtained with acceleromyography of ≥1.0 has been recommended to better guarantee complete recovery. What the authors of this report did not determine was T1 at the point that the train-of-four ratio had recovered to 1.0.[3] It would have been both interesting and important to know if these recovery variables occurred at the same time.

C. Lien, MD

References

1. de Boer HD, Driessen JJ, Marcus MA, Kerkkamp H, Heeringa M, Klimek M. Reversal of rocuronium-induced (1.2 mg/kg) profound neuromuscular blockade

by sugammadex: a multicenter, dose-finding and safety study. *Anesthesiology.* 2007;107:239-244.

2. Staals LM, Snoek MM, Driessen JJ, Flockton EA, Heeringa M, Hunter JM. Multicentre, parallel-group, comparative trial evaluating the efficacy and safety of sugammadex in patients with end-stage renal failure or normal renal function. *Br J Anaesth.* 2008;101:492-497.

3. Capron F, Alla F, Hottier C, Meistelman C, Fuchs-Buder T. Can acceleromyography detect low levels of residual paralysis? A probability approach to detect a mechanomyographic train-of-four ratio of 0.9. *Anesthesiology.* 2004;100:1119-1124.

Transcranial Doppler Detection of Cerebral Fat Emboli and Relation to Paradoxical Embolism: A Pilot Study

Forteza AM, Koch S, Campo-Bustillo I, et al (Univ of Miami Miller School of Medicine, FL)
Circulation 123:1947-1952, 2011

Background.—The fat embolism syndrome is clinically characterized by dyspnea, skin petechiae, and neurological dysfunction. It is associated mainly with long bone fracture and bone marrow fat passage to the systemic circulation. An intracardiac right-to-left shunt (RLS) could allow larger fat particles to reach the systemic circulation. Transcranial Doppler can be a useful tool to detect both RLS and the fat particles reaching the brain.

Methods and Results.—We prospectively studied patients with femur shaft fracture with RLS evaluation, daily transcranial Doppler with embolus detection studies, and neurological examinations to evaluate the relation of RLS and microembolic signals to the development of fat embolism syndrome. Forty-two patients were included; 14 had an RLS detected. Seven patients developed neurological symptoms; all of them had a positive RLS ($P=<0.001$). The patients with an RLS showed higher counts and higher intensities of microembolic signals ($P=<0.05$ and $P=<0.01$, respectively) compared with those who did not have an RLS identified. The presence of high microembolic signal counts and intensities in patients with RLS was strongly predictive of the occurrence of neurological symptoms (odds ratio, 204; 95% confidence interval, 11 to 3724; $P<0.001$) with a positive predictive value of 86% and negative predictive value of 97%.

Conclusions.—In patients with long bone fractures, the presence of an RLS is associated with larger and more frequent microembolic signals to the brain detected by transcranial Doppler study and can predict the development of neurological symptoms (Table 1).

▶ Ostensibly, this article bears little relevance to anesthesiologists, but the abstract doesn't tell the whole story. First, all patients with femoral shaft fractures show transcranial Doppler (TCD) evidence of cerebral embolization, with or without evidence supporting a right-to-left shunt (RLS). Second, one-third of this predominantly young adult male population had TCD evidence of an RLS. Third, half of the patients with RLS experienced neurologic dysfunction (Table 1). Fourth, embolic "load" peaked intraoperatively in patients with

TABLE 1.—Relationship Between the Presence of a Right-to-Left Shunt and Occurrence of Respiratory and Neurological Dysfunction

	All (n=42), n	RLS Present (n=14), n	RLS Absent (n=28), n
Respiratory dysfunction	20	9	11
Neurological dysfunction*	7	7	0

RLS indicates right-to-left shunt.
*Two patients with neurological symptoms developed respiratory dysfunction.

RLS and neurologic dysfunction. Unfortunately, there was no postdischarge follow-up, so the natural history of the neurologic dysfunction remains unclear. The authors suggest that patients experiencing femur fractures may benefit from some or all of the following interventions: (1) Preoperative assessment for RLS/patent foramen ovale, (2) early surgery if RLS is identified, (3) prophylactic preoperative patent foramen ovale closure if RLS is identified. It would be fascinating to perform a similar study on elderly patients with hip fractures, because one might surmise that those patients would be less neurologically resilient.

G. P. Gravlee, MD

4 Cardiothoracic and Vascular Anesthesia

A Randomized, Double-Blind Trial Comparing Continuous Thoracic Epidural Bupivacaine With and Without Opioid in Contrast to a Continuous Paravertebral Infusion of Bupivacaine for Post-thoracotomy Pain
Grider JS, Mullet TW, Saha SP, et al (Univ of Kentucky, Lexington)
J Cardiothorac Vasc Anesth 26:83-89, 2012

Objective.—To compare the results of continuous epidural bupivacaine analgesia with and without hydromorphone to continuous paravertebral analgesia with bupivcaine in patients with post-thoracotomy pain.

Design.—A prospective, randomized, double-blinded trial.

Setting.—A teaching hospital.

Participants.—Patients at a tertiary care teaching hospital undergoing throracotomy for lung cancer.

Interventions.—Subjects were assigned randomly to receive a continuous thoracic epidural or paravertebral infusion. Patients in the epidural group were randomized to receive either bupivacaine alone or in combination with hydromorphone. Visual analog scores as well as incentive spirometery results were obtained before and after thoracotomy.

Methods and Main Results.—Seventy-five consecutive patients presenting for thoracotomy were enrolled in this institutional review board—approved study. On the morning of surgery, subjects were randomized to either an epidural group receiving bupivicaine with and without hydromorphone or a paravertebral catheter—infused bupvicaine. Postoperative visual analog scores and incentive spirometry data were measured in the postanesthesia care unit, the evening of the first operative day, and daily thereafter until postoperative day 4. Analgesia on all postoperative days was superior in the thoracic epidural group receiving bupivacaine plus hydromorphone. Analgesia was similar in the epidural and continuous paravertebral groups receiving bupivacaine alone. No significant improvement was noted by combining the continuous infusion of bupivacaine via the paravertebral and epidural routes. Incentive spirometry goals were best achieved in the epidural bupivacaine and hydromorphone group and equal in the group receiving bupivacaine alone either via epidural or continuous paravertebral infusion.

Conclusions.—The current study provided data that fill gaps in the current literature in 3 important areas. First, this study found that thoracic epidural analgesia (TEA) with bupivacaine and a hydrophilic opioid, hydromorphone, may provide enhanced analgesia over TEA or continuous paravertebral infusion (CPI) with bupivacaine alone. Second, in the bupivacaine-alone group, the increased basal rates required to achieve analgesia resulted in hypotension more frequently than in the bupivacaine/hydromorphone combination group, underscoring the benefit of the synergistic activity. Finally, in agreement with previous retrospective studies, the current data suggest that CPI of local anesthetic appears to provide acceptable analgesia for post-thoracotomy pain.

▶ For post-thoracotomy acute analgesia, studies comparing continuous paravertebral and continuous epidural analgesia remain inconclusive. This study adds some new twists. First, the paravertebral catheters were used with an elastomeric OnQ system (iFlow Corp, Lake Forest, IL) for continuous infusion. Second, the opioid used for the epidural combined local anesthetic-opioid infusion was hydromorphone, which is intermediate in lipophilicity between fentanyl and morphine. The analgesic quality was best in the combined bupivacaine/hydromorphone group, but it was quite acceptable in the other 2 groups as well. The paravertebral catheter group required patient-controlled analgesia "rescue" significantly more often (5 of 23 patients) than the epidural bupivacaine/hydromorphone group (1 of 24 patients). More than 75% of patients in all 3 groups reached the designated incentive spirometry threshold of 2L by postoperative day 3. Post hoc data analysis revealed that the epidural bupivacaine patients required a higher basal infusion rate (median 5 mL/h) to maintain analgesia than did the epidural bupivacaine/hydromorphone group (median 3.5 mL/h). The authors speculate that this difference accounted for the observation that 3 patients in the epidural bupivacaine group experienced hypotension, which did not occur in the other 2 groups. It appears that all 3 approaches to postoperative analgesia are good ones, with a small efficacy advantage to an epidural bupivacaine/hydromorphone infusion.

G. P. Gravlee, MD

Acute Safety and 30-Day Outcome After Percutaneous Edge-to-Edge Repair of Mitral Regurgitation in Very High-Risk Patients
Pleger ST, Mereles D, Schulz-Schönhagen M, et al (Univ of Heidelberg, Germany)
Am J Cardiol 108:1478-1482, 2011

Percutaneous edge-to-edge mitral valve repair using the MitraClip device has evolved as a new tool for the treatment of severe mitral valve regurgitation. This technique has been evaluated in surgical low- and high-risk patients. Patients with advanced age, multiple morbidities, and heart failure will be the first to be considered for a nonsurgical approach. Thus safety and feasibility data in very high-risk patients are crucial for clinical decision making. The aim of this study was to assess short-term safety and clinical efficacy in high-risk patients with a Society of Thoracic Surgeons (STS) score >15% after MitraClip implantation (mean STS score 24 ± 4%). All relevant complications, mortality, echocardiographic improvement, and changes in brain natriuretic peptide, high-sensitive troponin T, 6-minute walk distance test, and New York Heart Association functional class were collected in patients within 30 days after MitraClip implantation. Mitral regurgitation had significantly decreased after 30 days from grade 2.9 ± 0.2 to 1.7 ± 0.7 (p < 0.0001). Accordingly, New York Heart Association functional class had significantly improved from 3.38 ± 0.59 to 2.2 ± 0.4 (p < 0.001). Objective parameters of clinical improvement showed a significant increase in 6-minute walk distance test (from 194 ± 44 to 300 ± 70 m, p < 0.01) and insignificant trends in brain natriuretic peptide (10,376 ± 1,996 vs 4,385 ± 1,266 ng/L, p = 0.06) and high-sensitive troponin T (43 ± 8.9 vs 36 ± 7.7 pg/L, p = 0.27) improvement. Thirty-day mortality was 0. Two patients developed a left atrial thrombus, 1 patient was on a ventilator for > 12 hours, and 1 patient had significant access site bleeding. In conclusion, this study shows that percutaneous edge-to-edge mitral valve repair can be safely performed even in surgical high-risk patients with an STS score >15. At 1-month follow-up most patients showed persistent improvement in mitral regurgitation and a clinical benefit.

▶ The authors report good short-term results with the MitraClip device, which uses a transcutaneous (from femoral vein transatrial septal) approach to place an "alligator jaw" device that approximates the middle portions of the anterior and posterior mitral leaflets. This is analogous to the Alfieri surgical repair, and similarly it creates a figure-of-eight mitral valve orifice. The short-term results are good in this high-risk population, but the reduction in mitral regurgitation is not as good as that seen following surgical mitral valve repair. The authors submit that these patients would experience high morbidity if not mortality if they were to undergo surgery, which may be true, yet review of the patient preoperative risk profiles does not suggest that an anesthesiologist would be shocked or surprised if they were to present for surgical mitral valve repair. Consequently, a prospective comparison with surgery is needed. No comments were made about anesthesia other than that general anesthesia was used. Both general anesthesia and sedation have been reported. In our local experience, the following factors lead us to a preference for general anesthesia: periods of apnea are required, the procedure lasts for 2 or more hours, a potential for hemodynamic instability from arrhythmias and even new mitral stenosis exists, and continuous transesophageal echocardiography is used.

G. P. Gravlee, MD

An Alternative Central Venous Route for Cardiac Surgery: Supraclavicular Subclavian Vein Catheterization

Kocum A, Sener M, Caliskan E, et al (Baskent Univ Faculty of Medicine, Ankara, Turkey)
J Cardiothorac Vasc Anesth 25:1018-1023, 2011

Objective.—To evaluate the clinical success rate, safety, and usefulness for intraoperative central venous pressure monitoring, and the intravenous access of the supraclavicular subclavian vein approach when compared with the infraclavicular subclavian vein approach and the internal jugular vein approach for central venous catheterization during open-chest cardiac surgery.

Design.—A prospective, randomized, single-center study.

Setting.—A university hospital.

Participants.—One hundred ninety-five patients scheduled for open-chest cardiac surgery.

Interventions.—The study population consisted of patients for whom central vein catheterization was intended during cardiac surgery. Patients were randomized to 3 groups according to the route of central vein catheterization: the supraclavicular group: the supraclavicular approach for the subclavian vein (n = 65); the infraclavicular group: the infraclavicular approach for the subclavian vein (n = 65); and the jugular group: the internal jugular vein approach (n = 65). After the induction of anesthesia, central venous catheterization was performed according to the assigned approach.

Measurements and Main Results.—The success rates for the assigned approach were 98%, 98%, and 92% for the supraclavicular, infraclavicular, and jugular groups, respectively ($p > 0.05$). The success rates in the first 3 attempts in patients who were catheterized successfully according to the assigned approach were 96%, 100%, and 96% for the supraclavicular, infraclavicular, and jugular groups, respectively ($p > 0.05$). There was no difference among groups in catheter insertion time ($p > 0.05$). After sternal retraction, central venous pressure trace loss and difficulty in fluid infusion were significantly more frequent in the infraclavicular group (21%) when compared with the supraclavicular (3%) and jugular groups (0%) ($p = 0.01$). There was no difference among groups in terms of catheter malposition, complications during catheterization, and rate of catheter-related infection.

Conclusion.—The supraclavicular approach for subclavian vein catheterization is an acceptable alternative for central venous access during cardiac surgery in terms of procedural success rate, ease of placement, rate of complications, and usability after sternal retractor expansion (Fig 1, Table 3).

▶ The internal jugular vein is cannulated more often than infraclavicular subclavian approach to avoid pneumothorax. However, inadvertent carotid artery puncture during internal jugular vein catheterization may lead to hematoma and serious neurological damage, especially in patients with severe atherosclerotic vacular

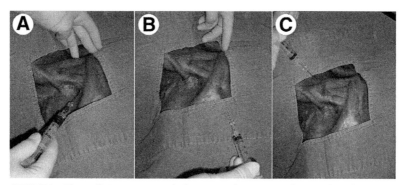

FIGURE 1.—The needle insertion site and advancement direction. (A) The supraclavicular subclavian. (B) The infraclavicular subclavian. (C) The internal jugular vein. (Reprinted from Kocum A, Sener M, Caliskan E, et al. An alternative central venous route for cardiac surgery: supraclavicular subclavian vein catheterization. *J Cardiothorac Vasc Anesth.* 2011;25:1018-1023, with permission Elsevier.)

TABLE 3.—Complications and Malpositioning During Catheterization

	Supraclavicular Group	Infraclavicular Group	Jugular Group	*p* Value
Complication during catheterization (%)	0	3	3	0.384
Inadvertent arterial puncture (n)	—	2	1	
Hematoma in the neck*	—	—	1	
Pneumothorax/hemothorax/hydrothorax	—	—	—	
Cardiac perforation/tamponade	—	—	—	
Air embolism	—	—	—	
Malpositioning during catheterization (n, %)	4 (2.1)	6 (3.2)	6 (3.2)	0.722
RA (n)	1	4	4	
RV (n)	—	1	1	
Left IV (n)	3	1	1	
LJV (n)	—	—	—	

Abbreviations: RA, right atrium; RV, right ventricle; IV, innominate vein; LJV, left jugular vein.
*Unrelated to inadvertent arterial puncture.

disease. Moreover, during cardiac surgery, CVP waveform of the infraclavicular subclavian vein may disappear during surgery due to excessive sternal retraction and mechanical compression at the level where the subclavian vein crosses the first rib. In the current study, the authors describe their experience in cannulating subclavian vein by supraclavicular approach, including success rate, ease of placement rate, and complications. In this prospective randomized study, the authors convincingly demonstrate that supraclavicular catheterization is an acceptable alternative approach for central venous access during cardiac surgery. The technical advantages of this approach include a wider target area for the insertion of the needle, a more direct route to the superior vena cava, and a more reliable constant surface landmark when using clavicular midpoint.

M. Mathru, MD

Anesthetic management of patients with Brugada syndrome: a case series and literature review

Kloesel B, Ackerman MJ, Sprung J, et al (Mayo Clinic, Rochester, MN)
Can J Anesth 58:824-836, 2011

Purpose.—To review the anesthetic management and perioperative outcomes of patients diagnosed with Brugada syndrome (BrS) who were treated at a single centre and to compare those results with a comprehensive review of the existing literature.

Clinical Features.—A retrospective chart review of anesthesia records from patients diagnosed with BrS at the Mayo Clinic was undertaken with the emphasis on administered drugs, ST segment changes, and occurrence of complications, including death, hemodynamic instability, and dysrhythmias. Eight patients were identified who underwent a total of 17 operative procedures from 2000 through 2010. A total of 20 significant ST segment elevations were recorded in four patients, several of which occurred in close temporal relation to anesthetic drug administration. These elevations resolved uneventfully. There were no recorded dysrhythmias, and recovery from anesthesia proceeded uneventfully. A literature review of patients with BrS yielded 52 anesthetics in 43 patients. The only recorded complications included unmasking of a Brugada ECG pattern, one episode of polymorphic ventricular tachycardia, which converted spontaneously to sinus rhythm, and one episode of postoperative ventricular fibrillation in the setting of epidural anesthesia.

Conclusions.—In this series and in the literature, BrS patients tolerated anesthesia without untoward disease-related complications. Propofol and local anesthetics carry a theoretical risk of arrhythmogenic potential in BrS patients, but clear evidence is lacking. However, awareness of their potential to induce arrhythmias warrants caution, especially with propofol infusions. Factors that might exacerbate ST segment elevations and subsequently lead to dysrhythmias (e.g., hyperthermia, bradycardia, and electrolyte imbalances, such as hyper- and hypokalemia and hypercalcemia) should be avoided or corrected (Fig 1).

▶ Anesthesiologists worldwide likely share the frustration of needing to anesthetize patients with uncommon diseases that may be exacerbated by anesthesia and surgery on short notice. Brugada syndrome is just such a disease. Its prevalence is approximately 1 in 5000 people. This retrospective case series mines the Mayo Clinic database to review 17 procedures in 8 patients with this autosomal dominant syndrome, which has several genotypes. Brugada syndrome is most often diagnosed in the fourth decade of life as a result of finding its characteristic baseline ST segment abnormalities (Fig 1), which may be asymptomatic or associated with a history of spontaneous or inducible ventricular tachycardia or fibrillation and their attendant association with syncope and sudden death. Most of the patients in the series experienced no perioperative difficulties, but a few episodes of ST segment elevation appeared in temporal association with propofol or oxymetazoline (topical alpha-adrenergic agonist) administration. Propofol

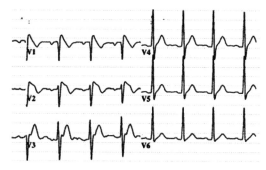

FIGURE 1.—Precordial lead tracing (Patient 3). Typical right precordial lead tracings (V1-V3) showing T wave abnormalities typically observed in patients with Brugada syndrome. (Reprinted from Kloesel B, Ackerman MJ, Sprung J, et al. Anesthetic management of patients with Brugada syndrome: a case series and literature review. *Can J Anesth*. 2011;58:824-836, Canadian Anesthesiologists' Society.)

avoidance is consistent with the very useful drug information Web site cited in the text (http://www.brugadadrugs.org); however, 6 of 7 patients who received propofol had no adverse event. Bupivacaine is rated as class IIa and propofol as class IIb among drugs to be avoided in Brugada syndrome. Lidocaine, ketamine, amiodarone, and propofol are also categorized as class IIb. Theoretically, all local anesthetic agents would be suspect in Brugada type 1 patients, because they share the undesired mechanism of sodium channel inhibition. Accordingly, isoproterenol and quinidine are the drugs recommended as first-line antiarrhythmics for these patients. ST segment changes typically appear in leads V1−V3. In a busy clinical practice, this syndrome merits advance notice so the anesthesia team can look up this syndrome and the Web site noted above.

G. P. Gravlee, MD

Anesthetic-induced Improvement of the Inflammatory Response to One-lung Ventilation

De Conno E, Steurer MP, Wittlinger M, et al (Univ of Zurich, Switzerland; et al)
Anesthesiology 110:1316-1326, 2009

Background.—Although one-lung ventilation (OLV) has become an established procedure during thoracic surgery, sparse data exist about inflammatory alterations in the deflated, reventilated lung. The aim of this study was to prospectively investigate the effect of OLV on the pulmonary inflammatory response and to assess possible immunomodulatory effects of the anesthetics propofol and sevoflurane.

Methods.—Fifty-four adults undergoing thoracic surgery with OLV were randomly assigned to receive either anesthesia with intravenously applied propofol or the volatile anesthetic sevoflurane. A bronchoalveolar lavage was performed before and after OLV on the lung side undergoing surgery. Inflammatory mediators (tumor necrosis factor α, interleukin 1β, interleukin 6, interleukin 8, monocyte chemoattractant protein 1) and cells were analyzed

TABLE 6.—Adverse Events

	Events	
	Propofol	Sevoflurane
Prolonged antibiosis	7	4
Pneumonia	3	2
Atelectasis	5	1
Fistula	3	1
Effusion	15	10
Reintubation	1	0
SIRS	1	0
Sepsis	1	0
ARDS	0	0
Surgical revision	4	0
Death	0	0
Total	40	18

ARDS = acute respiratory distress syndrome; SIRS = systemic inflammatory response syndrome.

in lavage fluid as the primary endpoint. The clinical outcome determined by postoperative adverse events was assessed as the secondary endpoint.

Results.—The increase of inflammatory mediators on OLV was significantly less pronounced in the sevoflurane group. No difference in neutrophil recruitment was found between the groups. A positive correlation between neutrophils and mediators was demonstrated in the propofol group, whereas this correlation was missing in the sevoflurane group. The number of composite adverse events was significantly lower in the sevoflurane group.

Conclusions.—This prospective, randomized clinical study suggests an immunomodulatory role for the volatile anesthetic sevoflurane in patients undergoing OLV for thoracic surgery with significant reduction of inflammatory mediators and a significantly better clinical outcome (defined by postoperative adverse events) during sevoflurane anesthesia (Table 6).

▶ This study adds to a growing clinical body of literature comparing organ-specific effects of volatile agents to intravenous agents (principally propofol) during surgical anesthesia. The differences in inflammatory mediators are interesting as primary outcomes, but the secondary outcomes (eg, pulmonary complications) will interest clinicians more than inflammatory markers. Sevoflurane anesthesia patients experienced 18 pulmonary complications, whereas propofol patients experienced 40. More than half of the 22-patient difference in observed complications fell into the categories of pleural effusions (15 propofol vs 10 sevoflurane), atelectasis (5 vs 1), and surgical revision (4 vs 0). No definition for surgical revision was provided, but presumably this means that the patient required a surgical reexploration before hospital discharge. Sevoflurane patients also spent significantly fewer days in the intensive care unit (0.87 ± 0.43 vs 1.52 ± 2.33). Taken collectively, the differences in inflammatory and pulmonary outcomes support the preferential use of volatile agents during 1-lung anesthesia. It seems unlikely that it would matter whether sevoflurane, desflurane, or isoflurane is chosen for this purpose.

G. P. Gravlee, MD

Association Between Postoperative Acute Kidney Injury and Duration of Cardiopulmonary Bypass: A Meta-Analysis

Kumar AB, Suneja M, Bayman EO, et al (Univ of Iowa Hosps and Clinics)

J Cardiothorac Vasc Anesth 26:64-69, 2012

Objective.—This meta-analysis examined the association between cardiopulmonary bypass (CPB) time and acute kidney injury (AKI).

Design.—Meta-analysis of previously published studies.

Setting.—Each single-center study was conducted in a surgical intensive care unit and/or academic or university hospital.

Participants.—Adult patients undergoing heart surgery with CPB.

Interventions.—A systematic literature review was conducted using PubMed, EMBASE, and Cochrane Library databases and Google Scholar from January 1980 through September 2009. Initial search results were refined to include human subjects, age >18 years, randomized controlled trials, and prospective and retrospective cohort studies, meet the Acute Kidney Injury Network definition of renal failure, and report times on CPB.

Measurements and Main Results.—The length of time on CPB has been implicated as an independent risk factor for development of AKI after CPB (AKI-CPB). The 9 independent studies included in the final meta-analysis had 12,466 patients who underwent CPB. Out of these, 756 patients (6.06%) developed AKI-CPB. In 7 of the 9 studies, the mean CPB times were statistically longer in the AKI-CPB cohort compared with the control group (cohort without AKI). The absolute mean differences in CPB time between the 2 groups were 25.65 minutes with the fixed-effects model and 23.18 minutes with the random-effects model.

Conclusions.—Longer CPB times are associated with a higher risk of developing AKI-CPB, which, in turn, has a significant effect on overall mortality as reported by the individual studies.

▶ This meta-analysis used rigorous study inclusion criteria that yielded just 9 studies, but the number of patients included in those studies was impressive. Four of them analyzed more than 1200 patients each. Unlike some previous studies, the authors did not seek a specific duration at which cardiopulmonary bypass (CPB) becomes an independent risk factor for acute kidney injury (AKI). In the 9 study cohorts, mean CPB durations in the non-AKI patients ranged from 82 to 130 minutes, and those for AKI patients ranged from 107 to 171 minutes. If the study with the longest CPB times is excluded, the highest mean CPB times for non-AKI and AKI patients drop to 113 and 139 minutes, respectively. Despite selection of the respected Acute Kidney Injury Network criteria for diagnosis of AKI, the definitions of AKI varied strikingly among the 9 studies analyzed, which may explain why the incidences of AKI did not appear to trend in the direction of CPB times across studies. This study reinforces a relationship between CPB time and renal injury that has been demonstrated repeatedly over the entire history of cardiac surgery with CPB, which will soon enter its seventh decade.

G. P. Gravlee, MD

Biventricular Circulatory Support With Two Miniaturized Implantable Assist Devices

Krabatsch T, Potapov E, Stepanenko A, et al (Deutsches Herzzentrum Berlin, Germany)
Circulation 124:S179-S186, 2011

Background.—Up to 30% of patients with end-stage heart failure experience biventricular failure that requires biventricular mechanical support. For these patients, only bulky extracorporeal or implantable displacement pumps or the total artificial heart have been available to date, which enables only limited quality of life for the patients. It was our goal to evaluate a method that would allow the use of 2 implantable centrifugal left ventricular assist devices as a biventricular assist system.

Methods and Results.—Seventeen patients have been implanted with 2 HeartWare HVAD pumps, 1 as a left ventricular assist device and 1 as a right ventricular assist device. Seventy-seven percent of the patients had idiopathic dilated or ischemic cardiomyopathy. Their age ranged from 29 to 73 years (mean 51.8 ± 14.5 years), and 11 (64.7%) received intravenous catecholamine support preoperatively. The right ventricular assist device pump was implanted into the right ventricular free wall. The afterload of this pump was artificially increased by local reduction of the outflow graft diameter, and the effective length of its inflow cannula was reduced by the addition of two 5-mm silicon suture rings to the original HVAD implantation ring. All right ventricular assist device devices could be operated in appropriate speed ranges and delivered a flow of between 3.0 and 5.5 L/min. Thirty-day survival was 82%, and 59% of the patients could be discharged home after recovering from the operation. There was no clinically relevant hemolysis in any of the patients.

Conclusions.—Two HeartWare HVAD pumps can be used as a biventricular assist system. This implantable biventricular support gives the patients more comfort and mobility than usual biventricular ventricular assist devices with large and noisy displacement pumps.

▶ Right ventricular failure is the bane of destination left ventricular assist device (LVAD) implantation, at least in the acute phase following implantation. Patients experiencing this complication may limp by with profound pharmacologic support (eg, nitric oxide, milrinone, dobutamine) or may require temporary right ventricular assist device (RVAD) support. This relatively small but highly innovative series used the deliberate strategy of biventricular support using compact, noiseless continuous-flow Heartware HVAD pumps. The 30-day survival of 82% and survival to discharge of 59% are encouraging in the context of these patients' very high-risk profiles. Placing this pump's inflow into the right ventricular free wall and connecting its outflow to the pulmonary artery imposed technical challenges to which the authors applied interesting solutions. This approach currently offers greater appeal than the unwieldy total artificial heart, yet reports of problems potentially attributable to the long-term use of nonpulsatile flow (eg, aortic insufficiency, gastrointestinal bleeding, acquired von Willebrand disease) cause concern.

G. P. Gravlee, MD

Blood transfusion after cardiac surgery: is it the patient or the transfusion that carries the risk?
Dardashti A, Ederoth P, Algotsson L, et al (Lund Univ, Sweden)
Acta Anaesthesiol Scand 55:952-961, 2011

Background.—The transfusion of red blood cells (RBCs) after cardiac surgery has been associated with increased long-term mortality. This study reexamines this hypothesis by including pre-operative hemoglobin (Hb) levels and renal function in the analysis.

Methods.—A retrospective single-center study was performed including 5261 coronary artery bypass grafting (CABG) patients in a Cox proportional hazard survival analysis. Patients with more than eight RBC transfusions, early death (7 days), and emergent cases were excluded. Patients were followed for 7.5 years. Previously known risk factors were entered into the analysis together with pre-operative Hb and estimated glomerular filtration rate (eGFR). In addition, subgroups were formed based on the patients' pre-operative renal function and Hb levels.

Results.—When classical risk factors were entered into the analysis, transfusion of RBCs was associated with reduced long-term survival. When pre-operative eGFR and Hb was entered into the analysis, however, transfusion of RBCs did not affect survival significantly. In the subgroups, transfusion of RBCs did not have any effect on long-term survival.

Conclusions.—When pre-operative Hb levels and renal function are taken into account, moderate transfusions of RBC after CABG surgery do not seem to be associated with reduced long-term survival (Fig 3).

▶ Both anemia and blood transfusion have been associated with adverse outcomes in cardiac surgery, which creates a chicken-versus-egg conundrum. Numerous retrospective studies have made herculean efforts to statistically isolate either anemia or transfusion, and typically whichever variable is isolated does correlate with increased morbidity and mortality. This study adds a new spin, which is to combine preoperative anemia and compromised renal function into a single comorbidity (called "study group" below) and then analyze this package as a single variable. Doing so appears to exonerate transfusion as an independent risk factor for mortality(Fig 3). I calculate that 60% of the study group received transfusion, whereas 35% of the "nonstudy" group did, hence preoperative anemia ostensibly affected transfusion prevalence. These authors did not assess preoperative anemia on a continuous scale but instead chose hemoglobin cutoff values to dichotomously define patients as anemic or non-anemic. This study does not resolve the chicken-versus-egg puzzle, but it

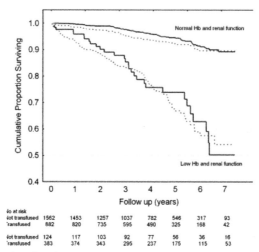

FIGURE 3.—Unadjusted Kaplan–Meier plot for two of the subgroups of patients depending on the pre-operative renal function and hemoglobin levels. The groups are divided into patients receiving red blood cell (RBC) transfusion (broken red line) and patients not receiving an RBC transfusion (solid blue line). (Reprinted from Dardashti A, Ederoth P, Algotsson L, et al. Blood transfusion after cardiac surgery: is it the patient or the transfusion that carries the risk? *Acta Anaesthesiol Scand.* 2011;55:952-961, with permission from publisher Wiley-Blackwell.)

attenuates concern about transfusion per se as a contributor to perioperative mortality in coronary artery bypass grafting patients.

G. P. Gravlee, MD

Blood transfusions recruit the microcirculation during cardiac surgery
Yuruk K, Almac E, Bezemer R, et al (Univ of Amsterdam, the Netherlands)
Transfusion 51:961-967, 2011

Background.—Perioperative red blood cell transfusions are commonly used in patients undergoing cardiac surgery to correct anemia caused by blood loss and hemodilution associated with cardiopulmonary bypass circulation. The aim of this investigation was to test the hypothesis that blood transfusion has beneficial effects on sublingual microcirculatory density, perfusion, and oxygenation. To this end, sidestream dark field (SDF) imaging and spectrophotometry were applied sublingually before and after blood transfusion during cardiac surgery.

Study Design and Methods.—Twenty-four adult patients undergoing on-pump cardiac surgery, including coronary artery bypass grafting, cardiac-valve surgery, or a combination of these two procedures, were included consecutively in this prospective, observational study. Sublingual microcirculatory density and perfusion were assessed using SDF imaging in 12 patients (Group A). Sublingual reflectance spectrophotometry was applied in 12 patients (Group B) to monitor microcirculatory oxygenation and hemoglobin (Hb) concentration.

Microcirculatory density

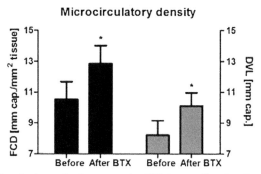

FIGURE 1.—Microcirculatory density, expressed as FCD (mm capillary [cap.]/mm² tissue) and DVL (mm capillary [cap.]), before and 30 minutes after blood transfusion (BTX). *p < 0.05 for before versus after BTX. (Reprinted from Yuruk K, Almac E, Bezemer R, et al. Blood transfusions recruit the microcirculation during cardiac surgery. *Transfusion.* 2011;51:961-967.)

Microcirculatory perfusion

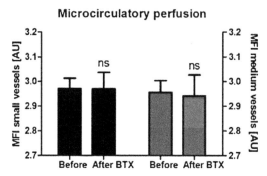

FIGURE 2.—Microcirculatory perfusion, expressed in MFI (AU), in small- and medium-sized vessels before and 30 minutes after blood transfusion (BTX). ns = not significant. (Reprinted from Yuruk K, Almac E, Bezemer R, et al. Blood transfusions recruit the microcirculation during cardiac surgery. *Transfusion.* 2011;51:961-967.)

Results.—Blood transfusion caused an increase in systemic Hb concentration (p < 0.01) and hematocrit (p < 0.01). At the microcirculatory level, blood transfusion resulted in increased microcirculatory density (from 10.5 ± 1.2 to 12.9 ± 1.2 mm capillary/mm² tissue, p < 0.01) as shown using SDF imaging. In concert with the SDF measurements, spectrophotometry showed that microcirculatory Hb content increased from 61.4 ± 5.9 to 70.0 ± 4.7 AU (p < 0.01) and that microcirculatory Hb oxygen saturation increased from 65.6 ± 8.3% to 68.6 ± 8.4% (p = 0.06).

Conclusion.—In this study we have shown that blood transfusion: 1) improves the systemic circulation and oxygen-carrying capacity, 2) improves sublingual microcirculatory density but not perfusion velocity, and 3) improves microcirculatory oxygen saturation (Figs 1-3).

▶ Although red blood cell (RBC) transfusion is a necessity in the presence of severe anemia, several studies have shown that it might have adverse effects, including increased incidence of infection, renal failure, and increased hospital

Microcirculatory Hb

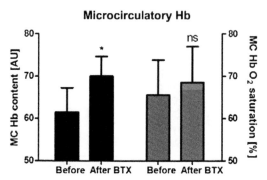

FIGURE 3.—Microcirculatory Hb (MC Hb) content [AU] en saturation [%] before and 30 minutes after blood transfusion (BTX). *p < 0.05 for before versus after BTX. (Reprinted from Yuruk K, Almac E, Bezemer R, et al. Blood transfusions recruit the microcirculation during cardiac surgery. *Transfusion.* 2011;51:961-967.)

length of stay. The precise mechanism responsible for these adverse effects is not known. Perturbations in microcirculation following RBC transfusion have been speculated to cause the adverse effects associated with transfusion. One of the primary goals of RBC transfusion is to improve oxygen delivery at the microcirculatory level and thus improve tissue oxygenation. The effect of RBC transfusion at the microcirculation is controversial, and few clinical studies have addressed this issue. Previous studies addressing this issue were done in septic patients. However, in sepsis structural alterations occurring in microcirculation (damage to the endothelium and glycocalyx) could have confounded their results. In this study, the authors examined the effect of RBC transfusion in nonseptic cardiac surgery patients. Microcirculation was examined by using sublingual sidestream dark field imaging. Their results show that leukoreduced RBC transfusion improves microcirculatory density and oxygenation. Decreased intercapillary diffusion distance after transfusion (ie, increased capillary density) enhances oxygen transport from the microcirculation to the tissues.

M. Mathru, MD

Central Airway Stabilization for Tracheobronchomalacia Improves Quality of Life in Patients With COPD
Ernst A, Odell DD, Michaud G, et al (St Elizabeth's Med Ctr, Boston, MA; Harvard Med School, Boston, MA; et al)
Chest 140:1162-1168, 2011

Background.—Tracheobronchomalacia (TBM) is characterized by excessive collapsibility of the central airways, typically during expiration. TBM may be present in as many as 50% of patients evaluated for COPD. The impact of central airway stabilization on symptom pattern and quality of life is poorly understood in this patient population.

Methods.—Patients with documented COPD were identified from a cohort of 238 patients assessed for TBM at our complex airway referral center. Pulmonary function testing, exercise tolerance, and health-related quality-of-life (HRQOL) measures were assessed at baseline and 2 to 4 weeks following tracheal stent placement/operative tracheobroncho-plasty (TBP). Severity of COPD was classified according to the GOLD (Global Initiative for Chronic Obstructive Lung Disease) staging system.

Results.—One hundred three patients (48 women) with COPD and moderately severe to severe TBM were identified. Statistically and clinically significant improvements were seen in HRQOL measures, including the transitional dyspnea index (stent, $P = .001$; TBP, $P = .008$), the St. George Respiratory Questionnaire (stent, $P = .002$; TBP, $P < .0001$), and the Karnofsky performance score (stent, $P = .163$; TBP, $P < .0001$). The improvement appeared greatest following TBP and was seen in all GOLD stages. Clinical improvement was also seen in measured FEV_1 and exercise capacity as assessed by 6-min walk test.

Conclusions.—Central airway stabilization may provide symptomatic benefit for patients with severe COPD and concomitant severe airway malacia. Operative airway stabilization appears to impart the greatest advantage. Long-term follow-up study is needed to fully ascertain the ultimate efficacy of both stenting and surgical airway stabilization in this patient group.

Trial Registry.—ClinicalTrials.gov; No.: NCT00550602; URL: www.clinicaltrials.gov.

▶ This article was selected in part because it and similar reports may explain the gradual increase in tracheobronchoplasty (TBP) procedures observed in my own clinical practice. In contradistinction to the current report, our pulmonologists and thoracic surgeons typically eschew tracheal stents and proceed directly to TBP in patients with severe tracheobronchomalacia (TBM) obstruction. TBP poses significant anesthetic challenges locally, because our surgeons typically desire tracheal and mainstem bronchial "stillness" but dislike the bulk of a double-lumen endobronchial tube as well as the mucosal drying and/or injury potentially imposed by several hours of jet or high-frequency ventilation. Consequently, we tend to use extra-long, fairly narrow (6–7 mm internal diameter) single-lumen endotracheal tubes that are typically advanced into the left mainstem bronchus under fiberoptic guidance. The other reason for including this article is to raise awareness of TBM among anesthesiologists caring for patients with advanced or highly symptomatic chronic obstructive pulmonary disorder (COPD). One should have a high index of suspicion for undiagnosed TBM in patients with frequent COPD exacerbations who are responding poorly to maximal bronchodilator therapy. The reported incidence of TBM in such patients is as high as 44%. These patients usually respond favorably to bilevel positive airway pressure (BiPAP), continuous positive airway pressure (CPAP), or standard positive pressure ventilation (PPV) because these interventions stent their collapsing membranous trachea. Plausible scenario: a patient with severe COPD has done unexpectedly well during general anesthesia with PPV but is struggling in the postanesthesia care unit and continues to wheeze despite bronchodilator nebulizer treatments. If you should see this, consider an empiric trial of

CPAP or BiPAP. If the patient responds well, strongly suggest a diagnostic bronchoscopy or dynamic CT scan emphasizing proximal airways.

G. P. Gravlee, MD

Cerebral Protection During Surgery for Acute Aortic Dissection Type A: Results of the German Registry for Acute Aortic Dissection Type A (GERAADA)

Krüger T, on behalf of the GERAADA Investigators (Univ Hosp Tübingen, Germany; et al)
Circulation 124:434-443, 2011

Background.—Cerebral protection during surgery for acute aortic dissection type A relies on hypothermic circulatory arrest, either alone or in conjunction with cerebral perfusion.

Methods and Results.—The perioperative and intraoperative conditions of 1558 patients submitted from 44 cardiac surgery centers in German-speaking countries were analyzed. Among patients with acute aortic dissection type A, 355 (22.8%) underwent surgery with hypothermic circulatory arrest alone. In 1115 patients (71.6%), cerebral perfusion was used: Unilateral antegrade cerebral perfusion (ACP) in 628 (40.3%), bilateral ACP in 453 (29.1%), and retrograde perfusion in 34 patients (2.2%). For 88 patients with acute aortic dissection type A (5.6%), no circulatory arrest and arch intervention were reported (cardiopulmonary bypass—only group). End points of the study were 30-day mortality (15.9% overall) and mortality-corrected permanent neurological dysfunction (10.5% overall). The respective values for the cardiopulmonary bypass—only group were 11.4% and 9.1%. Hypothermic circulatory arrest alone resulted in a 30-day mortality rate of 19.4% and a mortality-corrected permanent neurological dysfunction rate of 11.5%, whereas the rates were 13.9% and 10.0%, respectively, for unilateral ACP and 15.9% and 11.0%, respectively, for bilateral ACP. In contrast with the ACP groups, there was a profound increase in mortality when systemic circulatory arrest times exceeded 30 minutes in the hypothermic circulatory arrest group ($P<0.001$). Mortality-corrected permanent neurological dysfunction correlated significantly with perfusion pressure in the ACP groups.

Conclusions.—This study reflects current surgical practice for acute aortic dissection type A in Central Europe. For arrest times less than 30 minutes, hypothermic circulatory arrest and ACP lead to similar results. For longer arrest periods, ACP with sufficient pressure is advisable. Outcomes with unilateral and bilateral ACP were equivalent (Fig 1).

▶ This retrospective database analysis confirms the writer's bedside observation that an ever-diminishing proportion of type A dissections are performed with distal ascending aortic cross-clamping and traditional cardiopulmonary bypass (Fig 1). It also confirms numerous studies associating longer circulatory arrest times with higher mortality and that over the years acceptable circulatory arrest time has decreased from 45 minutes to 30 minutes, circumstances permitting. Antegrade cerebral perfusion (ACP) has thankfully replaced a brief period of fascination

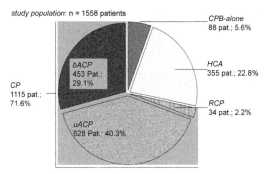

FIGURE 1.—Frequency distribution of cerebral protection techniques. CP indicates cerebral perfusion; CPB, cardiopulmonary bypass; HCA, hypothermic circulatory arrest; bACP and uACP, bilateral and unilateral antegrade cerebral perfusion, respectively; RCP, retrograde cerebral perfusion; and pat., patients. (Reprinted from Krüger T, on behalf of the GERAADA Investigators. Cerebral protection during surgery for acute aortic dissection type A: results of the German registry for acute aortic dissection type A (GERAADA). *Circulation.* 2011;124:434-443, with permission from American Heart Association.)

with retrograde cerebral perfusion. This writer has observed far more unilateral than bilateral antegrade perfusions and was surprised to read that more than 40% of ACPs in the current series were performed bilaterally, with no outcome advantage. This study could not comprehensively account for all anatomic complexities nor for surgeon factors, such as experience or technical facility. Although cerebral perfusion pressures exceeding 60 mm Hg appeared favorable, the more important issue was avoidance of circulatory arrest times exceeding 30 minutes.

G. P. Gravlee, MD

Clinical Strategies and Outcomes in Advanced Heart Failure Patients Older Than 70 Years of Age Receiving the HeartMate II Left Ventricular Assist Device: A Community Hospital Experience

Adamson RM, Stahovich M, Chillcott S, et al (Sharp Memorial Hosp, San Diego, CA)
J Am Coll Cardiol 57:2487-2495, 2011

Objectives.—The primary objective of this study was to determine outcomes in left ventricular assist device (LVAD) patients older than age 70 years.

Background.—Food and Drug Administration approval of the Heart-Mate II (Thoratec Corporation, Pleasanton, California) LVAD for destination therapy has provided an attractive option for older patients with advanced heart failure.

Methods.—Fifty-five patients received the HeartMate II LVAD between October 5, 2005, and January 1, 2010, as part of either the bridge to transplantation or destination therapy trials at a community hospital. Patients were divided into 2 age groups: ≥ 70 years of age (n = 30) and < 70 years of age (n = 25). Outcome measures including survival, length of hospital stay, adverse events, and quality of life were compared between the 2 groups.

Results.—Pre-operatively, all patients were in New York Heart Association functional class IV refractory to maximal medical therapy. Kaplan-Meier survival for patients ≥ 70 years of age (97% at 1 month, 75% at 1 year, and 70% at 2 years) was not statistically different from patients <70 years of age (96% 1 month, 72% at 1 year, and 65% at 2 years, $p = 0.806$). Average length of hospital stay for the ≥ 70-year age group was 24 ± 15 days, similar to that of the < 70-year age group (23 ± 14 days, $p = 0.805$). There were no differences in the incidence of adverse events between the 2 groups. Quality of life and functional status improved significantly in both groups.

Conclusions.—The LVAD patients ≥ 70 years of age have good functional recovery, survival, and quality of life at 2 years. Advanced age should not be used as an independent contraindication when selecting a patient for LVAD therapy at experienced centers.

▶ This retrospective analysis shows that very carefully selected New York Heart Association Class IV heart failure patients older than 70 years can safely undergo destination left ventricular assist device (LVAD) placement. In fact, this group's outcome measures were comparable to those for the comparison group, which had a mean age 20 years younger (56 vs 76 years). Preoperatively, the older group had a lower incidence of ventilator support (0% vs 20%), a higher incidence of angiotensin-converting enzyme use (43% vs 8%) and a trend toward a higher incidence of ischemic cardiomyopathy (80% vs 60%). Postoperative outcomes were virtually identical. The authors argue that these patients may in some ways be better VAD candidates than the younger population, suggesting that they may tend to be more highly motivated if screened appropriately for cognitive function. They even report a few self-referrals from hospice care! We will likely be seeing more elderly LVAD patients in the future unless the Center for Medicare and Medicaid Services decides to curtail this trend by restricting reimbursement.

G. P. Gravlee, MD

Cognitive function after sevoflurane- *vs* propofol-based anaesthesia for on-pump cardiac surgery: a randomized controlled trial

Schoen J, Husemann L, Tiemeyer C, et al (Univ of Luebeck, Germany)
Br J Anaesth 106:840-850, 2011

Background.—Cognitive dysfunction is a frequent complication after cardiac surgery and has been found to be associated with decreases in cerebral oxygen saturation (Sco_2) measured with near-infrared spectroscopy. Sevoflurane has neuroprotective properties *in vitro* and in animal models. This study was designed to determine cognitive and clinical outcomes after sevoflurane- compared with propofol-based anaesthesia for on-pump cardiac surgery and the impact of decreases in Sco_2 under different anaesthesia regimens.

Methods.—One hundred and twenty-eight patients were randomly assigned to either i.v. anaesthesia with propofol- (PROP) or sevoflurane-based anaesthesia (SEVO). An intraoperative Sco_2 <50% was defined as desaturation. The Abbreviated Mental Test, Stroop Test, Trail-Making Test, Word Lists, and mood-assessment tests were performed before, 2, 4, and 6 days after cardiac surgery. Markers of general outcome were obtained.

Results.—The analysis groups had differences in baseline cognitive performance. Analysis of variance for repeated measures (incorporating covariance of baseline scores) showed that in three of four cognitive tests, patients with cerebral desaturation showed worse results than patients without desaturation. Patients assigned to sevoflurane-based anaesthesia showed better results in all cognitive tests than patients after propofol. Interactions between the anaesthetic regimen and desaturation were found in all four cognitive tests. There were no differences in markers of organ dysfunction or general clinical outcome.

Conclusions.—Patients with impaired cognitive performance before operation may be at particular risk for intraoperative cerebral insult. A sevoflurane-based anaesthesia was associated with better short-term postoperative cognitive performance than propofol.

▶ Substantial and growing evidence supports the presence of a preconditioning effect for volatile anesthetics. Some evidence of preconditioning also exists for propofol, the difference being a lesser number of clinical outcome studies and the possibility that propofol's protective effect requires supraclinical doses, whereas the volatile agent effect clearly occurs at 0.5–1 monitored anesthesia care doses. Most of the volatile agent studies show cardiac protection, so this one assessing cerebral protection is a welcome addition. Of note, sevoflurane was not administered during cardiopulmonary bypass even in the sevoflurane group (propofol was), but the protection still occurred, which is consistent with preconditioning. Also of interest is the association of low cerebral oxygen saturation values with neurocognitive dysfunction and sevoflurane's reduced incidence of this association. The absence of long-term follow-up causes concern, as all or most of the observed neurocognitive changes could have resolved over weeks to months, and none were associated with prolonged intensive care unit or hospital lengths of stay.

G. P. Gravlee, MD

Colchicine prevents early postoperative pericardial and pleural effusions
Imazio M, Brucato A, Rovere ME, et al (Maria Vittoria Hosp, Torino, Italy; Ospedali Riuniti, Bergamo, Italy; Ospedale Mauriziano, Torino, Italy; et al)
Am Heart J 162:527-532.e1, 2011

Background.—No preventive pharmacologic strategies have been proven efficacious for the prevention of postoperative effusions after cardiac surgery. Colchicine is safe and efficacious for the prevention of pericarditis. On this basis, we realized a substudy of the COPPS trial to assess the efficacy and safety of colchicine for the prevention of postoperative pericardial and pleural effusions.

Methods.—The COPPS is a multicenter, double-blind, randomized trial, where 360 consecutive patients (mean age 65.7 ± 12.3 years, 66% men), 180 in each treatment arm, were randomized on the third postoperative day to receive placebo or colchicine for 1 month (1.0 mg twice daily for the first day, followed by a maintenance dose of 0.5 mg twice daily in patients ≥70 kg, and halved doses for patients <70 kg). The incidence of postoperative effusions was evaluated in each study group.

Results.—Despite similar baseline features, colchicine significantly reduced the incidence of postoperative pericardial (12.8% vs 22.8%, $P = .019$, relative risk reduction 43.9%, no. of patients needed to treat 10) and pleural effusions (12.2% vs 25.6%, $P = .002$, relative risk reduction 52.3%, no. of patients needed to treat 8). The rate of side effects (only gastrointestinal intolerance) and drug withdrawal was similar in the study groups with a trend toward an increased rate of both events for colchicine. In multivariable analysis, female gender (hazard ratio 1.76, 95% CI 1.03-3.03, $P = .040$) and pleura incision (hazard ratio 2.58, 95% CI 1.53-4.53, $P < .001$) were risk factors for postoperative effusions.

Conclusions.—Colchicine is safe and efficacious for the primary prevention of postoperative effusions after cardiac surgery.

▶ Pleural and/or pericardial effusions occur postoperatively in 10% to 30% of patients undergoing cardiac surgery. In this blinded, prospective study, prophylactic postoperative colchicine approximately halved the incidence of effusions and virtually eliminated the occurrence of moderate to large pericardial effusions (5% for placebo vs 0.6% for colchicine, $P < .01$). Nevertheless, in the placebo group, only 3 of 180 patients had a large effusion, and only 1 experienced cardiac tamponade. The authors did not report the size or clinical consequences of the pleural effusions they found. The colchicine group had a small but significant reduction in hospital length of stay (mean of 10 vs 9 days, SD 4 days for each group). Side effects were few and mainly gastrointestinal, but the authors ideally should have followed blood counts more closely, because colchicine has been associated with myelosuppression. Although the results are impressive, the clinical significance is dubious, because one could argue that only 1 of 60 patients was prevented from having a clinically important pericardial effusion.

G. P. Gravlee, MD

Cost and cost-effectiveness of cardiac surgery in elderly patients

Gelsomino S, Lorusso R, Livi U, et al (Careggi Hosp, Florence, Italy; Civic Hosp, Brescia, Italy; General Hosp S. Maria della Misericordia, Udine, Italy; et al)
J Thorac Cardiovasc Surg 142:1062-1073, 2011

Objective.—Cost-effectiveness of heart surgery for elderly patients is still poorly defined. We evaluated outcome, quality of life (QoL), cost, and cost-effectiveness of octogenarians undergoing cardiac surgery.

Methods.—One thousand six hundred forty octogenarians undergoing various cardiac surgical procedures were prospectively studied between January 1998 and January 2009 and compared with similar patients aged 70 to 79 years. Several questionnaires were used to assess QoL. Six hundred age- and sex- matched healthy octogenarians and three hundred forty patients older than 80 years with medically treated valvular or coronary artery disease were healthy and unoperated control groups, respectively. In-hospital costs were obtained from the hospital's financial accounting department and cost-effectiveness was estimated and expressed as cost/ QoL-adjusted life year (QALY) and cost-effectiveness ratio.

Results.—Significant improvements occurred in elderly patients in Role Physical ($P < .001$), Bodily Pain ($P < .001$), General Health ($P = .004$), Social Functioning ($P < .001$), and Role Emotional ($P < .001$), whereas Physical Functioning, Vitality, and Mental Health did not change (difference not significant). Total direct costs were $5293 higher in the octogenarian group. Cost-effectiveness was $1391/QALY for elderly surgical patients, $516/QALY for younger cardiac surgical patients ($P < .001$ vs elderly), $897/QALY for untreated control group, and $641/QALY for healthy control group ($P < .001$ vs elderly surgical patients). The cost-effectiveness ratio for octogenarians was $94,426.

Conclusions.—Our findings confirm that cardiac surgery in elderly patients remains controversial from a cost-effectiveness standpoint, making econometric analysis an important component for any future evaluation of novel cardiovascular therapies. Our findings need to be confirmed by additional multicenter studies.

▶ The patient population represents that from 3 hospitals in Italy, which has one of the highest proportions of octogenarians in the world. The comparison groups included cardiac surgical octogenarians, nonsurgical octogenarians with comparable cardiac disease (although not randomly assigned), cardiac surgical septuagenarians, and "healthy" octogenarians. In general, cardiac surgery in the septuagenarians met or exceeded fairly rigorous cost-effectiveness and quality-adjusted life-year standards, whereas for octogenarians, attainment of these standards was inconsistent. Operations on the thoracic aorta and combined coronary bypass/valve procedures in octogenarians fell short of cost efficacy, and all cardiac surgical procedures in that age group were marginally cost-effective at best (Fig 1 in the original article). Any analysis of this type requires a set of actuarial life-span and future cost-of-care projections and assumptions that amount to educated guesswork, perhaps more so when applied to narrowly defined patient groups such as octogenarians who have undergone cardiac surgery. There can be no doubt that the acute costs of hospital care and the cost per quality-adjusted life year (Fig 1 in the original article) were higher in octogenarian than septuagenarian cardiac surgical patients. Tough societal decisions lie ahead, as the number of octogenarians (and older) will continue to rise at least through 2050.

G. P. Gravlee, MD

Current Concepts in the Management of Esophageal Perforations: A Twenty-Seven Year Canadian Experience

Bhatia P, Fortin D, Inculet RI, et al (The Univ of Western Ontario, London, Ontario, Canada)
Ann Thorac Surg 92:209-215, 2011

Background.—Perforation of the esophagus remains a challenging clinical problem.

Methods.—A retrospective review was performed of patients diagnosed with an esophageal perforation admitted to the London Health Sciences Centre from 1981 to 2007. Univariate and multivariate logistic regression was used to determine which factors had a statistically significant effect on mortality.

Results.—There were 119 patients; 15 with cervical, 95 with thoracic, and 9 with abdominal perforations. Fifty-one percent of all the perforations were iatrogenic and 33% were spontaneous. Multivariate logistic regression analysis revealed that patients with preoperative respiratory failure requiring mechanical ventilation had a mortality odds ratio of 32.4 (95% confidence interval [CI] 3.1 to 272.0), followed by malignant perforations with 20.2 (95% CI 5.4 to 115.6), a Charlson comorbidity index of 7.1 or greater with 19.6 (95% CI 4.8 to 84.9), the presence of a pulmonary comorbidity with 13.9 (95% CI 2.9 to 97.4), and sepsis with 3.1 (95% CI 1.0 to 10.1). A wait time of greater than 24 hours was not associated with an increased risk of mortality ($p = 0.52$).

Conclusions.—Malignant perforations, sepsis, mechanical ventilation at presentation, a higher overall burden of comorbidity, and a pulmonary comorbidity have a significant impact on the overall survival. Time to treatment is not as important. Restoration of intestinal continuity, either by primary repair or by excision and reanastomosis can be attempted even in patients with a greater time from perforation to treatment with respectable morbidity and mortality rates.

▶ The authors challenge the longstanding axiom that rapid intervention following esophageal perforation improves outcome. This challenge is not posed so much in the sense of buying time for patient preoperative stabilization as it is in the sense of accepting the patient for surgery even if the interval between perforation and diagnosis is substantial. Presumably, the authors performed urgent or emergent surgery once the patients presented to them, but this was not specified. The different types of perforation had strikingly different times to clinical presentation, ranging from 19 hours for abdominal perforations to 129 hours for malignant thoracic perforations. The 30-day mortality rate for malignant thoracic perforations was 63%, suggesting the possibility that these patients might be best served by conservative measures, such as closed-chest thoracostomy, palliative diversion, or stenting, especially if comorbidity is substantial.

G. P. Gravlee, MD

Development and Validation of a Risk Calculator for Prediction of Cardiac Risk After Surgery

Gupta PK, Gupta H, Sundaram A, et al (Creighton Univ, Omaha, NE; et al)
Circulation 124:381-387, 2011

Background.—Perioperative myocardial infarction or cardiac arrest is associated with significant morbidity and mortality. The Revised Cardiac Risk Index is currently the most commonly used cardiac risk stratification tool; however, it has several limitations, one of which is its relatively low discriminative ability. The objective of the present study was to develop and validate a predictive cardiac risk calculator.

Methods and Results.—Patients who underwent surgery were identified from the American College of Surgeons' 2007 National Surgical Quality Improvement Program database, a multicenter (>250 hospitals) prospective database. Of the 211 410 patients, 1371 (0.65%) developed perioperative myocardial infarction or cardiac arrest. On multivariate logistic regression analysis, 5 predictors of perioperative myocardial infarction or cardiac arrest were identified: type of surgery, dependent functional status, abnormal creatinine, American Society of Anesthesiologists' class, and increasing age. The risk model based on the 2007 data set was subsequently validated on the 2008 data set (n = 257 385). The model performance was very similar between the 2007 and 2008 data sets, with C statistics (also known as area under the receiver operating characteristic curve) of 0.884 and 0.874, respectively. Application of the Revised Cardiac Risk Index to the 2008 National Surgical Quality Improvement Program data set yielded a relatively lower C statistic (0.747). The risk model was used to develop an interactive risk calculator.

Conclusions.—The cardiac risk calculator provides a risk estimate of perioperative myocardial infarction or cardiac arrest and is anticipated to

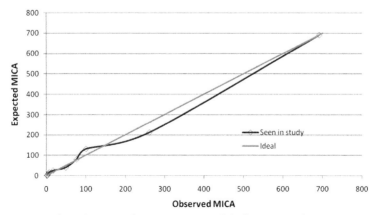

FIGURE 1.—Observed vs expected perioperative myocardial infarction or cardiac arrest (MICA): calibration of predictions in the training set. (Reprinted from Gupta PK, Gupta H, Sundaram A, et al. Development and validation of a risk calculator for prediction of cardiac risk after surgery. *Circulation.* 2011;124:381-387, with permission from American Heart Association, Inc.)

simplify the informed consent process. Its predictive performance surpasses that of the Revised Cardiac Risk Index (Fig 1).

▶ The Revised Cardiac Risk Index (RCRI) is the most commonly used bedside tool for cardiac risk stratification. However, it is limited by the following: the scoring system was derived from a very small cohort of patients. Furthermore, categorization of surgeries used in RCRI are no longer relevant today. Finally, RCRI lacks discriminative/predictive ability. In the current study, the authors describe a new model for the prediction of cardiac risk after noncardiac surgery. To create this model, the authors used the American College of Surgeons National Surgical Improvement Program Database. This is a landmark study because it convincingly demonstrates the use of a current, validated model to predict, with the use of a calculator by clinicians for real time point-of-patient care, the likelihood of perioperative cardiac events in patients undergoing noncardiac surgery. The scheme provided by the author would be very helpful in objectively influencing whether or not to operate on a patient, and if so, whether to attempt to create an optimal cardiac status before surgery.

M. Mathru, MD

Effects of Donor Pre-Treatment With Dopamine on Survival After Heart Transplantation: A Cohort Study of Heart Transplant Recipients Nested in a Randomized Controlled Multicenter Trial

Benck U, Hoeger S, Brinkkoetter PT, et al (Univ Med Centre Mannheim, Germany; Univ of Cologne, Germany; et al)
J Am Coll Cardiol 58:1768-1777, 2011

Objectives.—We determined the outcome of cardiac allografts from multiorgan donors enrolled in a randomized trial of donor pre-treatment with dopamine.

Background.—Treatment of the brain-dead donor with low-dose dopamine improves immediate graft function after kidney transplantation.

Methods.—A cohort study of 93 heart transplants from 21 European centers was undertaken between March 2004 and August 2007. We assessed post-transplant left ventricular function (LVF), requirement of a left ventricular assist device (LVAD) or biventricular assist device (BVAD), need for hemofiltration, acute rejection, and survival of recipients of a dopamine-treated versus untreated graft.

Results.—Donor dopamine was associated with improved survival 3 years after transplantation (87.0% vs. 67.8%, p = 0.03). Fewer recipients of a pre-treated graft required hemofiltration after transplant (21.7% vs. 40.4%, p = 0.05). Impaired LVF (15.2% vs. 21.3%, p = 0.59), requirement of a LVAD (4.4% vs. 10.6%, p = 0.44), and biopsy-proven acute rejection (19.6% vs. 14.9%, p = 0.59) were not statistically different between groups. Post-transplant impaired LVF (hazard ratio [HR]: 4.95; 95% confidence interval [CI]: 2.08 to 11.79; p < 0.001), requirement of LVAD (HR:

6.65; 95% CI: 2.40 to 18.45; p < 0.001), and hemofiltration (HR: 2.83; 95% CI: 1.20 to 6.69; p = 0.02) were predictive of death. The survival benefit remained (HR: 0.33; 95% CI: 0.12 to 0.89; p = 0.03) after adjustment for various risks affecting mortality, including pre-transplant LVAD/BVAD, inotropic support, and impaired kidney function.

Conclusions.—Treatment of brain-dead donors with dopamine of 4 μg/kg/min will not harm cardiac allografts but appears to improve the clinical course of the heart allograft recipient. (Prospective Randomized Trial to Evaluate the Efficacy of Donor Preconditioning With Dopamine on Initial Graft Function After Kidney Transplantation; NCT00115115).

▶ This is the first evidence I have seen for dopamine-induced organ protection since the scientifically driven demise of its incorrectly assumed renal protective effect. The authors probably correctly attribute the apparent dopamine renoprotective effect (as judged by the lower incidence of hemofiltration) in these heart transplant recipients to a lower incidence of posttransplant cardiac dysfunction. Why would pretreating a donor heart with dopamine improve its posttransplant function? If anything, anecdotal evidence to the contrary has been previously proposed. The authors propose that dopamine in sufficient doses to induce tachycardia may indeed damage the donor heart, while also citing in vitro evidence that dopamine lessens the accumulation of intracellular calcium and scavenges reactive oxygen species. As the authors suggest, this study needs confirmation. If dopamine indeed protects against myocardial ischemia, then a host of other questions arise, such as whether the protective mechanism derives from a dopaminergic effect, an adrenergic effect, or some yet-undetermined mechanism.

G. P. Gravlee, MD

High-Dose Tranexamic Acid Is an Independent Predictor of Early Seizure After Cardiopulmonary Bypass

Kalavrouziotis D, Voisine P, Mohammadi S, et al (Laval Univ, Quebec, Canada)
Ann Thorac Surg 93:148-155, 2012

Background.—Risk factors associated with early seizure after cardiopulmonary bypass (CPB) were examined. The role of tranexamic acid in seizure development was evaluated.

Methods.—Early seizure was defined as a seizure occurring within 24 hours of CPB, without neurologic deficit or new lesion on brain imaging. Independent determinants of early seizure were examined by multivariate logistic regression modelling.

Results.—Between 2004 and 2009, early seizure occurred in 119 of 8,929 patients (1.3%). A significant increase in the yearly rate of early seizure was observed in 2004 (0.73%) vs 2009 (1.97%; $p < 0.0001$). Multivariate analysis showed the following variables were independent predictors of early seizure: age older than 75 years (adjusted odds ratio [OR], 2.1; $p = 0.0001$), open heart procedure (OR, 12.0; $p < 0.0001$), preoperative renal failure (OR, 3.2;

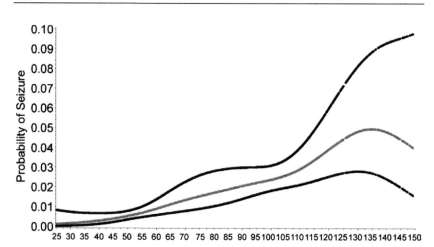

FIGURE 2.—The risk of early seizure according to total dose of tranexamic acid. The estimated risk is shown in red along with the 95% confidence intervals in black. For interpretation of the references to color in this figure legend, the reader is referred to web version of this article. (This article was published in the Annals of Thoracic Surgery, Kalavrouziotis D, Voisine P, Mohammadi S, et al. High-dose tranexamic acid is an independent predictor of early seizure after cardiopulmonary bypass. *Ann Thorac Surg.* 93:148-155. Copyright The Society of Thoracic Surgeons 2012.)

$p < 0.0001$), peripheral vascular disease (OR, 1.8; $p = 0.02$), and total tranexamic acid dose of 100 mg/kg or more (OR, 2.6; $p < 0.0001$). Risk of seizure was related to tranexamic acid in a dose-dependent fashion, with higher doses associated with increased risk of seizure. The use of CO_2 in a subset of patients undergoing open heart procedures did not decrease the incidence of early seizure (4.8% vs 2.5% for no CO_2; $p = 0.27$). Postoperative chest tube drainage and blood product use were similar between patients receiving low-dose and high-dose tranexamic acid.

Conclusions.—High-dose tranexamic acid (≥ 100 mg/kg) is independently associated with an increased risk of early seizure. Future tranexamic acid trials should assess the blood-conserving effect of tranexamic acid at a lower dosage and specifically monitor for seizure occurrence (Fig 2).

▶ This single-center retrospective study confirms other recent studies associating tranexamic acid prophylaxis with postoperative seizures. Because aprotinin's demise (at least in the United States), aminocaproic acid has ostensibly become the dominant prophylactic lysine analogue in cardiac surgery, even though the scientific literature supports tranexamic more strongly for that purpose. Recent American shortages of aminocaproic acid have caused centers to stock tranexamic acid, and one of the challenges they then face is selection of an appropriate tranexamic dose for prophylaxis. This process is complicated by the wide-ranging dosing used for tranexamic acid in previous studies. Although this study does show a dose-related effect of tranexamic acid (Fig 2), the retrospective nature of the data and the low overall incidence of seizures even in the high-risk group temper concerns about this relationship. However, because several studies strongly support a hemostatic effect of lower doses of tranexamic acid, the best current recommendation is to avoid high-dose tranexamic acid prophylaxis. A loading dose of 10 to 15 mg/kg followed by a maintenance dose of 1 to 1.5 mg/kg/hour for the remainder of surgery should suffice for that purpose.

G. P. Gravlee, MD

Influence of Low Tidal Volume Ventilation on Time to Extubation in Cardiac Surgical Patients

Sundar S, Novack V, Jervis K, et al (Beth Israel Deaconess Med Ctr, Boston, MA; et al)

Anesthesiology 114:1102-1110, 2011

Background.—Low tidal volumes have been associated with improved outcomes in patients with established acute lung injury. The role of low tidal volume ventilation in patients without lung injury is still unresolved. We hypothesized that such a strategy in patients undergoing elective surgery would reduce ventilator-associated lung injury and that this improvement would lead to a shortened time to extubation.

Methods.—A single-center randomized controlled trial was undertaken in 149 patients undergoing elective cardiac surgery. Ventilation with 6 *versus* 10 ml/kg tidal volume was compared. Ventilator settings were applied immediately after anesthesia induction and continued throughout surgery and the subsequent intensive care unit stay. The primary endpoint of the study was time to extubation. Secondary endpoints included the proportion of patients extubated at 6 h and indices of lung mechanics and gas exchange as well as patient clinical outcomes.

Results.—Median ventilation time was not significantly different in the low tidal volume group; a median (interquartile range) of 450 (264−1,044) min was achieved compared with 643 (417−1,032) min in the control group ($P = 0.10$). However, a higher proportion of patients in the low tidal volume group was free of any ventilation at 6 h: 37.3% compared with 20.3% in the control group ($P = 0.02$). In addition, fewer patients in the low tidal volume group required reintubation (1.3 *vs.* 9.5%; $P = 0.03$).

Conclusions.—Although reduction of tidal volume in mechanically ventilated patients undergoing elective cardiac surgery did not significantly shorten time to extubation, several improvements were observed in secondary outcomes. When these data are combined with a lack of observed complications, a strategy of reduced tidal volume could still be beneficial in this patient population.

▶ The initial studies showing an advantage when using low tidal volumes to ventilate patients with pulmonary disease were as much about inspiratory pressures as tidal volume.[1,2] Avoidance of peak inspiratory pressures less than 40 cm H_2O were a major component of the original trials. In this report of the potential benefit of low tidal volumes in cardiac surgical patients, plateau pressures were below 20 cm H_2O in both study groups and, not unexpectedly, compliance was indistinguishable between the low tidal volume and conventional respiratory therapy groups.

Given these similarities in the study groups, is there any significance to the study's findings? The lack of difference in average duration of ventilation in the study groups is just one component of this study's results. The investigators found that, in cardiac surgical patients, ventilation with small tidal volumes, 6 mL/kg (ideal body weight), did have advantages. Fewer of the patients ventilated with 6 mL/kg when compared with those ventilated with 10 mL/kg, required ventilator support 6 hours after admission to the intensive care unit, and they required re-intubation less frequently than the patients intubated with larger tidal volumes. Perhaps most importantly, there were no adverse effects associated with ventilating patients with smaller tidal volumes. Positive end expiratory pressure used in both study groups was similar, as was PaO_2 at all points through the course of the study. While not problematic in this study, the degree of hypercarbia in the low tidal volume group found on admission to the intensive care unit may be a concern in some patients.

Larger studies of the impact of ventilation with small tidal volumes on patient outcomes, in patients not at risk for acute lung injury, are necessary to determine its safety as well as the potential utility of application of this ventilatory strategy in other patients.

C. Lien, MD

References

1. Amato MB, Barbas CS, Medeiros DM, et al. Effect of a protective-ventilation strategy on mortality in the acute respiratory distress syndrome. *N Engl J Med.* 1998;338:347-354.
2. Amato MB, Barbas CS, Medeiros DM, et al. Beneficial effects of the "open lung approach" with low distending pressures in acute respiratory distress syndrome. A prospective randomized study on mechanical ventilation. *Am J Respir Crit Care Med.* 1995;152:1835-1846.

Lack of Effectiveness of the Pulmonary Artery Catheter in Cardiac Surgery

Schwann NM, Hillel Z, Hoeft A, et al (Lehigh Valley Health Network, Allentown, PA; St Luke's—Roosevelt Hosp Ctr, NY; Bonn Univ, Germany; et al)
Anesth Analg 113:994-1002, 2011

Background.—The pulmonary artery catheter (PAC) continues to be used for monitoring of hemodynamics in patients undergoing coronary artery bypass graft (CABG) surgery despite concerns raised in other settings regarding both effectiveness and safety. Given the relative paucity of data regarding its use in CABG patients, and given entrenched practice patterns, we assessed the impact of PAC use on fatal and nonfatal CABG outcomes as practiced at a diverse set of medical centers.

Methods.—Using a formal prospective observational study design, 5065 CABG patients from 70 centers were enrolled between November 1996 and June 2000 using a systemic sampling protocol. Propensity score matched-pair analysis was used to adjust for differences in likelihood of PAC insertion. The predefined composite endpoint was the occurrence of any of the following: death (any cause), cardiac dysfunction (myocardial infarction or congestive heart failure), cerebral dysfunction (stroke or encephalopathy), renal dysfunction (dysfunction or failure), or pulmonary dysfunction (acute respiratory distress syndrome). Secondary variables included treatment indices (inotrope use, fluid administration), duration of postoperative intubation, and intensive care unit length of stay. After categorization based on PAC and transesophageal echocardiography use (both, neither, PAC only, transesophageal echocardiography only), we performed the primary analysis contrasting PAC only and neither (total, 3321 patients), from which propensity paring yielded 1273 matched pairs.

Results.—The primary endpoint occurred in 271 PAC patients versus 196 without PAC (21.3% vs. 15.4%; adjusted odds ratio [AOR], 1.68; 95% confidence interval [CI], 1.24 to 2.26; $P < 0.001$). The PAC group had an increased risk of all-cause mortality, 3.5% vs 1.7% (AOR, 2.08; 95% CI, 1.11 to 3.88; $P = 0.02$) and an increased risk of cardiac (AOR, 1.58; 95% CI, 1.14 to 2.20; $P = 0.007$), cerebral (AOR, 2.02; 95% CI, 1.08 to 3.77; $P = 0.03$) and renal (AOR, 2.47; 95% CI, 1.68 to 3.62; $P < 0.001$) morbid outcomes. PAC patients received inotropic drugs more frequently (57.8% vs 50.0%; $P < 0.001$), had a larger positive IV fluid balance after surgery (3220 mL vs 3022 mL; $P = 0.003$), and experienced longer time to tracheal extubation (15.40 hours [11.28/20.80] versus 13.18 hours [9.58/19.33], median plus Q1/Q3 interquartile range; $P < 0.0001$). Use of PAC was also associated with prolonged intensive care unit stay (14.5% vs 10.1%; AOR, 1.55; 95% CI, 1.06 to 2.27; $P = 0.02$).

Conclusions.—Use of a PAC during CABG surgery was associated with increased mortality and a higher risk of severe end-organ complications in this propensity-matched observational study. A randomized controlled trial with defined hemodynamic goals would be ideal to either confirm or refute our findings.

▶ This international multicenter study retrospectively correlates pulmonary artery (PA) catheter use to increased morbidity and mortality in cardiac surgery. This conclusion was reached using a somewhat controversial statistical technique called propensity analysis. The study is highly provocative and may influence clinical practice, but it does have some potentially important limitations. First, patients who underwent transesophageal echocardiography were excluded; the rationale for this exclusion is unclear. Second, the 70 centers varied from 1% to 99% in their use of PA catheters. Although the authors contend that they incorporated this variation into their statistical analysis, I am skeptical that a variation of that magnitude among centers can be effectively incorporated into a retrospective database analysis, so there should be some concern about the comparability of the patient groups. Although it seems unlikely that PA catheters intrinsically contribute to the morbidities incorporated into this analysis, this article raises legitimate concern about the decisions being made from the data generated by PA catheters. Their data suggest the possibility of overintervention with inotropic support. Some previous evidence casts doubt on the ability of bedside caregivers to correctly interpret PA catheter data.[1] In recent years, one of the PA catheter's alleged strengths, that is, approximation of left atrial filling pressure, has been largely discredited as a useful measurement of left ventricular preload. The article is accompanied by a good editorial that suggests the need for randomized prospective trials. My view is that this is unlikely to happen and that we should simply become more selective in the use of PA catheters. Patients with pulmonary hypertension or right ventricular dysfunction might benefit from their use more than patients who lack these characteristics. Less invasive measurements of cardiac output continue to develop, and some critical care literature supports continuous monitoring of central venous oxygen saturation in place of the true mixed venous oxygen saturation that can be measured best in the PA.

G. P. Gravlee, MD

Reference

1. Hessel EA, Apostolidou I. Pulmonary artery catheter for coronary artery bypass graft: does it harm our patients? Primum non nocere. *Anesth Analg.* 2011;113: 987-989.

Low-dose desmopressin improves hypothermia-induced impairment of primary haemostasis in healthy volunteers

Ng KFJ, Cheung CW, Lee Y, et al (The Univ of Hong Kong, China)
Anaesthesia 66:999-1005, 2011

Mild hypothermia (34–35 °C) increases peri-operative blood loss. We have previously demonstrated the beneficial effect of in vitro desmopressin on impairment of primary haemostasis associated with hypothermia. This study evaluated subcutaneous desmopressin in 52 healthy volunteers, randomly assigned to receive either normal saline or desmopressin 1.5, 5 or 15 μg (with 13 in each group). Blood samples were collected before and 2 h after drug administration and incubated at 32 and 37 °C. Platelet function analyser PFA-100® closure times were measured. Hypothermia at 32 °C prolonged mean (95% CI) closure times (for adenosine diphosphate/collagen by 11.3% (7.5–15.2%) and for adrenaline/collagen by 16.2% (11.3–21.2%); these changes were reversed by desmopressin. A very small dose was found to be effective (1.5 μg); this dose did not significantly change closure times at 37 °C, but fully prevented its prolongation at 32 °C. Subcutaneous desmopressin prevents the development of hypothermia-induced impairment of primary haemostasis.

▶ This study investigates the dose-ranging effect of subcutaneously administered desmopressin on platelet aggregation in the blood of healthy volunteers that was made hypothermic in vitro. Desmopressin uniformly reversed hypothermia-induced platelet dysfunction at doses too small even to induce an increase in plasma von Willebrand factor level. The finding deserves further study, but the clinical implication is that a very small dose of desmopressin administered subcutaneously might correct or reduce coagulopathy associated with hypothermia. By inference, a similarly small (1.5 µg) intravenous dose would have a faster onset and would be equally effective. That dose seems unlikely to induce either hypotension or a hypercoagulable state. Clinical studies in hypothermic coagulopathic patients are needed, but, in the meantime, it seems reasonable to try this therapy if rapid rewarming is infeasible.

G. P. Gravlee, MD

Mixed venous oxygen saturation predicts short- and long-term outcome after coronary artery bypass grafting surgery: a retrospective cohort analysis
Holm J, Håkanson E, Vánky F, et al (Linköping Univ, Sweden)
Br J Anaesth 107:344-350, 2011

Background.—Complications of an inadequate haemodynamic state are a leading cause of morbidity and mortality after cardiac surgery. Unfortunately, commonly used methods to assess haemodynamic status are not well documented with respect to outcome. The aim of this study was to investigate Svo_2 as a prognostic marker for short- and long-term outcome in a large unselected coronary artery bypass grafting (CABG) cohort and in subgroups with or without treatment for intraoperative heart failure.

Methods.—Two thousand seven hundred and fifty-five consecutive CABG patients and subgroups comprising 344 patients with and 2411 patients without intraoperative heart failure, respectively, were investigated. Svo_2 was routinely measured on admission to the intensive care unit (ICU). The mean (SD) follow-up was 10.2 (1.5) yr.

Results.—The best cut-off for 30 day mortality related to heart failure based on receiver-operating characteristic analysis was Svo_2 60.1%. Patients with Svo_2 <60% had higher 30 day mortality (5.4% *vs* 1.0%; $P<0.0001$) and lower 5 yr survival (81.4% *vs* 90.5%; $P<0.0001$). The incidences of perioperative myocardial infarction, renal failure, and stroke were also significantly higher, leading to a longer ICU stay. Similar prognostic information was obtained in the subgroups that were admitted to ICU with or without treatment for intraoperative heart failure. In patients admitted to ICU without treatment for intraoperative heart failure and $Svo_2 \geq 60\%$, 30 day mortality was 0.5% and 5 yr survival 92.1%.

Conclusions.—Svo_2 <60% on admission to ICU was related to worse short- and long-term outcome after CABG, regardless of whether the patients were admitted to ICU with or without treatment for intraoperative heart failure.

▶ There are remarkably few data relating venous oxygen saturation (Svo_2) measurements to cardiac surgical outcomes. This retrospective but very large observational study yields a pretty impressive inflection point at Svo_2 values below 60% in patients with coronary artery bypass graft (CABG) at the time of arrival in the intensive care unit (ICU) (Fig 1 in the original article). The usual risk factor suspects, such as female gender, low left ventricular ejection fraction, older age, and longer aortic cross-clamp and cardiopulmonary bypass times, and the use of inotropic support were statistically associated with low Svo_2 at ICU arrival. The association held up for an impressive 5-year follow-up period. The authors appropriately note that their data are fairly old (collection ended in 2000) and that the study lacked any interventions based on Svo_2 data. They suggest that efforts to maintain Svo_2 values above 60% in patients with CABG appear desirable. Despite the study's limitations, it is difficult to argue against that conclusion.

G. P. Gravlee, MD

Mortality and Readmission of Patients With Heart Failure, Atrial Fibrillation, or Coronary Artery Disease Undergoing Noncardiac Surgery: An Analysis of 38 047 Patients
van Diepen S, Bakal JA, McAlister FA, et al (Univ of Alberta, Edmonton, Canada)
Circulation 124:289-296, 2011

Background.—The postoperative risks for patients with coronary artery disease (CAD) undergoing noncardiac surgery are well described. However, the risks of noncardiac surgery in patients with heart failure (HF) and atrial fibrillation (AF) are less well known. The purpose of this study is to compare the postoperative mortality of patients with HF, AF, or CAD undergoing major and minor noncardiac surgery.

Methods and Results.—Population-based data were used to create 4 cohorts of consecutive patients with either nonischemic HF (NIHF; n = 7700), ischemic HF (IHF; n = 12 249), CAD (n = 13 786), or AF (n = 4312) who underwent noncardiac surgery between April 1, 1999, and September 31, 2006, in Alberta, Canada. The main outcome was 30-day postoperative mortality. The unadjusted 30-day postoperative mortality was 9.3% in NIHF, 9.2% in IHF, 2.9% in CAD, and 6.4% in AF (each versus CAD, *P* < 0.0001). Among patients undergoing minor surgical procedures, the 30-day postoperative mortality was 8.5% in NIHF, 8.1% in IHF, 2.3% in CAD, and 5.7% in AF (*P* < 0.0001). After multivariable adjustment, postoperative mortality remained higher in NIHF, IHF, and AF patients than in those with CAD (NIHF versus CAD: odds ratio 2.92; 95% confidence interval 2.44 to 3.48; IHF versus CAD: odds ratio 1.98; 95% confidence interval 1.70 to 2.31; AF versus CAD: odds ratio 1.69; 95% confidence interval 1.34 to 2.14).

Conclusions.—Although current perioperative risk prediction models place greater emphasis on CAD than HF or AF, patients with HF or AF have a significantly higher risk of postoperative mortality than patients with CAD, and even minor procedures carry a risk higher than previously appreciated.

▶ This observational study used an extensive administrative database to assess a variety of characteristics in patients who had major or minor surgery following previous hospitalization for heart failure, coronary artery disease (CAD), or atrial fibrillation. The authors arguably overstate surprise at the importance of heart failure as a risk factor in view of the fact that patients who have been hospitalized for heart failure are more likely to fall into a category of poorly controlled heart failure than those who have been managed as outpatients. However, because a majority of patients with new-onset atrial fibrillation would likely be hospitalized for initial management, such bias might be less prevalent in the atrial fibrillation subgroup. The most striking findings were that even minor procedures (eg, cystoscopy, bronchoscopy, colonoscopy; often done without general anesthesia) performed within 30 days of hospitalization for heart failure or atrial fibrillation carry a surprisingly high risk for 30-day mortality. The message may be that elective noncardiac procedures are unwise within 30 days of previous hospitalization for heart failure or atrial fibrillation. To a lesser degree, this applies to hospitalization for CAD as well.

G. P. Gravlee, MD

One-Year Outcomes of Cohort 1 in the Edwards SAPIEN Aortic Bioprosthesis European Outcome (SOURCE) Registry: The European Registry of Transcatheter Aortic Valve Implantation Using the Edwards SAPIEN Valve
Thomas M, Schymik G, Walther T, et al (King's Health Partners, London, UK; Städtisches Klinikum und Herzklinik, Karlsruhe, Germany; Herzzentrum, Leipzig, Germany; et al)
Circulation 124:425-433, 2011

Background.—Transcatheter aortic valve implantation was developed to provide a therapeutic option for patients considered to be ineligible for, and to mitigate mortality and morbidity associated with, high-risk surgical aortic valve replacement.

Methods and Results.—The Edwards SAPIEN Aortic Bioprosthesis European Outcome (SOURCE) Registry was designed to assess initial post commercial clinical transcatheter aortic valve implantation results of the Edwards SAPIEN valve in consecutive patients in Europe. Cohort 1 consists of 1038 patients enrolled at 32 centers. One-year outcomes are presented. Patients with the transapical approach (n = 575) suffered more comorbidities than transfemoral patients (n = 463) with a significantly higher logistic EuroSCORE (29% versus 25.8%; $P = 0.007$). These groups are different; therefore, outcomes cannot be directly compared. Total Kaplan Meier 1-year survival was 76.1% overall, 72.1% for transapical and 81.1% for transfemoral patients, and 73.5% of surviving patients were in New York Heart Association (NYHA) class I or II at 1 year. Combined transapical and transfemoral causes of death were cardiac in 25.1%, noncardiac in 49.2%, and unknown in 25.7%. Pulmonary complications (23.9%), renal failure (12.5%), cancer (11.4%), and stroke (10.2%) were the most frequent noncardiac causes of death. Multivariable analysis identified logistic EuroSCORE, renal disease, liver disease, and smoking as variables with the highest hazard ratios for 1-year mortality whereas carotid artery stenosis, hyperlipidemia, and hypertension were associated with lower mortality.

Conclusion.—The SOURCE Registry is the largest consecutively enrolled registry for transcatheter aortic valve implantation procedures. It demonstrates that with new transcatheter aortic techniques excellent 1-year survival in high-risk and inoperable patients is achievable and provides a benchmark against which future transcatheter aortic valve implantation cohorts and devices can be measured.

▶ This is the largest series reported to date on transcatheter aortic valve implantation (TAVI). The principal reported outcome in this high-risk population was 1-year mortality, which approximated 100 minus the EuroSCORE. In other words, the 1-year mortality following TAVI approximated the predicted 30-day mortality for surgical aortic valve replacement (AVR). On its surface, this appears to make TAVI a prohibitive favorite over surgical AVR in this patient population, but one never knows until a prospective comparison occurs. For example, the vast majority of surgical morbidity and mortality occurs in the first 30 days, whereas that for interventional cardiology procedures occurs predominantly between 30 days and 1 year. To complicate matters further, only 25% of TAVI mortality between 30 days and 1 year was definitely cardiac, whereas 50% was noncardiac and 25% was of undetermined cause that might have been cardiac. TAVI is expanding fairly rapidly in the United States, so cardiac anesthesiologists are likely to see quite a bit more of it in the next few years. Most TAVIs are performed with general anesthesia.

G. P. Gravlee, MD

Postoperative hypothermia and patient outcomes after elective cardiac surgery
Karalapillai D, Story D, Hart GK, et al (Austin Health, Heidelberg, Australia; et al)
Anaesthesia 66:780-784, 2011

Hypothermia after elective cardiac surgery is an important physiological abnormality and is associated with increased morbidity and mortality. The Australian and New Zealand intensive care adult patient database was studied to obtain the lowest and highest temperature in the first 24 h after surgery. Hypothermia was defined as core temperature < 36 °C; transient hypothermia as temperature < 36 °C that was corrected within 24 h; and persistent hypothermia as hypothermia that was not corrected within 24 h. Hypothermia occurred in 28 587 out of a total of 43 158 consecutive patients (66%) and was persistent in 111 (0.3%). Transient hypothermia was not independently associated with increased hospital mortality (OR = 0.9, 95% CI 0.8−1.1), whereas persistent hypothermia was associated with markedly increased risk of death (OR = 6.3, 95% CI = 3.3−12.0). Hypothermia is common in postoperative cardiac surgery patients during the first 24 h after ICU admission but, if transient, is not independently associated with an increased risk of death.

▶ This retrospective database review included more than 43 000 cardiac surgical patients. The incidence of transient hypothermia was unsurprising in view of the general inability of traditional rewarming techniques during cardiopulmonary bypass (CPB) to "repay" the total caloric deficit without risking cerebral hyperthermia. That this occurrence was benign in terms of outcomes is encouraging, but it invokes concern about the wisdom of extubating patients "on the table," that is, before transport to the intensive care unit. Only a small percentage of patients (approximately 0.3%) experienced persistent hypothermia for the first 24 hours after surgery, and the only striking demographic distinctions of those patients were higher APACHE scores and a higher prevalence of operations other than coronary revascularization and/or valve procedures. Circulatory arrest patients were excluded from analysis, so this could not explain the persistent hypothermia. It seems likely that these patients had some combination of moderate hypothermia during cardiopulmonary bypass (lowest temperature between 28° and 33°C), insufficient rewarming at the conclusion of CPB, and a low cardiac output state in the first 24 hours following surgery (potentially rendering rewarming efforts ineffective). Should hypothermia persist at 6 to 12 hours after cardiac surgery, the findings suggest a need to expeditiously seek and correct its cause.

G. P. Gravlee, MD

Prevalence and Risk of Preexisting Heparin-Induced Thrombocytopenia Antibodies in Patients With Acute VTE
Warkentin TE, Davidson BL, Büller HR, et al (McMaster Univ, Hamilton, Ontario, Canada; Univ of Washington, School of Medicine, Seattle; Academic Med Ctr, Amsterdam, The Netherlands; et al)
Chest 140:366-373, 2011

Background.—Some patients with acute VTE who may previously have been exposed to heparin products have unrecognized antibodies implicated in heparin-induced thrombocytopenia (HIT). Antibody prevalence and patient consequences upon exposure to heparin, low-molecular-weight heparin, and fondaparinux are uncertain.

Methods.—In this secondary analysis, we tested patients in the Matisse VTE studies at study entry for heparin-dependent antibodies and further tested patients with enzyme-linked immunosorbent assay (ELISA)-positive results for platelet-activating antibodies. We compared the risk of HIT (>50% fall in platelet count, heparin-dependent antibodies, no contradicting features) between patients treated with heparin (either unfractionated or low molecular weight [enoxaparin]) vs those who received fondaparinux. Comparison groups for thrombocytopenia occurrence comprised patients with ELISA-positive, platelet-activating, antibody-positive results;

ELISA-positive, but platelet-activating antibody-negative results; and randomly selected antibody-negative results.

Results.—A total of 127 of 3,994 patients (3.2%) had ELISA-positive results at baseline, but only 14 (0.4%; 95% CI, 0.2%-0.6%) had platelet-activating antibodies. Among these 14, four treated with unfractionated or low-molecular-weight heparin developed HIT compared with zero of 10 fondaparinux-treated patients (OR, 95; 95% CI, 8-1,123; *P* < .001). This frequency (four of four, 100%) significantly differed from that of both heparin-treated patients whose results were ELISA positive but platelet-activating antibody negative and from heparin-treated antibody-negative control subjects (zero of 15 and zero of 27, respectively; *P* < .001 for both).

Conclusions.—Of patients with VTE, 0.4% had pathologic platelet-activating heparin-dependent antibodies rather than the 3.2% detected by the recommended cutoff of the commercial ELISA. Among study patients with acute VTE who had platelet-activating antibodies, treatment with fondaparinux reduced the risk of precipitating rapid-onset HIT.

▶ The authors took a deep vein thrombosis (DVT) patient population that was ostensibly free of heparin-induced thrombocytopenia (HIT) and analyzed its patients for occult DVT. Because the patients were treated for DVT with some type of heparin while HIT antibody diagnosis was ongoing, this afforded the opportunity to assess the diagnostic specificity of HIT tests as well as the potential for development of clinical HIT when unfractionated heparin, low molecular weight heparin (LMWH), or fondaparinux was given to DVT patients who had unrecognized heparin-dependent antibodies. The study confirms the author's previous documentation that ELISA positivity for heparin-dependent platelet-activating antibodies is sensitive but nonspecific for clinical HIT. This problem is only partially attenuated by setting a diagnostic threshold higher than the ELISA assay manufacturer recommends (1.0 U instead of 0.4 U). The gold-standard (but seldom available) serotonin-release assay performs much better, so the tendency is to overdiagnose HIT with the readily available ELISA test. Although patient numbers were small, all 4 patients with serotonin assay—positive heparin antibodies developed HIT when given either unfractionated heparin or LMWH, but 0 of 10 developed HIT when given fondaparinux. This makes sense in view of the fact that fondaparinux contains only a 5-saccharide chain, which is considered too short to initiate an antibody response and perhaps even to bind an existing antibody. Anesthesiologists are advised to seek more than an ELISA-positive test (eg, serotonin-release assay or a platelet-aggregation test) before committing patients to the use of an anticoagulant other than unfractionated heparin for surgical anticoagulation.

G. P. Gravlee, MD

Protection by remote ischemic preconditioning during coronary artery bypass graft surgery with isoflurane but not propofol – a clinical trial
Kottenberg E, Thielmann M, Bergmann L, et al (Universitätsklinikum Essen, Germany)
Acta Anaesthesiol Scand 56:30-38, 2012

Background.—Remote ischemic preconditioning (RIPC) of the myocardium by limb ischemia/reperfusion may mitigate cardiac damage, but its interaction with the anesthetic regimen is unknown. We tested whether RIPC is associated with differential effects depending on background anesthesia. Specifically, we hypothesized that RIPC during isoflurane anesthesia attenuates myocardial injury in patients undergoing coronary artery bypass graft (CABG) surgery, and that effects may be different during propofol anesthesia.

Methods.—In a randomized, single-blinded, placebo-controlled prospective study, serum troponin I concentration (cTnI) (baseline, and 1, 6, 12, 24, 48, and 72 h postoperatively) were measured during isoflurane/sufentanil or propofol/sufentanil anesthesia with or without RIPC (three 5-min periods of intermittent left upper arm ischemia with 5 min reperfusion each) in non-diabetic patients ($n = 72$) with three-vessel coronary artery disease (ClinicalTrials.gov(http://ClinicalTrials.gov)NCT01406678).

Results.—RIPC during isoflurane anesthesia ($n = 20$) decreased the area under the cTnI time curve (cTnI AUC) (-50%, 190 $\pm$ 105 ng/ml $\times$ 72 h vs. 383 $\pm$ 262 ng/ml $\times$ 72 h, $P = 0.004$), and the peak (7.3 $\pm$ 3.6 ng/ml vs. 11.8 $\pm$ 5.5, $P = 0.004$) and serial ($P < 0.041$) postoperative cTnI when compared to isoflurane alone ($n = 19$). In contrast, RIPC during propofol anesthesia ($n = 14$) did not alter the cTnI AUC [263 $\pm$ 157 ng/ml $\times$ 72 h vs. 372 $\pm$ 376 ng/ml $\times$ 72 h ($n = 19$), $P = 0.318$] or peak postoperative cTnI (10.1 $\pm$ 4.5 ng/ml vs. 12 $\pm$ 8.2, $P = 0.444$). None of the patients experienced harm or side effects from the intermittent left arm ischemia.

Conclusion.—Thus, RIPC during isoflurane but not during propofol anesthesia decreased myocardial damage in patients undergoing CABG surgery. Accordingly, effects of RIPC evoked by upper limb ischemia/reperfusion depend on background anesthesia, with combined RIPC/isoflurane exerting greater beneficial effects under conditions studied.

▶ Preconditioning has an ever-expanding range of techniques, but the fundamental principle is to do something that reduces the injury resulting from an ischemic event. One of the most interesting applications is remote preconditioning, in which creating ischemia in one vascular bed confers protection against subsequent ischemia in another vascular bed. This study combines the concepts of remote preconditioning and anesthetic preconditioning. In essence, the authors show that upper extremity in the presence of isoflurane activated cardiac preconditioning, whereas neither isoflurane or propofol alone nor propofol with remote preconditioning did so (Fig 1 in the original article). The study did not assess outcomes such as length of hospital stay, use of inotropes after cardiopulmonary bypass, or long-term cardiac morbidity. As the authors note, these findings should be considered preliminary, and follow-up studies are anticipated.

G. P. Gravlee, MD

Risk Factors and Early Outcomes of Multiple Reoperations in Adults With Congenital Heart Disease

Holst KA, Dearani JA, Burkhart HM, et al (Mayo Clinic and Foundation, Rochester, MN)

Ann Thorac Surg 92:122-130, 2011

Background.—Advances in treatment of congenital heart disease (CHD) have resulted in most patients surviving to adulthood. Despite surgical "correction," the need for reoperation(s) persists, and there are few outcome data. This study examined early postoperative results to determine risk factors for cardiac injury and early death in adults with CHD undergoing repeat median sternotomy.

Methods.—Data from the most recent median sternotomy of 984 adults (49% male) with CHD were analyzed. Mean age at operation was 36.4 years. Diagnoses were conotruncal anomaly, 361 (37%); Ebstein/Tricuspid valve, 174 (18%); pulmonary stenosis/right ventricular outflow tract obstruction, 92 (9%); single ventricle, 71 (7%); atrioventricular septal defect, 64 (7%); subaortic stenosis, 62 (6%); aortic arch abnormalities, 23 (2%); anomalous pulmonary vein, 21 (2%); Marfan syndrome, 14 (1%); and other, 102 (10%).

Results.—Overall early mortality was 3.6%: including 2%, 6%, 7%, and 0% at sternotomy 2 (n = 597), 3 (n = 284), 4 (n = 72), and 5+ (n = 31), respectively. Cardiac injury occurred in 6%. Independent predictors of cardiac injury were single-ventricle diagnosis and increased number of prior sternotomies. Increased time from previous sternotomy decreased the incidence of cardiac injury. Independent risk factors for early death were urgent operation, single-ventricle diagnosis, and longer bypass time. Increased preoperative ejection fraction decreased early mortality.

Conclusions.—Subsequent sternotomy showed increased early mortality, yet neither sternotomy number nor cardiac injury was an independent predictor of early death. Two variables were protective: early mortality was reduced with increased ejection fraction and cardiac injury was less likely with increased interval from the previous sternotomy.

▶ This is a retrospective single-center analysis of nearly 1000 adult patients undergoing reoperative sternotomy for congenital heart disease. For many, if not most adult cardiac anesthesiologists, this constitutes a growing segment of our clinical practices. In descending order of frequency, the "target" area for the reoperation was the pulmonic valve, the tricuspid valve, the aortic valve, and the mitral valve. After the 4 valves, the next most common indication for surgery was arrhythmia. The authors provide excellent advice about surgical approaches and note the need to anticipate unwanted invasion of cardiac chambers and mediastinal great vessels (as well as coronary arteries) during sternotomy and mediastinal dissection before cardiopulmonary bypass. They liberally used preoperative magnetic resonance and ultrasound imaging to identify areas of concern and also often performed ultrasound imaging of the femoral and cervical arteries and veins to assess the patency of potential cannulation sites for either surgeons or anesthesiologists. The risk factors for early death were not surprising, and the overall surgical mortality was low even after multiple sternotomies.

G. P. Gravlee, MD

'Safe' methaemoglobin concentrations are a mortality risk factor in patients receiving inhaled nitric oxide
Rolley L, Bandeshe H, Boots RJ (Univ of Queensland, Brisbane, Australia)
Anaesth Intensive Care 39:919-925, 2011

Inhaled nitric oxide (iNO) can reduce pulmonary arterial hypertension and improve oxygenation in some patients with severe respiratory or heart failure. Despite this, iNO has not been found to improve survival.

This study aimed to perform a local practice audit to assess the mortality predictors of critically ill patients who had received iNO as therapy for pulmonary hypertension and respiratory or heart failure. A retrospective audit in a single tertiary centre intensive care unit of patients receiving iNO was conducted between 2004 and 2009. The indications for iNO use, comorbidities, severity of illness, organ function, oxygenation, Sequential Organ Failure Assessment scores, patterns of iNO use, adverse events and outcomes were reviewed.

In 215 patients receiving iNO, improvement in oxygenation after one hour from iNO commencement did not predict either intensive care unit ($P = 0.36$) or hospital ($P = 0.72$) mortality. The independent risk factors for intensive care unit mortality were worsening Sequential Organ Failure Assessment scores within 24 hours of commencing iNO (adjusted odds ratio 1.07, 95% confidence interval 1.05 to 1.18), the Charlson Comorbidity Score (adjusted odds ratio 1.49, 95% confidence interval 1.16 to 1.91) and the peak methaemoglobin concentration in arterial blood while receiving iNO (adjusted odds ratio 2.67, 95% confidence interval 1.42 to 4.96).

Inhaled nitric oxide as salvage therapy for severe respiratory failure in critically ill patients is not routinely justified. Increased methaemoglobin concentration during iNO therapy, even when predominantly less than 3%, is associated with increased mortality.

▶ Identifying the appropriate use of highly expensive inhaled nitric oxide (iNO) challenges both cardiothoracic anesthesiologists and intensivists. In the former group, a tendency toward a low threshold for iNO administration in the presence of moderately elevated pulmonary vascular resistance appears prevalent in many centers, especially for patients undergoing orthotopic cardiac transplantation and left ventricular assist device placement. For intensivists, the debate centers around appropriate use of iNO in patients with acute respiratory distress syndrome, which comprised more than two-thirds of the present study population. The absence of a favorable impact of iNO on survival is consistent with previous studies. Identification of an association between peak methemoglobin concentrations during iNO therapy and increased mortality is new. This association is surprising in view of the presumed innocuousness of methemoglobin concentrations below 5% and the presence of just 5 patients who had methemoglobin concentrations exceeding 3%. The data suggest a possible threshold of concern at 1.5% methemoglobin, but the authors concede that this may simply be a surrogate marker for adverse outcomes. Further studies appear warranted, but close monitoring of methemoglobin levels in patients receiving iNO also appears warranted, as does avoidance of methemoglobin concentrations exceeding 3% in critically ill patients.

G. P. Gravlee, MD

The Effect of Nasogastric Tube Application During Cardiac Surgery on Postoperative Nausea and Vomiting—A Randomized Trial

Lavi R, Katznelson R, Cheng D, et al (Univ of Toronto, Ontario, Canada)
J Cardiothorac Vasc Anesth 25:105-109, 2011

Objective.—Postoperative nausea and vomiting (PONV) are significant morbidities following cardiac surgery. The purpose of this study was to determine if application of a nasogastric (NG) tube during cardiac surgery can reduce the prevalence of postoperative PONV.

Design.—This study was a prospective randomized controlled trial.

Setting.—University tertiary referral center.

Participants.—Two hundred two patients undergoing elective cardiac procedures.

Interventions.—Patients were prospectively enrolled and randomized to either receive or not receive an NG tube after induction of anesthesia. Standard anesthetic technique and postoperative care were employed in all patients. Preoperative demographic data, pain score, nausea score and incidence of vomiting were recorded early (0-8 hours) and late (8-16 hours) following extubation. Antiemetic and analgesic medications were compared between the 2 groups.

Measurements and Main Results.—One hundred three patients were randomized to no an NG tube (controls) and 99 received an NG tube as part of their perioperative management. Demographic data and surgical characteristics were similar between the 2 groups. However, the control group had more smokers. Incidence and severity of nausea, pain scores, and analgesic requirements were similar between the 2 groups. Prevalence of vomiting was more frequent in the control group (24%) than in the NG tube group (10%, $p = 0.007$), and was more frequent in patients who underwent valve and redo procedures.

Conclusions.—Use of an NG tube during cardiac surgery may reduce the incidence of postoperative vomiting.

▶ Although the results of this study did demonstrate that insertion of a nasogastric tube was associated with a decreased incidence of vomiting, other studies have not found similar results.[1,2] There was no difference in the incidence of nausea between the 2 study groups and no difference in the rate of antiemetic use. Differences in vomiting were small in the first 8 hours after surgery (24% vs 10%) and disappeared when measured at 8 to 16 hours.

It is unclear why the type of surgery would have resulted in a different frequency of vomiting. Valvular surgery and repeat operations were associated with a greater frequency of vomiting in both single predictor models and multivariate models. The duration of cardiopulmonary bypass and cross-clamp times, however, were not. Pain scores and postoperative use of morphine also did not contribute to the observed difference in the frequency of vomiting in the study groups.

As noted, the difference in vomiting in the study groups was small. The results of this trial may have been more compelling had the primary anesthetic administered been something other than propofol, which will decrease postoperative nausea and vomiting and may not be typically administered to patients undergoing cardiac surgery. Additionally, there is a difference in the study groups relative to whether or not patients smoked. There were more smokers in the control group, and this may have contributed to the low incidence of vomiting in these patients.[3-5] In spite of the potential adverse impact of nausea and vomiting on patients who have had cardiac surgery, better-controlled and better-designed studies will be required to recommend routine placement of nasogastric tubes.

C. Lien, MD

References

1. Nelson R, Edwards S, Tse B. Prophylactic nasogastric decompression after abdominal surgery. *Cochrane Database Syst Rev.* 2007;18. CD004929.
2. Kerger KH, Mascha E, Steinbrecher B, et al; IMPACT Investigators. Routine use of nasogastric tubes does not reduce postoperative nausea and vomiting. *Anesth Analg.* 2009;109:768-773.
3. Gan TJ, Meyer TA, Apfel CC, et al; Society for Ambulatory Anesthesia. Society for Ambulatory Anesthesia guidelines for the management of postoperative nausea and vomiting. *Anesth Analg.* 2007;105:1615-1628.
4. Stadler M, Bardiau F, Seidel L, Albert A, Boogaerts JG. Difference in risk factors for postoperative nausea and vomiting. *Anesthesiology.* 2003;98:46-52.
5. Cohen MM, Duncan PG, DeBoer DP, Tweed WA. The postoperative interview: assessing risk factors for nausea and vomiting. *Anesth Analg.* 1994;78:7-16.

The Impact of Immediate Extubation in the Operating Room After Cardiac Surgery on Intensive Care and Hospital Lengths of Stay

Chamchad D, Horrow JC, Nachamchik L, et al (Lankenau Inst of Med Res, Wynnewood, PA; et al)
J Cardiothorac Vasc Anesth 24:780-784, 2010

Objective.—To determine if lengths of stay in intensive care and the hospital are associated with extubation in the operating room at the conclusion of cardiac surgery.

Design.—A nonrandomized, observational study with propensity score—guided case-control matching of prospectively collected data.

Setting.—Three interrelated, university-affiliated, community hospitals.

Participants.—Three thousand three hundred seventeen patients undergoing elective or urgent coronary artery, valve repair or replacement, or combined surgery between 2000 and 2006.

Interventions.—Tracheal extubation occurred, based on history and intraoperative events, either immediately in the operating room or in the intensive care unit.

Measurements and Main Results.—Of 3,317 patients in the institutions' Society of Thoracic Surgeons database, 3,089 were extubated within 24 hours, 69% of them in the operating room. Only 0.6% of patients extubated in the operating room required reintubation, compared with 5.9% extubated in the intensive care unit ($p < 0.0001$). By logistic regression, 12 of 25 preoperative and intraoperative factors generated a propensity score for each of the 2,595 patients with complete data, representing the likelihood of immediate extubation (c-statistic = 0.727). A "greedy 5 to 1" propensity score-matching technique created 713 matched pairs of patients by extubation pathway. Those undergoing immediate extubation had reductions in intensive care duration by 23 hours on average (median from 46 to 27 hours, $p < 0.0001$) and in hospital length of stay by 0.8 days on average (median = 6 for each, $p < 0.0001$). Cox regression, using matched pairs as strata, identified the following independent predictors of length of stay in the intensive care unit and hospital: immediate extubation in the operating room, need for reintubation, postoperative renal failure, and postoperative atrial fibrillation.

Conclusions.—Selection of patients for immediate extubation in the operating room by experienced clinicians was associated with shorter ICU and hospital stays. Immediate extubation rarely resulted in tracheal re-intubation.

▶ As shown in this study, healthier patients undergoing cardiac vascular bypass or valvular surgery or those having off-pump procedures are more likely to be immediately extubated in the operating room after surgery if they have a shorter cross-clamp time, have a shorter bypass time, or do not require an intraortic balloon pump. When compared with patients extubated within 24 hours, these patients were less likely to require reintubation or have postoperative bleeding or atrial fibrillation. Not surprisingly, they also had shorter stays in the intensive care unit (ICU) and the hospital.

This leads to the question of whether it was the early extubation, the patient's comorbidities, or the less-complex perioperative course that resulted in the shorter hospital and ICU stay. When examining data from a matched control group, in which the only significant difference was for the patients in the immediate extubation group to have been prior smokers, ICU stays remained significantly shorter in the patients extubated in the operating room.

This work confirms the results of a previous study that found that patients extubated in the operating room do not have a higher reintubation rate.[1] Other factors that increased the length of hospital stay included atrial fibrillation and the use of β-blockers. The development of renal failure increased the duration of a patient's ICU stay. One can easily understand why renal failure or an arrhythmia would cause a patient to require a longer course of medical treatment. What is it, though, about intubation that might prolong a hospital course?

To begin to understand this, we would have to know how being intubated on admission to the ICU caused their perioperative course to be different from those of patients who were not intubated. Any of several factors may contribute to this and would include prolonged sedation, negative impact of mechanical ventilation on hemodynamics, decreased patient mobility, and less aggressive attention on other patient care issues as medical attention was focused on weaning and extubation. Additional work needs to be done in this area, but based on the results of this study, patients who are appropriate candidates for early extubation should be extubated in the operating room. The risk of their requiring of reintubation is not increased by doing so, and ICU and hospital stays will be shorter.

C. Lien, MD

Reference

1. Royse CF, Royse AG, Soeding PF. Routine immediate extubation after cardiac operation: a review of our first 100 patients. *Ann Thorac Surg.* 1999;68:1326-1329.

5 Pediatric Anesthesia

A Comparison of Dexmedetomidine with Propofol for Magnetic Resonance Imaging Sleep Studies in Children

Mahmoud M, Gunter J, Donnelly LF, et al (Cincinnati Children's Hosp Med Center, OH)
Anesth Analg 109:745-753, 2009

Background.—Magnetic resonance imaging (MRI) sleep studies can be used to guide management of children with obstructive sleep apnea (OSA) refractory to conservative therapy. Because children with OSA are sensitive to the respiratory-depressant effects of sedatives and anesthetics, provision of anesthesia for imaging studies in this patient population can be challenging. Dexmedetomidine has been shown to have pharmacological properties simulating natural sleep with minimal respiratory depression. We hypothesized that, compared with propofol, dexmedetomidine would have less effect on upper airway tone and airway collapsibility, provide more favorable conditions during dynamic MRI airway imaging in children with OSA, have fewer scan interruptions, and require less aggressive airway interventions.

Methods.—In this retrospective descriptive study, we reviewed the records of 52 children receiving dexmedetomidine and 30 children receiving propofol for anesthesia during MRI sleep studies between July 2006 and March 2008. Documentation of the severity of OSA by overnight polysomnography was available for 67 of the 82 subjects, who were analyzed separately. Data analyzed included demographics, severity of OSA, comorbidities, hemodynamic changes, use of artificial airways, additional airway maneuvers, and successful completion of the MRI scan.

Results.—Demographics, OSA severity by polysomnography, anesthetic induction, and baseline hemodynamics were comparable in both groups. An interpretable MRI sleep study was obtained for 98% of children in the dexmedetomidine group and 100% in the propofol group. Of 82 children, MRI sleep studies were successfully completed without the use of artificial airways in 46 children (88.5%) in the dexmedetomidine group versus 21 children (70%) in the propofol group ($P = 0.03$). An artificial airway was required to complete the study in five children (12%) in the dexmedetomidine group versus nine children (35%) in the propofol group ($P < 0.06$). Additional airway maneuvers (chin lift and shoulder roll) were required to complete the study in one child (2%) in the dexmedetomidine group and three children (10%) in the propofol group ($P < 0.14$). Children in the dexmedetomidine group experienced reductions in heart rate, whereas those in

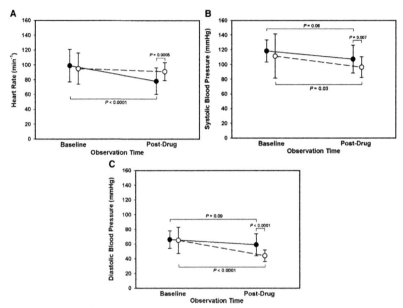

FIGURE 1.—Baseline and postbolus hemodynamics. Closed circles represent dexmedetomidine group and open circles represent propofol group. In the x axis, the first data point is the mean baseline hemodynamic value and the second data point is the mean hemodynamic value after the drug bolus. (A) Comparison of baseline and postdrug heart rates: baseline mean heart rate in beats per minute (bpm) in the dexmedetomidine group (99 ± 22 bpm) and the propofol group (95 ± 21 bpm) were comparable (P = 0.47). Compared with baseline, use of propofol did not change mean heart rate significantly but use of dexmedetomidine decreased mean heart rate (P < 0.0001). Postdrug mean heart rate in the dexmedetomidine group (78 ± 18 bpm) was significantly lower than in the propofol group (91 ± 12 bpm; P < 0.0005). (B) Comparison of baseline and postdrug systolic blood pressures: baseline mean systolic blood pressure in the dexmedetomidine group (118 ± 15 mm Hg) and the propofol group (111 ± 30 mm Hg) was comparable (P = 0.28). Compared with baseline, use of propofol (P = 0.03) decreased mean systolic blood pressure and the reduction after dexmedetomidine was not statistically significant (P = 0.06). Postdrug mean systolic blood pressure in the propofol group (96 ± 14 mm Hg) was significantly lower than the dexmedetomidine group (107 ± 19 mm Hg; P < 0.007). (C) Comparison of baseline and postdrug diastolic blood pressures: baseline mean diastolic blood pressure (in mm Hg) in the dexmedetomidine group (66 ± 12 mm Hg) and the propofol group (65 ± 18 mm Hg) was comparable (P = 0.83). Compared with baseline, use of propofol (P < 0.0001) significantly decreased mean diastolic blood pressure. Postdrug mean diastolic blood pressure in the propofol group (44 ± 8 mm Hg) was significantly lower than the dexmedetomidine group (59 ± 15 mm Hg; P < 0.0001). (Reprinted from Mahmoud M, Gunter J, Donnelly LF, et al. A comparison of dexmedetomidine with propofol for magnetic resonance imaging sleep studies in children. *Anesth Analg.* 2009;109:745-753, with permission from International Anesthesia Research Society.)

the propofol group experienced reductions in arterial blood pressure; these reductions were statistically, but not clinically, significant.

Conclusions.—Dexmedetomidine provided an acceptable level of anesthesia for MRI sleep studies in children with OSA, producing a high yield of interpretable studies of the patient's native airway. The need for artificial airway support during the MRI sleep study was significantly less with dexmedetomidine than with propofol. Dexmedetomidine may be the preferred drug for anesthesia during MRI sleep studies in children with a history of severe OSA and may offer benefits to children with

TABLE 2.—Airway Interventions During MRI Sleep Study

	All Subjects Dexmedetomidine (N = 52)	Propofol (N = 30)	P	Subjects with Polysomnography Study Available Dexmedetomidine (N = 41)	Propofol (N = 26)	P
Artificial airway N (%)			0.03			0.04
None	47 (90)	21 (70)		36 (88)	17 (65)	
Intermittent	5 (10)	9 (30)		5 (12)	9 (35)	
Chin lift or shoulder roll, N (%)	1 (2)	3 (10)	0.14	1 (2)	3 (12)	0.29
Any airway intervention, N (%)	6 (12)	12 (40)	0.005	6 (15)	12 (46)	0.01
Interpretable MRI scan, N (%)	51 (98)	30 (100)	1	40 (98)	26 (100)	1
With native airway, N (%)	46 (88)	21 (70)	0.03	35 (85)	17 (65)	0.06
With artificial airway, N (%)	5 (10)	9 (30)		5 (12)	9 (35)	

Fisher's exact test was used to calculate the P values.
MRI = magnetic resonance imaging.

TABLE 3.—Requirement for Artificial Airway by Severity of OSA as Documented by Polysomnography

OSA severity	Dexmedetomidine	Propofol	P
Mild	N = 16	N = 8	
Obstructive index (events/h)	2.7 ± 1.9	3.1 ± 1.3	0.53*
Respiratory disturbance index (events/h)	3.6 ± 1.9	4.4 ± 1.7	0.30*
Needed artificial airway, N (%)	2 (13)	1 (13)	1[†]
Room air Spo_2 nadir (%)	91 (89, 94)	92 (88, 96)	0.54[‡]
Moderate	N = 11	N = 9	
Obstructive index (events/h)	10.2 ± 5.8	8.8 ± 3.8	0.54*
Respiratory disturbance index (events/h)	11.0 ± 5.8	10.9 ± 4.3	0.96*
Needed artificial airway, N (%)	2 (18)	3 (33)	0.62[†]
Room air Spo_2 nadir (%)	86 (85, 87)	86 (84, 89)	0.91[‡]
Severe	N = 14	N = 9	
Obstructive index (events/h)	21.8 ± 11.3	23.6 ± 13.5	0.74*
Respiratory disturbance index (events/h)	23.8 ± 11.2	24.9 ± 13.1	0.83*
Needed artificial airway, N (%)	1 (7)	5 (56)	0.02[†]
Room air Spo_2 nadir (%)	84 (77, 88)	86 (82, 92)	0.45[‡]

The obstructive index is the number of obstructive apneas per hour of sleep. The respiratory disturbance index is the number of apneas including both central and obstructive components and hypoapneic episodes per hour of sleep. The severity of OSA was defined as follows normal = obstructive index <1; mild OSA = obstructive index 1–5; moderate OSA = obstructive index >5–10; and severe OSA = obstructive index >10. The obstructive index and the respiratory disturbance index values were reported as mean ± SD. Need for artificial airway and successful MRI completions were reported by N (percentages). Room air SpO_2 nadir from preprocedure polysomnography was reported as 50% (25%, 75%) percentiles.
OSA = obstructive sleep apnea; MRI = magnetic resonance imaging.
*Two-sample t-test was used.
[†]Fisher's exact test was used.
[‡]Wilcoxon's rank sum test was used. $P < 0.05$ was considered statistically significant.

sleep-disordered breathing requiring anesthesia or anesthesia for other diagnostic imaging studies (Fig 1, Tables 2 and 3).

▶ This retrospective study of just over 80 children having MRI sleep studies with either propofol or dexmedetomidine sedation identifies advantages to dexmedetomidine in this clinical scenario. In Table 2, rate of successful imaging is shown to be similar with both drugs. However, artificial airways were required more frequently in the patients receiving propofol. In Table 3, it is shown that the advantage to dexmedetomidine is more apparent in children with severe obstructive sleep apnea. There are differences in the hemodynamic effects of the agents as shown in Fig 1, with propofol causing decreases in blood pressure and dexmedetomidine causing heart rate decreases. Neither was clinically significant. Use of dexmedetomidine in children requiring sleep studies may be more efficacious and safer.

S. Black, MD

Cardiovascular Effects of Dexmedetomidine Sedation in Children
Wong J, Steil GM, Curtis M, et al (Children's Hosp Boston and Harvard Med School, MA; Children's Hosp Boston, MA)
Anesth Analg 114:193-199, 2012

Background.—Dexmedetomidine (DEX) affects heart rate (HR), mean arterial blood pressure, cardiac index (CI), stroke index (SI), and systemic vascular resistance index (SVRI) in adults. In this study we sought to determine whether similar effects occur in children undergoing DEX sedation.

Methods.—Hemodynamic changes in children were followed during IV DEX sedation for radiological procedures. One group of 8 patients (DEX-brief) received a bolus (2 mcg/kg bolus over 10 minutes) and completed the procedure within 10 minutes. The second group of 9 patients (DEX-prolong) received the bolus plus additional DEX as needed to maintain sedation for procedures lasting longer than 10 minutes (additional 1 mcg/kg/hr infusion with second bolus if needed). CI, SI, and SVRI were measured using a continuous noninvasive cardiac output monitor. Changes in hemodynamic variables at minutes 10, 20, and discharge (time at which patient achieved Aldrete Score $\geq$9) were compared to baseline by repeated measures ANOVA with effect sizes reported as mean [95% confidence interval].

Results.—Data were obtained during 8 DEX-brief and 9 DEX-prolong procedures. In DEX-brief, HR and CI decreased (18.9 [2.3 to 35.5] bpm and 0.74 [0.15 to 1.33] L/min/m^2; respectively) at T1. There was no change in any other hemodynamic variables and all hemodynamic variables returned to baseline at recovery. In DEX-prolong, both HR and CI remained decreased (24.0 [8.3 to 39.6] bpm, 1.51 [0.95 to 2.06] L/min/m^2; respectively) at recovery. In addition, SI was decreased (8.01 [1.71 to 14.31] mL/m^2) and SVRI was increased (776.0 [271.9 to 1280.4] dynes-sec/cm^5/m^2) at recovery in the DEX-prolong group. There were no significant changes in mean arterial blood pressure in either group.

Conclusion.—DEX decreases CI in children and has a cumulative effect. For patients undergoing prolonged procedures HR and CI remained decreased at the time of discharge together with a decrease in SI and an increase in SVRI (Figs 1 and 2).

▶ In this prospective study, the authors investigated the hemodynamic effects of sedative doses of dexmedetomidine in pediatric patients. Children ranged in age from infants to young school-age children. As in adults, dexmedetomidine caused

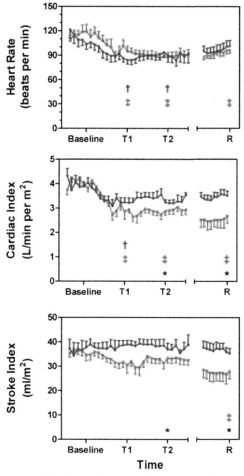

FIGURE 1.—Time course of the effects of dexmedetomidine (DEX) on heart rate (HR; mean ± SEM), cardiac index (CI), and stroke index (SI) in children undergoing brief (DEX-brief; Blue; ≤10 min) and prolonged (DEX-prolong; Red, >10 min) procedures. Time course is in minutes with baseline (BL) defined as minute 0 (start of DEX bolus; 2 mcg/kg over 10 min); T1 defined as minute 10; T2 defined as minute 20 (end of second bolus or 1 mcg/kg/h infusion as needed), and R defined at the time at which discharge criteria was met (varies by patient). Differences from BL are indicted by † (DEX-brief) and ‡ (DEX-prolong); differences between groups by *($P < 0.05$, 2-way repeated measures ANOVA with least significant difference post hoc analysis). For interpretation of the references to color in this figure legend, the reader is referred to web version of this article. (Reprinted from Wong J, Steil GM, Curtis M, et al. Cardiovascular effects of dexmedetomidine sedation in children. *Anesth Analg.* 2012;114:193-199, with permission from International Anesthesia Research Society.)

decreases in heart rate, cardiac index and stroke index and an increase in systemic vascular resistance (Figs 1 and 2). Interestingly, in pediatric patients who received brief exposure (<10 minutes), the only significant change was a decrease in heart rate that returned to baseline at recovery. In children with more prolonged exposure, decreases in heart rate, cardiac index, and stroke index occurred and persisted more than 1 hour after termination of the infusion. These findings are

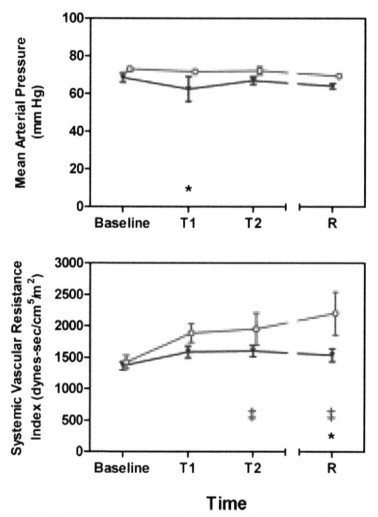

FIGURE 2.—Effects of dexmedetomidine (DEX) on mean arterial blood pressure (MAP; mean ± SEM) and systemic vascular resistance index (SVRI) in the DEX-brief (Blue) and DEX-prolong (Red) groups. Baseline (BL) defined as minute 0 (start of dexmedetomidine bolus; 2 mcg/kg over 10 min); T1 defined as minute 10; T2 defined as minute 20 (end of second bolus or 1 mcg/kg/h infusion as needed), and R defined at the time at which discharge criteria was met (varies by patient). Differences from BL are indicted by † (DEX-brief) and ‡ (DEX-prolong); differences between groups by *($P < 0.05$, 2-way repeated measures ANOVA with least significant difference post hoc analysis). For interpretation of the references to color in this figure legend, the reader is referred to web version of this article. (Reprinted from Wong J, Steil GM, Curtis M, et al. Cardiovascular effects of dexmedetomidine sedation in children. *Anesth Analg.* 2012;114:193-199, with permission from International Anesthesia Research Society.)

similar to those in adults and suggest dexmedetomidine can be used safely for sedation in pediatric patients. Of note, no other sedatives were administered. This should be taken into account when considering using dexmedetomidine in children.

S. Black, MD

Consistency between guidelines and reported practice for reducing the risk of catheter-related infection in British paediatric intensive care units
Harron K, on behalf of the CATCH team (UCL Inst of Child Health, UK)
Intensive Care Med 37:1641-1647, 2011

Purpose.—Optimal strategies for reducing catheter-related blood stream infection (CR-BSI) differ for adults and children. National guidelines do not make child-specific recommendations. We determined whether evidence explained the inconsistencies between guidelines and reported practice in paediatric intensive care units (PICUs).

Methods.—We conducted a survey of eight interventions for reducing CR-BSI in all 25 British PICUs in 2009. Interventions were categorised as requiring child-specific evidence, generalisable to adults and children, or organisational recommendations.

Results.—Twenty-four of the 25 PICUs responded. For child-specific interventions, practice diverged from guidelines for "Insert into subclavian/ jugular veins" (18 PICUs frequently used femoral veins, supported by observational evidence for increased safety in children). Practice reflected guidelines for "Use standard but consider antimicrobial-impregnated central venous catheters (CVCs) for high-risk patients" (14 used standard only, 3 used standard and antimicrobial-impregnated despite no randomised controlled trial (RCT) evidence for antimicrobial-impregnated CVCs in children, 7 used heparin-bonded for some or all children); "Use 2% chlorhexidine for skin preparation" (20 PICUs); "Avoid routine CVC replacement" (20 PICUs). For generalisable interventions, practice was consistent with guidelines for "Administration set replacement" (21 PICUs) but deviated for "Maintenance of CVC asepsis" (11 PICUs used alcohol due to inconclusive

---

TABLE 1.—Guidelines and Categorisation for Eight Interventions

Intervention	Guideline [13, 14]	Categorisation
1 Insertion site	Use subclavian or internal jugular veins—avoid femoral	Child-specific
2 Type of CVC	Use standard CVC but consider antimicrobial impregnated catheter if duration 1 to 3 weeks or risk of CR-BSI high	Child-specific
3 Skin preparation	Use 2% chlorhexidine gluconate in 70% isopropyl alcohol and allow to dry	Child-specific
4 Avoid routine catheter replacement	Check if still required daily	Child-specific
5 Administration set replacement	Replace administration set following total parenteral nutrition—after 24 h (72 h if no lipid). With other fluid sets—replace after a maximum of 72 h	Generalisable
6 Maintenance of CVC asepsis	Use aseptic technique and swab ports or hub with 2% chlorhexidine gluconate in 70% isopropyl alcohol prior to accessing the line for administering fluids or injections	Generalisable
7 Training in CVC care	Healthcare workers caring for a patient with a central venous access device should be trained and assessed	Organisational
8 Monitor BSI rates	Monitor BSI rates to identify lapses in infection-control practices	Organisational

Editor's Note: Please refer to original journal article for full references.

TABLE 2.—Evidence, Reported Practice and Guidelines Relating to Interventions

	Reported Practice	Evidence	Consistency	
Clinical interventions requiring child-specific evidence				
1. Insertion site	In emergency patients, the femoral site was used more than 50% of the time in 18/21 PICUs. In post-operative patients, the internal jugular site was used more than 50% of the time in 12/20 PICUs	Systematic reviews found no RCTs comparing subclavian, jugular and femoral sites for CRBSI or venous thrombosis in children (one RCT favoured the subclavian site compared with the femoral for adults) [19–21]. In children, observational studies suggest a similar risk of infection with femoral and nonfemoral catheters, increased safety with femoral insertion sites compared with subclavian or jugular sites and greater ease of insertion in emergency situations [22–24]	**Evidence:** RCT evidence of benefit for adults, weak observational evidence of harm for children. **Guideline:** Does not follow best available evidence for children. **Practice:** Majority (18/21) of PICUs were consistent with best available evidence but inconsistent with guidelines	+
2. Type of CVC	Standard CVCs were used for all patients in 14/24 PICUs. A further 3/24 PICUs used standard and antibiotic-impregnated CVCs. Heparin-bonded CVCs were used for all patients in 3/24 PICUs. A further 4/24 PICUs used standard and heparin-bonded CVCs	Systematic reviews of RCTs show antibiotic-impregnated CVCs significantly reduce CRBSI in adults, but there are no RCTs of antibiotic-impregnated CVCs in children [25]. RCTs and cost-effectiveness studies have shown large benefits of heparin-bonded CVCs regardless of risk status [25]	**Evidence:** Strong RCT evidence of benefit for antibiotic-impregnated CVCs in adults but a lack of evidence for children. Strong RCT evidence of benefit for heparin-bonded CVCs in children. **Guideline:** Does not follow best evidence for children. **Practice:** Majority of PICUs (17/24) were consistent with guidelines. 3/24 PICUs consistent with best available evidence contrary to the guidelines	↘
3. Skin preparation	19 and 20/24 responders in emergency and postoperative admissions respectively used 2% chlorhexidine to clean the skin prior to CVC insertion. Practice for neonates was not separately recorded	A meta-analysis of RCTs indicated that use of chlorhexidine reduced the risk of CR-BSI by an estimated 49% for short-term catheterisation compared with povidone–iodine [26, 27]. Evidence for paediatric patients is lacking [28].	**Evidence:** Strong RCT evidence of benefit for adults, weak RCT evidence of benefit for children and observational evidence of harm for preterm and very low birth weight babies. **Guideline:** Follows best evidence for adults and children, but does not address harms for neonates	↘

4. Avoid routine replacement	CVCs were not routinely replaced after 7 days by 20/24 PICUs unless under special circumstances. CVCs were routinely replaced after 7 days in 4/24 PICUs. Only 12/24 responders reported a system for daily recording of the need for CVC	One RCT in neonates found chlorhexidine gluconate more effective than povidone–iodine in reducing CVC tip colonization in neonatal intensive care units (NICUs), and an observational study found chlorhexidine to be more effective than povidone–iodine in children on long-term haemodialysis [29, 30]. Cases of skin irritation have been reported with 2% chlorhexidine for preterm and very low birth weight neonates [31, 32]	**Practice:** Majority of PICUs (20/24) were consistent with guidelines and best available evidence. Consistency with evidence is unknown for neonates ✓
		Systematic reviews of RCTs show no benefit of routine replacement of CVCs to reduce infection in children or adults [33, 34]	**Evidence:** Strong RCT evidence of no benefit of routine replacement for adults or children. **Guideline:** Follows best evidence for adults and children. **Practice:** Majority of PICUs (20/24) were consistent with evidence and guidelines ✓
Clinical interventions generalisable to adults and children			
5. Administration set replacement	Administration sets for total parenteral nutrition were reported to be changed every 24 h by almost all (21/24) responders, every 48 h by 1/24, every 72 h by 1/24, and routinely less often than 72 h by 1/24. Administration sets for fluids and medications were reported to be changed every 24 h by 20/24 responders, every 48 h by 1/24 and every 72 h by 3/24	A Cochrane review found that administration sets that do not contain lipids, blood or blood products may be left in place for up to 96 h, and administration sets which contain lipids should be changed every 24 h, with no differences between children and adults [35]	**Evidence:** Strong RCT evidence of benefit. **Guideline:** Follows best available evidence. **Practice:** Majority of PICUs (21/24) were consistent with evidence and guidelines. ✓
6. Maintenance of CVC asepsis	12/24 PICUs used 2% chlorhexidine in alcohol to clean hubs prior to CVC access; 1 PICU used 0.5% chlorhexidine; 11 used alcohol	Guidelines are based on one RCT in adults that found needle-less connectors disinfected with alcohol had significantly higher rates of contamination compared with those disinfected with chlorhexidine/alcohol or povidone–iodine (69.2, 30.8 and 41.6% respectively) [36]	**Evidence:** Inconclusive evidence of benefit. **Guideline:** Based on inconclusive evidence. **Practice:** Half (12/24) of the PICUs were consistent with guidelines ✗

(Continued)

Table 2.—(*Continued*)

	Reported Practice	Evidence	Consistency
Organisational interventions			
7. Training in CVC care	A small proportion of responders held specific training sessions on CVC insertion for doctors (9 and 7/24 responders for emergency and post-operative admissions respectively), whilst 22/23 responders had dedicated training sessions on CVC care for nurses	The effectiveness of training in insertion and maintenance of CVCs for reducing complications relating to CVCs has been well documented through observational studies. Before-after studies have shown systematic interventions of education in combination with care bundles reduced infection rates by 23–37% in paediatric settings [9, 37]	**Evidence:** Strong observational evidence for benefit X **Guideline:** Follows best available evidence **Practice:** Less than half (9/24) of the PICUs were consistent with available evidence and guidelines for doctors; the majority (22/24) were consistent for nurses
8. Monitoring BSI	Six PICUs monitored BSI rates by catheter-day (ranging from 0 to 6.3 per 1,000 catheter-days) and a further 2 PICUs monitored BSI per patient (0.5–11.8% of patients). There was no routine recording of BSI rates in the remaining 16/24 PICUs. Nine responders stated that rates had remained the same over the past 2 years; 13 thought rates had decreased; the remaining 2 did not know	Guidelines are based on the National Nosocomial Infections Surveillance (NNIS) at the Centers for Disease Control and Prevention (CDC) [38]. This system has shown substantial improvements in infection control within NNIS hospitals. Surveillance systems have been shown to improve quality of care and to be critical for assessing effectiveness of interventions, although they have also been associated with higher rates of BSI in PICUs [39–42]	**Evidence:** Inconclusive observational evidence for benefit X **Guideline:** Follows best available evidence **Practice:** Majority (16/24) of PICUs were inconsistent with best available evidence and guidelines

Editor's Note: Please refer to original journal article for full references.

┌ reported practice consistent with guidelines.
x reported practice diverged from guidelines.
† reported practice diverged from guidelines but consistent with best available evidence.

evidence for chlorhexidine). Practice diverged from guidelines for organisational interventions: "Train healthcare workers in CVC care" (9 PICUs); "Monitor blood stream infection (BSI) rates" (8 PICUs).

Conclusions.—Guidelines should explicitly address paediatric practice and report the quality of evidence and strength of recommendations. Organisations should ensure doctors are trained in CVC insertion and invest in BSI monitoring, especially in PICUs. The type of CVC and insertion site are important gaps in evidence for children (Tables 1 and 2).

▶ In this survey of 25 pediatric intensive care units in Great Britain, the authors investigate compliance with guidelines for central line placement and maintenance. They divided the guidelines into those in which the best evidence for pediatric patients was consistent with the general recommendations generated for adult patients and those in which the best evidence for pediatrics was not supportive of the general guidelines (Table 1). In particular, for site of placement and type of placement, the practice consistently deviated from the general guidelines but was consistent with best evidence in pediatric patients. For maintenance guidelines in which best evidence in pediatric patients is consistent with general guidelines, most pediatric intensive care units consistently followed guidelines. However, guidelines related to institutional activities in which best evidence for pediatric patients was consistent with the general guidelines, there was substantial noncompliance (Table 2). Development of pediatric-specific guidelines and improved institutional support would be helpful in further decreasing central line—related infections.

S. Black, MD

Dexmedetomidine in Children: Current Knowledge and Future Applications
Mason KP, Lerman J (Children's Hosp Boston, MA; Univ of Rochester, NY)
Anesth Analg 113:1129-1142, 2011

More than 200 studies and reports have been published regarding the use of dexmedetomidine in infants and children. We reviewed the English literature to summarize the current state of knowledge of this drug in children for the practicing anesthesiologist. Dexmedetomidine is an effective sedative for infants and children that only minimally depresses the respiratory system while maintaining a patent airway. However, dexmedetomidine does depress the cardiovascular system. Specifically, bradycardia, hypotension, and hypertension occur to varying degrees depending on the age of the child. Hypertension is more prevalent when larger doses of dexmedetomidine are given to infants. Consistent with its 2-hour elimination half-life, recovery after dexmedetomidine may be protracted in comparison with other sedatives. Dexmedetomidine provides and augments analgesia and diminishes shivering as well as agitation postoperatively. The safety record of dexmedetomidine suggests that it can be

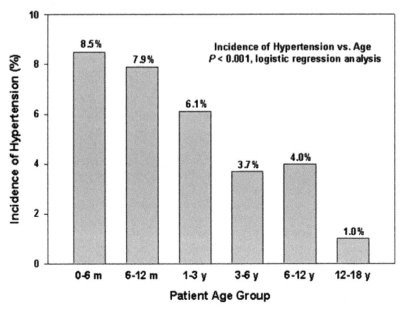

FIGURE 4.—Three-thousand five-hundred twenty-two children received dexmedetomidine per protocol: initial bolus of 3 μg/kg dexmedetomidine over 10 minutes, followed by a continuous infusion of 2 μg/kg/h to maintain a Ramsay Sedation Score (RSS) of 4. If at any point during the sedation, the child failed to achieve or maintain RSS 4, this bolus could be repeated up to 2 more times. The most frequent incidence of hypertension occurred in children <1 year of age who received more than 1 bolus (P < 0.001). From Mason,[53] publisher permission obtained. *Editor's Note*: Please refer to original journal article for full references. (Reprinted from Mason KP, Lerman J. Dexmedetomidine in children: current knowledge and future applications. *Anesth Analg.* 2011;113:1129-1142, with permission from International Anesthesia Research Society.)

used effectively and safely in children, with appropriate monitoring and interventions to manage cardiovascular sequelae (Fig 4).

▶ This excellent review article thoroughly covers use of dexmedetomidine in children, in the operating room, preoperatively, postoperatively, in the intensive care units, and for procedures outside the operating room. As dexmedetomidine gains in popularity and use, this is an important resource to the anesthesiologist. As in adults, dexmedetomidine is a safe and effective agent for sedation or as an adjunct to general anesthesia. The article points out some unique effects in children, such as hypertension in young children (Fig 4), especially with the use of glycopyrrolate for bradycardia and hypothermia in infants.

S. Black, MD

Early Childhood Exposure to Anesthesia and Risk of Developmental and Behavioral Disorders in a Sibling Birth Cohort

DiMaggio C, Sun LS, Li G (Columbia Univ, NY)

Anesth Analg 113:1143-1151, 2011

Background.—In vitro and in vivo studies of anesthetics have demonstrated serious neurotoxic effects on the developing brain. However, the clinical relevance of these findings to children undergoing anesthesia remains unclear. Using data from a sibling birth cohort, we assessed the association between exposure to anesthesia in the setting of surgery in patients younger than 3 years and the risk of developmental and behavioral disorders.

Methods.—We constructed a retrospective cohort of 10,450 siblings who were born between 1999 and 2005 and who were enrolled in the New York State Medicaid program. The exposed group was 304 children without a history of developmental or behavioral disorders who underwent surgery when they were younger than 3 years. The unexposed group was 10,146 children who did not receive any surgical procedures when they were younger than 3 years. Exposed children were entered into analysis at the date of surgery. Unexposed children were entered into analysis at age 10 months (the mean age at which exposed children underwent surgery). Both exposed and unexposed children were followed until diagnosis with a developmental or behavioral disorder, loss to follow-up, or the end of 2005. The association of exposure to anesthesia with subsequent developmental and behavioral disorders was assessed with both proportional hazards modeling, and pair-matched analysis.

Results.—The incidence of developmental and behavioral disorders was 128.2 diagnoses per 1000 person-years for the exposed cohort and 56.3 diagnoses per 1000 person-years for the unexposed cohort. With adjustment for sex and history of birth-related medical complications, and clustering by sibling status, the estimated hazard ratio of developmental or behavioral disorders associated with any exposure to anesthesia when they were younger than 3 years was 1.6 (95% confidence interval [CI]: 1.4, 1.8). The risk increased from 1.1 (95% CI: 0.8, 1.4) for 1 operation to 2.9 (94% CI: 2.5, 3.1) for 2 operations and 4.0 (95% CI: 3.5, 4.5) for $\geq$3 operations. The relative risk in a matched analysis of 138 sibling pairs was 0.9 (95% CI: 0.6, 1.4).

Conclusion.—The risk of being subsequently diagnosed with developmental and behavioral disorders in children who were enrolled in a state Medicaid program and who had surgery when they were younger than 3 years was 60% greater than that of a similar group of siblings who did not undergo surgery. More tightly matched pairwise analyses indicate that the extent to which the excess risk is causally attributable to anesthesia or mediated by unmeasured factors remains to be determined (Tables 2 and 3).

▶ This large retrospective study using the Medicaid database sheds light on the question of relationship between anesthetic exposure before age 3 and risk of

TABLE 2.—Frequency and Proportion of Behavioral/ Developmental Diagnoses Among 304 Children Exposed to Surgery/Anesthesia with No History of Behavioral/Developmental Diagnoses Versus 10,982 Unexposed Children Followed from Age 10 Months

Diagnosis	Exposed	Unexposed
Development delay	62 (82.7%)	692 (77.2%)
Language disorder	5 (6.7%)	127 (14.2%)
Attention deficit	4 (5.3%)	30 (3.3%)
Coordination disorder	1 (1.3%)	14 (1.6%)
Conduct disorder	1 (1.3%)	20 (2.2%)
Other[a]	2 (2.7%)	13 (1.5%)
Total	75 (100%)	896 (100%)

Data based on New York State Medicaid Analytic Extract Files, 1999–2005.

TABLE 3.—Hazard Ratios and 95% Confidence Intervals of Behavioral/Developmental Outcomes in Children Exposed to Surgery/Anesthesia Before Age 3 Years, Adjusted for Clustering by Sibling Status

	Hazard Ratio (95% CI)
No. of operations at <3 y of age	
0	1
1	1.1 (0.8, 1.4)
2	2.8 (2.5, 3.1)
≥3	4.0 (3.5, 4.5)
History of complication at birth	
No	1
Yes	1.5 (1.3, 1.6)
Gender	
Female	1
Male	1.4 (1.3, 1.5)

Based on New York State Medicaid Data, 1999–2005.

developmental or behavioral disorders. Comparing children exposed to anesthetics (although no data were available as to type of anesthetic or duration of exposure) with matched children with no exposure, developmental or behavioral disorders occurred in almost 25% of children who underwent anesthetic and surgical procedure compared with only just less than 9% in unexposed children (Table 2). These results cannot separate the risk associated with surgery or the underlying disease from that associated with the anesthetic. A number of other observations are important to consider (Table 3). First, exposure to a single anesthetic and surgical procedure was not associated with increased risk. Second, investigation of twin siblings, which would control for differences in genetic predisposition and effects of environment, shows no increased risk with exposure to surgery and anesthesia. This study does not answer the question of neurotoxicity from general anesthetics in infants and young children but does support the current recommendations that indicated surgery should not be delayed in infants and young children.

S. Black, MD

FDA Considers Data on Potential Risks of Anesthesia Use in Infants, Children
Kuehn BM
JAMA 305:1749-1750, 2011

Background.—The Food and Drug Administration (FDA) has voiced concern over whether anesthesia may harm infants or young children, producing later developmental or emotional problems. Much of the evidence comes from animal studies and suggests that developing brains may be damaged by anesthetic agents, causing lasting behavioral and cognitive deficits. Clinical studies suggest that later cognitive deficits may develop after pediatric patients are exposed to anesthetics under some conditions, but not others. However, no conclusive evidence links exposure to anesthesia or sedative drugs to neurotoxicity or neurodevelopmental abnormalities. Without such evidence, the FDA panel meeting has concluded that it is unethical to have a child undergo a fear-producing or painful procedure without sedation.

Animal Studies.—When animals are exposed to anesthetics during critical stages of brain development, they experience widespread brain cell death, with resulting long-term effects on behavior, cognition, or both. No specific anesthetic agent or regimen has been proven safer than others. However, it is difficult to translate the window of vulnerability from rats to humans because rat brains develop over a relatively short time compared to human brain patterns. When young primates are tested, however, the results were similar to those found with rats. Studies indicate it is likely there are doses and levels that can be used without risking adverse effects. A study involving the exposure of fetal and neonatal rhesus monkeys to isoflurane, ketamine, or propofol indicated that ketamine was most toxic for fetuses, isoflurane was more toxic for neonates, and propofol had the least toxicity. Neurotoxicity has also varied depending on the effects of other drugs, such as caffeine. Many factors can complicate the outcomes of studies on the effects of anesthesia. The neurologic changes that result from exposure to anesthesia early in life can have lasting effects on cognition and behavior. Studies of rhesus monkeys have shown that ketamine exposure can alter the motivation and capacity to work for food and the ability to perform cognitive tasks. These results were permanent.

Clinical Results.—Concerns with these primate models have not been well-supported by clinical evidence. The evidence base has been too limited to provide conclusive findings. Some studies also produce conflicting results. For example, a study of 1143 twin pairs found that a twin exposed to anesthesia before age 3 years had more cognitive problems and worse school performance than a twin not exposed, but within twin pairs discordant for anesthesia exposure, educational and cognitive outcomes were similar. The anesthesia may not be causing the problem; vulnerability for such difficulties may predate the exposure. Some studies show brief perinatal exposure does not affect developmental progression. Others find learning disabilities are more likely with multiple exposures, with no difference between children with a single early anesthesia exposure or no exposure. Associations have also been found between multiple anesthesia exposures and learning disabilities but not with emotional and behavioral disorders.

Conclusions.—Ongoing studies may help to clarify the situation and provide more definitive answers. Currently the evidence for anesthesia neurotoxicity is not conclusive enough to support warning parents about the potential risk.

▶ This article reviews, although briefly, clinical and laboratory research related to neurotoxicity of anesthetic agents administered to neonates, infants, and children less than 3 years of age. While the animal evidence indicates neuronal injury and neural developmental abnormalities, many of the studies utilize very long exposure in very young animals. Generalizing these results to short single procedures in patients would clearly be premature. Clinical evidence is varied, with some showing cognitive and behavioral problems in children who required anesthetics compared with those who did not, while others fail to do so. Perhaps the most consistent data to date are those that show that children who require multiple procedures under anesthesia have an increased risk of cognitive, developmental, or behavioral abnormalities. This could be due to the surgical stress, underlying pathology, or psychosocial factors related to repeated illnesses and surgeries. Ongoing animal and clinical research will add further data. However, it is important to counsel parents regarding this issue carefully. Delaying necessary procedures or inappropriately limiting the use of general anesthesia for procedures is likely to do more harm than good.

S. Black, MD

Neurotoxicity of Anesthetic Drugs in the Developing Brain
Stratmann G (Univ of California San Francisco)
Anesth Analg 113:1170-1179, 2011

Anesthesia kills neurons in the brain of infantile animals, including primates, and causes permanent and progressive neurocognitive decline. The anesthesia community and regulatory authorities alike are concerned that is also true in humans. In this review, I summarize what we currently know about the risks of pediatric anesthesia to long-term cognitive function. If anesthesia is discovered to cause cognitive decline in humans, we need to know how to prevent and treat it. Prevention requires knowledge of the mechanisms of anesthesia-induced cognitive decline. This review gives an overview of some of the mechanisms that have been proposed for anesthesia-induced cognitive decline and discusses possible treatment options. If anesthesia induces cognitive decline in humans, we need to know what type and duration of anesthetic is safe, and which, if any, is not safe. This review discusses early results of comparative animal studies of anesthetic neurotoxicity. Until we know if and how pediatric anesthesia affects cognition in humans, a change in anesthetic practice would be premature, not guided by evidence of better alternatives, and therefore potentially dangerous. The SmartTots initiative jointly supported by the International Anesthesia Research Society and the Food and Drug Administration aims to fund research designed to shed light on these issues that are of high priority to the anesthesia community and the public alike and therefore deserves the full support of these interest groups.

▶ This excellent review article is important for all anesthesiologists, especially those who anesthetize children. With increasing awareness in the press of the potential for neurotoxicity of anesthetics in the developing brain, it will become an increasing concern for our patients and pediatric patients' parents. This article nicely reviews the human data, concluding that there is no consistent clinical evidence that exposure to anesthetics in children causes cognitive abnormalities. In particular, there appears to be relatively consistent evidence that at least a single anesthetic administered not longer than an hour or 2 is not associated with evidence of neural injury. On the other hand, animal data are consistent that anesthetics administered to young animals of many species cause neurodegeneration. The authors argue that at this time it is important to focus research on the relationship between neurodegeneration and cognitive decline, if it exists, the mechanism of the neural injury, and what can be done to prevent or lessen the effect. Likewise, they argue that there is no support for changing current practice, as there is no clear evidence of human cognitive decline related to exposure to anesthetics at a young age, and there is no identified safe alternative. The SmartTots joint initiative (International Anesthesia Research Society and the US Food and Drug Administration) is an example of physicians leading the way to improve patient safety.

S. Black, MD

Paediatric MRI under sedation: is it necessary? What is the evidence for the alternatives?
Edwards AD, Arthurs OJ (Cambridge Univ Hosps NHS Foundation Trust, UK)
Pediatr Radiol 41:1353-1364, 2011

To achieve diagnostic images during MRI examinations, small children need to lie still to avoid movement artefact. To reduce patient motion, obviate the need for voluntary immobilisation or breath-holding and therefore obtain high-quality images, MRI of infants is frequently carried out under sedation or general anaesthesia, but this is not without risk and expense. However, many other techniques are available for preparing children for MRI, which have not been fully evaluated. Here, we evaluate the advantages and disadvantage of sedation and anaesthesia for MRI. We then evaluate the alternatives, which include neonatal comforting techniques, sleep manipulation, and appropriate adaptation of the physical environment. We summarize the evidence for their use according to an established hierarchy. Lastly, we

TABLE 2.—Summary of Evidence Available for Each Preparation Strategy. A Summary of the Level of Evidence During Imaging Studies is Provided, as Well as Studies Evaluating the Effectiveness in Other Clinical Situations

Preparation	Level Evidence	Imaging Studies	Level Evidence	Non-Imaging Studies
Sedation / general anaesthesia	3	Retrospective study [9, 12, 16, 17, 19, 23, 79]; Prospective study [13, 25]; Opinion [8, 10, 11, 51]	1	Systematic review of sedation during paediatric dentistry [3]; Retrospective study of sedation during PEG insertion / ERCP [4]; Opinion of sedation during emergency department procedures [5]
Pacifiers	—	None available	2	RCT during painful procedure, e.g. venepuncture [26, 36, 37]; RCT during ophthalmology screening [27]; Consensus statement [30]
Sucrose	—	None available	1	Systematic review [29, 31, 34]; DBRCT during painful procedure, e.g. venepuncture [28, 32]; RCT during painful procedure, e.g. venepuncture [28, 36, 37]
Sucrose and pacifier in conjunction	—	None available	2	RCT during painful procedure [26, 36, 37]
Swaddling	5	Anecdotal evidence only	1	RCT during ophthalmology screening [44]; Consensus statement [30]; Systematic review of swaddling during painful procedures [46]; Observation of swaddling during painful procedure [40]; Trial of swaddling for normal sleep [41, 42]; Opinion on swaddling for neonatal abstinence syndrome [43]; Consensus statement [30]
Feed and sleep/wrap	4	Retrospective study during MRI [52]; Opinion / anecdotal evidence [50, 51, 53]	—	None available
Sleep deprivation	4	Retrospective study of sleep deprivation during MRI [55, 56]	5	Sleep deprivation during normal sleep [57]

Intervention				
Melatonin	2	DBRCT melatonin prior to sedation for MRI [61] Observational study with sleep deprivation [59]	5	Opinion [58]
Hypnosis and distraction	2	RCT hypnosis with sedation versus sedation alone [66] Observational study of audio / visual system [82] Observational study of watching DVD during MR scan [54]	1	Systematic review of hypnosis for reducing procedure-related pain [64] Systematic review of hypnosis during anaesthetic induction [63] RCT of guided imagery for progressive muscle relaxation [69]
Physical environment	5	Retrospective study of physical environment [72]	—	Anecdotal evidence only
Play therapy	3	RCT of photo book [77] Retrospective study [71] Observational study [22]	1	Meta-analysis of play therapy [73] Prospective study [74, 75] Opinion [76] None available
Practice MRI	4	Observational study of short training session [78] Observational study of MRI habituation [54] Retrospective study of mock scanner [78, 79]	—	
Parental involvement	5	RCT of photo book with parental involvement [77]	—	Anecdotal evidence only

Editor's Note: Please refer to original journal article for full references.

discuss several factors that will influence the choice of imaging preparation, including patient factors, imaging factors and service provision. The choice of approach to paediatric MRI is multi-factorial, with limited scientific evidence for many of the current approaches. These considerations may enable others to image children using MRI under different circumstances (Table 2).

▶ In this review article, options for management of pediatric patients during magnetic resonance imaging (MRI) are evaluated. The authors' review reports of sedation, general anesthesia, and alternative techniques for MRI as well as in other procedures, some painful (Table 2). While it is imperative to facilitate obtaining good-quality images, ability to avoid the use of sedative and anesthetic drugs in children would have many benefits. These include decreased cost in terms of drugs but also in terms of hospital stay and manpower costs related to prolonged recovery time with the use of sedation and general anesthesia. In addition, sedation and general anesthesia are associated with a small risk of immediate morbidity. Finally, increasing concern about the impact of general anesthesia in children under 3 on long-term cognitive and behavioral development emphasizes the importance of reserving this technique for situations in which it is truly indicated. Low-risk techniques, such as swaddling, pacifiers, preparation with play therapy, environmental manipulation (eg, lighting, distraction) may have a place. Sleep manipulation with sleep deprivation or melatonin may be beneficial used independently but may delay discharge when combined with sedation. Ideally, age-specific protocols could be developed for each institution regarding best alternative techniques, their use, and indications.

S. Black, MD

Simulation-based Assessment of Pediatric Anesthesia Skills

Fehr JJ, Boulet JR, Waldrop WB, et al (Washington Univ School of Medicine, St Louis, MO; Foundation for Advancement of International Med Education and Res, Philadelphia, PA)
Anesthesiology 115:1308-1315, 2011

Background.—Assessment of pediatric anesthesia trainees is complicated by the random nature of adverse patient events and the vagaries of clinical exposure. However, assessment is critical to improve patient safety. In previous studies, a multiple scenario assessment provided reliable and valid measures of the abilities of anesthesia residents. The purpose of this study was to develop a set of relevant simulated pediatric perioperative scenarios and to determine their effectiveness in the assessment of anesthesia residents and pediatric anesthesia fellows.

Methods.—Ten simulation scenarios were designed to reflect situations encountered in perioperative pediatric anesthesia care. Anesthesiology residents and fellows consented to participate and were debriefed after each scenario. Two pediatric anesthesiologists scored each scenario by

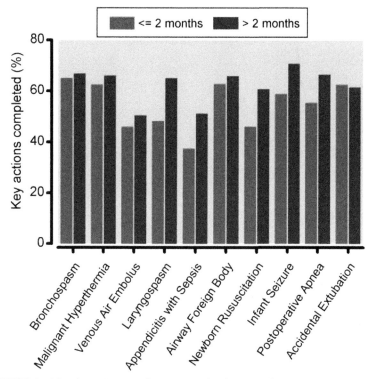

FIGURE 1.—Mean key action scores by scenario and pediatric anesthesia experience. The total key action scores out of 100% for the simulation scenarios for each group of trainees with either less (*red bars*) or more (*blue bars*) than 2 months of pediatric anesthesia training. For interpretation of the references to color in this figure legend, the reader is referred to web version of this article. (Reprinted from Fehr JJ, Boulet JR, Waldrop WB, et al. Simulation-based assessment of pediatric anesthesia skills. *Anesthesiology*. 2011;115:1308-1315, with permission from the American Society of Anesthesiologists, Inc.)

key action checklist. The psychometric properties (reliability, validity) of the scores were studied.

Results.—Thirty-five anesthesiology residents and pediatric anesthesia fellows participated. The participants with greater experience administering pediatric anesthetics generally outperformed those with less experience. Score variance attributable to raters was low, yielding a high interrater reliability.

Conclusions.—A multiple-scenario, simulation-based assessment of pediatric perioperative care was designed and administered to residents and fellows. The scores obtained from the assessment indicated the content was relevant and that raters could reliably score the scenarios. Participants with more training achieved higher scores, but there was a wide range of ability among subjects. This method has the potential to contribute to pediatric anesthesia performance assessment, but additional measures of validity

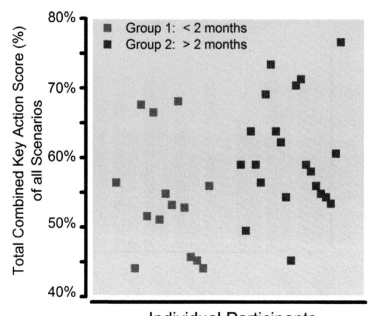

FIGURE 2.—Total key action score by participant. The total key action scores achieved by each trainee with either less (*red squares*) or more (*blue squares*) than 2 months of pediatric anesthesia training. Each point represents a specific trainee's percent overall score. The scores are scattered to highlight both the overlap and the score variation that occurs among individuals within and between groups. For interpretation of the references to color in this figure legend, the reader is referred to web version of this article. (Reprinted from Fehr JJ, Boulet JR, Waldrop WB, et al. Simulation-based assessment of pediatric anesthesia skills. *Anesthesiology.* 2011;115:1308-1315, with permission from the American Society of Anesthesiologists, Inc.)

including correlations with more direct measures of clinical performance are needed to establish the utility of this approach (Figs 1 and 2, Table 1).

▶ The authors investigate the use of simulation to access skills in pediatric anesthesiology among anesthesiology residents and pediatric anesthesiology fellows. The majority of scenarios chosen are those that an anesthesiologist might face in a general practice (Table 1). The results are interesting on several fronts. After 2 months of experience in pediatrics, additional experience in pediatrics did not result in significant improvement in performance on the scenarios (Fig 1). As the authors point out, if more complex cases were included as would be seen in a pediatric hospital, a difference in performance with increasing experience beyond the 2 months might well be apparent. Nonetheless, the study is reassuring that the current training requirements for pediatric experience during anesthesiology core training are appropriate. Secondly, the results validate what has long been observed, acquisition of skills proceeds at varying rates among trainees. Some people are better with less than 2 months of experience in pediatrics than other trainees with more experience (Fig 2). Finally, it supports the use of simulation as 1 potential tool in maintenance of certification.

S. Black, MD

TABLE 1.—Pediatric Anesthesia Simulation Scenarios

Scenario	Scenario Descriptor	Scoring Items
Bronchospasm	5-yr-old, 20-kg child with asthma is wheezing after extremity fracture repair	Administer oxygen, auscultate lungs, review past medical history, inquire about intraoperative events, recognize wheezing, administer albuterol, confirm chest x-ray has been done, communicate with surgeons
Malignant hyperthermia	During inguinal hernia repair in a 6-yr-old, 20-kg child, MH occurs with elevated carbon dioxide, tachycardia	Give 100% oxygen, state diagnosis, discontinue volatile anesthetic, hyperventilate, call for malignant hyperthermia cart, administer dantrolene, administer bicarbonate, cool patient, order laboratory studies, call for ICU bed
Venous air embolus	Intraoperative resection of a Wilms tumor in a 6-yr-old, 20-kg child, complicated by sudden desaturation and decrease in end-tidal carbon dioxide	Recognize decreased end-tidal carbon dioxide, administer 100% oxygen, state diagnosis, notify surgeon, ask surgeon to flood surgical field, position patient in left lateral decubitus position, bolus fluid, administer epinephrine, arrange for ICU bed
Laryngospasm	At the beginning of strabismus surgery with a laryngeal mask airway in place, a 5-yr-old, 20-kg child loses end-tidal carbon dioxide	Auscultate in <60 s, administer 100% oxygen, remove laryngeal mask airway, attempt bag-mask ventilation, call for help, deepen anesthetic, administer muscle relaxant, intubate patient, confirm end-tidal carbon dioxide, auscultate bilateral breath sounds
Appendicitis with sepsis	A 7-yr-old, 30-kg child with appendicitis is ill, appearing with heart rate 136, respiratory rate 38, and blood pressure 72/48	Check laboratory results, inquire about pain, check blood pressure before induction, bolus fluid, state diagnosis of possible sepsis, prepare suction, preoxygenate, rapid sequence induction with cricoid, decrease dose of induction agent, confirm end-tidal carbon dioxide
Airway foreign body	A 4-yr-old, 15-kg child preoperative for myringotomy tubes has a cough. Nurse is concerned. Mannequin with unilateral breath sounds and not on monitor	Ask for vital signs, administer oxygen, obtain past medical history, obtain history of cough, auscultate chest, obtain chest x-ray, state diagnosis, consult otolaryngology, plan for induction with maintenance of spontaneous respiration
Newborn resuscitation	Resuscitation of 2-kg newborn who was born less than 1 min ago: no respiratory effort, decreased tone, heart rate <60, and poor perfusion. The special care nurse and pediatrician have not yet arrived	Dry patient, stimulate and warm baby, suction mouth, begin bag-mask ventilation, call for help, start chest compressions for heart rate <60 after 30 s, intubate, request umbilical venous line, request bed in the NICU
Infant seizure	Called to evaluate 7-wk-old, 4.8-kg infant found seizing on the general pediatrics ward	Recognize seizure, give oxygen, place intraosseous needle when can't get an intravenous line, give anticonvulsant, recognize apnea, bag-mask ventilation, call for help, intubate patient, check glucose and electrolytes, request ICU bed
Postoperative apnea	2-month-old, 2.8-kg former 32-week premature infant having apnea and bradycardia in PACU after cleft lip repair; had been given an excessive dose of narcotic	Inquire about neonatal history, inquire about intraoperative course, recognize desaturation, apply oxygen, recognize apnea, inquire about narcotic dose, administer naloxone or intubates, consider caffeine, arrange monitored bed and/or alerts surgeon
Accidental extubation	3-month-old, 5-kg infant is brought to the ICU after colostomy takedown has accidental extubation	Recognize desaturation, auscultate and/or check endotracheal tube position, remove endotracheal tube if SpO$_2$<90%, recognize tube out before SpO$_2$<80%, bag-mask ventilate, call for help, reintubate, verify bilateral breath sounds, request end-tidal carbon dioxide confirmation

ICU = intensive care unit; MH = malignant hyperthermia; NICU = neonatal intensive care unit; PACU = postanesthesia care unit.

6 Head Injury and Neuroanesthesia

A Comparison of Three Types of Postoperative Pain Control After Posterior Lumbar Spinal Surgery

Wu M-H, Wong C-H, Niu C-C, et al (Chang Gung Memorial Hosp at Chiayi, Taiwan; Chang Gung Memorial Hosp at Linkou, Taoyuan, Taiwan)
Spine 36:2224-2231, 2011

Study Design.—Retrospective, nonrandomized, comparative study.

Objective.—This study compared the early postoperative analgesic effects and the postoperative nausea and vomiting (PONV) associated with three methods of pain control after posterior lumbar spinal surgery.

Summary of Background Data.—The use of opioids for postoperative pain control is common after spinal surgery; however, PONV is the most frequently encountered side effect, and it is yet to be overcome. The effectiveness of the use of an absorbable low-dose morphine-soaked microfibrillar collagen hemostatic sponge placed on the surface of the dural sac (epidural MMCHS) was compared to patient-controlled analgesia (PCA) and intermittent intramuscular bolus injection of meperidine for postoperative pain control after spine surgery.

Methods.—One hundred sixty-five patients who underwent short-segment posterior lumbar spinal decompression and fusion surgery between January 2007 and July 2007 in the orthopedic department of a medical center were enrolled. For postoperative pain control, 40 patients received epidural MMCHS, 48 patients received PCA, and 77 patients received meperidine injection. Patient ratings of pain intensity (visual analog scale score from 0 [no pain] to 10 [most severe pain]), nausea (from 0 [no nausea] to 5 [severe nausea]), and vomiting (from 0 [no vomiting] to 5 [severe vomiting]) were recorded at 4 hours postoperation and on postoperative days 1, 2, and 3.

Results.—The analgesic effect was enhanced significantly in both epidural MMCHS group and the PCA group as compared with the meperidine group on postoperative days 1 and 2 ($P < 0.05$). On postoperative days 1, 2, and 3, PONV was more severe in the PCA group than in the other two groups ($P < 0.05$). The side effects of epidural MMCHS were nausea (25%), pruritus (12.5%), vomiting (5%), and hypotension (2.5%).

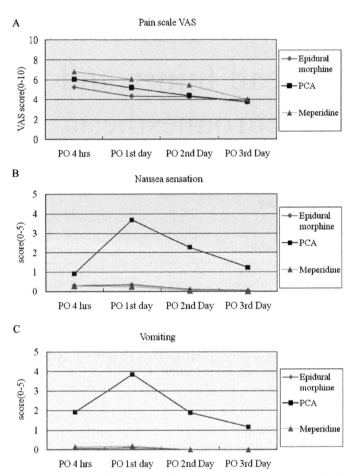

FIGURE 3.—(**A**) The scoring of pain intensity showed better postoperative pain control in the epidural MMCHS group and in the PCA group at 4 hours postoperation, and on postoperative days 1 and 2. (**B**) Nausea was significantly higher in the PCA group, peaking on day 1 postoperation. (**C**) Vomiting showed a similar pattern to nausea. (Reprinted from Wu M-H, Wong C-H, Niu C-C, et al. A comparison of three types of postoperative pain control after posterior lumbar spinal surgery. *Spine.* 2011;36:2224-2231, with permission from Lippincott Williams & Wilkins.)

Conclusion.—A single low-dose epidural MMCHS is effective for postoperative pain control and minimizes the occurrence of PONV after posterior lumbar spinal surgery (Fig 3, Table 2).

▶ This retrospective study compares 3 techniques for postoperative pain management after lumbar spine surgery. Not surprisingly, intermittent narcotic administration was less effective than patient-controlled analgesia (PCA) or epidural administration of morphine via a morphine-soaked microfibrillar collagen hemostatic sponge placed on the dura. What is encouraging is the high quality of pain control with a lower incidence of nausea and vomiting

TABLE 2.—Preoperative and Postoperative Pain Rating (Visual Analog Scale)

	Epidural MMCHS (N = 40)	PCA (N = 46)	Meperidine (N = 76)	P	Scheffe
Preoperation	7.03 (1.143)	7.15 (1.154)	7.38 (1.177)	0.257	(1) = (2) = (3)
4 h postoperation	5.25 (1.020)	6.08 (1.671)	6.82 (1.411)	0.008*	(3) > (1) = (2)
1 day postoperation	4.35 (0.875)	5.19 (1.132)	6.05 (1.165)	0.005*	(3) > (2) > (1)
2 days postoperation	4.30 (0.820)	4.38 (0.983)	5.46 (1.371)	0.037*	(3) > (1) = (2)
3 days postoperation	3.75 (1.259)	3.80 (1.296)	4.00 (1.200)	0.310	(1) = (2) = (3)

Graded from 0 to 10 points (0 is no pain, 10 is the most severe pain possible). Data are presented as the mean (standard deviation). The rank of pain rating is listed in the Scheffe.
MMCHS indicates morphine-soaked microfibrillar collagen hemostatic sponge; PCA, patient controlled analgesia.
†P < 0.05.
*P < 0.01.

associated with the epidural morphine in the surgical field compared with PCA morphine (Table 2, Fig 3). Epidural narcotic administered in the field in the form of morphine was used in the past. However, this technique fell into disfavor due to concern over an increased risk of infection.

S. Black, MD

Air elimination capability in rapid infusion systems
Zoremba N, Gruenewald C, Zoremba M, et al (Univ Hosp RWTH Aachen, Germany; Med Ctr Marienhöhe Würselen, Germany; Univ Hosp Marburg, Germany)
Anaesthesia 66:1031-1034, 2011

Pressure infusion devices are used in clinical practice to apply large volumes of fluid over a short period of time. Although air infusion is a major complication, they have limited capability to detect and remove air during pressure infusion. In this investigation, we tested the air elimination capabilities of the Fluido® (The Surgical Company), Level 1® (Level 1 Technologies Inc.) and Ranger® (Augustine Medical GmbH) pressure infusion devices. Measurements were undertaken with a crystalloid solution during an infusion flow of 100, 200, 400 and 800 ml.min^{-1}. Four different volumes of air (25, 50, 100 and 200 ml) were injected as boluses in one experimental setting, or infused continuously over the time needed to perfuse 2 l saline in the other setting. The perfusion fluid was collected in an airtight infusion bag and the amount of air obtained in the bag was measured. The delivered air volume was negligible and would not cause any significant air embolism in all experiments. In our experimental setting, we found, during high flow, an increased amount of uneliminated air in all used devices compared with lower perfusion flows. All tested devices had a good air elimination capability. The use of ultrasonic air detection coupled

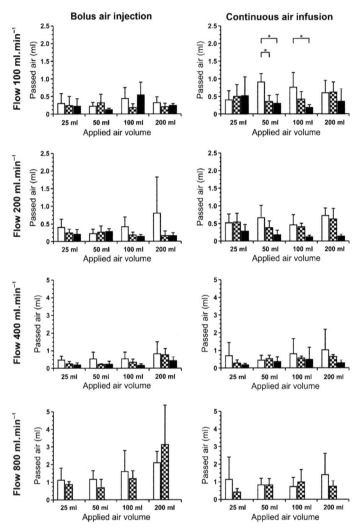

FIGURE 1.—Mean volume of air passed through the Fluido (□), Level 1 (▨) and Ranger (■) pressure infusion devices at different flow rates, during bolus (left) and continuous (right) injection of air. (In the Ranger, a flow of 800 ml.min^{-1} was not tested because this exceeded the maximum infusion flow of 500 ml.min^{-1}). Error bars represent SD. *$p<0.05$. (Reprinted from Zoremba N, Gruenewald C, Zoremba M, et al. Air elimination capability in rapid infusion systems. *Anaesthesia.* 2011;66:1031-1034, with permission from The Authors.)

with an automatic shutoff is a significant safety improvement and can reliably prevent accidental air embolism at rapid flows (Fig 1, Table 1).

▶ In this study, the authors measured the efficacy of 3 different fluid warming devices in delivering high-volume fluids while eliminating air from the infusions into the patients. They studied both steady entrainment of air into the system as well as boluses of air. Each of these circumstances can occur in the clinical setting.

TABLE 1.—Maximum Volume of Air Passed Through the Fluido, Level 1 and Ranger Pressure Infusion Devices, During Bolus and Continuous Injection of Air. Values are Mean (SD)

Air Application	Fluido	Maximum Volume; ml Level 1	Ranger
25 ml			
Bolus	1.1 (0.7)	0.9 (0.2)	0.2 (0.2)
Continuous	1.1 (1.3)	0.5 (0.3)	0.5 (0.5)
50 ml			
Bolus	1.2 (0.5)	0.7 (0.5)	0.3 (0.1)
Continuous	0.9 (0.2)	0.8 (0.4)	0.4 (0.3)
100 ml			
Bolus	1.6 (1.2)	1.2 (0.5)	0.5 (0.4)
Continuous	0.8 (0.9)	1.0 (0.7)	0.5 (0.7)
200 ml			
Bolus	2.1 (0.6)	3.1 (2.7)	0.4 (0.2)
Continuous	1.4 (1.2)	0.7 (0.2)	0.4 (0.4)

If the delivery systems lack an effective mechanism to eliminate the air or detect the air and stop infusion, patients would be a risk for hemodynamically significant venous air embolism episodes. Indeed, such events have been reported and have resulted in morbidity and mortality. In this study, all 3 devices were effective at preventing the infusion of significant volumes of air as shown in Fig 1 and Table 1. Of note is the Ranger system, which does not have an air detection device as tested when used correctly - with the device below the level of the patient. Its efficacy in preventing air infusion cannot be assumed if the device is used incorrectly, being placed at or above the level of the patient. This study shows the improvements in patient safety that have come with improvements in technology. Nonetheless, vigilance of the anesthesiologists remains paramount in ensuring patent safety. With the 2 devices with air detection and flow cutoff mechanisms, proper vigilance is needed to ensure that life-sustaining rapid infusions continue. And with the Ranger system, without a cutoff or detection mechanism, proper use of the device in a chaining clinical situation is the responsibility of the anesthesiologist. Both technology and human vigilance are required for safe rapid infusions.

S. Black, MD

Airway management in the patient with potential cervical spine instability: Continuing Professional Development
Robitaille A (Centre Hospitalier de l'Université de Montréal, Quebec, Canada)
Can J Anaesth 58:1125-1139, 2011

Purpose.—Securing the airway of a patient with a potentially unstable cervical spine (C-spine) is a complex and challenging task. The objective of this continuing professional development module is to review the current knowledge essential for airway management in the face of potential C-spine instability and, at the same time, to underline areas of uncertainty and limitations in the literature.

Principal Findings.—In low-risk patients—defined by strict criteria derived from large multicentre studies—the C-spine can be considered stable or "cleared" without imaging. In all other patients, at least a thin-section computed tomographic examination of the spine from the occiput to T1 should be obtained, including sagittal and coronal multiplanar reconstructed images. Until the C-spine is cleared, it should be immobilized in the neutral position using a rigid cervical collar, sandbags, tape, and a backboard. During airway management, the anterior part of the cervical collar should be removed, and manual in-line stabilization should be applied. Some airway techniques, such as fibreoptic bronchoscopy and the Trachlight®, have been shown to induce less C-spine movement than direct laryngoscopy; however, the impact of such airway management on outcome is uncertain.

Conclusion.—Adequate airway management in the patient with potential C-spine injury demands an understanding of C-spine anatomy, the criteria required to clear the C-spine, and the indications, techniques, and pitfalls of C-spine immobilization. When choosing an airway technique, minimization of C-spine motion should be considered, but the method of choice should also incorporate the broader clinical context (Table 2).

▶ This excellent review article covers all aspects important in airway management of patients with known or suspected cervical spine instability including anatomy, immobilization, diagnosis, and airway management. Multiple studies are reviewed, and several concrete recommendations are made. First, in low-risk patients, history and examination are adequate to clear the cervical spine. Second, in higher-risk patients based on mechanism of injury, thin-slice CT scans are effective at establishing risk of instability. Third, multiple devices, including hard cervical collars, are

TABLE 2.—Characteristics of Different Airway Techniques in the Patient with a Potentially Injured Cervical Spine (C-Spine)

Technique	Characteristics
Basic airway maneuvres	C-spine movement is comparable with or less than direct laryngoscopy.
Direct laryngoscopy (DL)	- ease of use
	- rapidity
	- fewer concerns for secretions in the airway
	- C-spine movement may be greater than with alternative techniques, such as the fibreoptic bronchoscope and the Trachlight®
	- glottic visualization may be limited with manual in-line stabilization (MILS)
GlideScope videolaryngoscope	- C-spine movement similar to direct laryngoscopy
	- better glottic visualization
	- takes more time to secure the airway than with DL
Trachlight® lighted stylet	- minimizes C-spine motion
	- immune to secretions in the airway
	- can be performed with cervical collar in place
	- contraindicated in patients with airway trauma or a deformed airway
Fibreoptic bronchoscope	- minimizes C-spine motion in patients under general anesthesia
	- preferred technique in the awake patient
	- more difficult and slower to perform than DL in unconscious patients and in patients with blood or secretions in the airway
Laryngeal mask airway device	- movement similar to direct laryngoscopy
	- relatively contraindicated in patients with a full stomach

effective to immobilize the spine. Fourth, to secure the airway, the front of hard collars should be removed, and manual in-line stabilization is effective. Finally, no single intubation technique is superior (Table 2), and the choice of which to use should be made based on the clinical situation and experience of the anesthesiologist.

S. Black, MD

Anesthetic Neurotoxicity: A Difficult Dragon to Slay

Thomas J, Crosby G, Drummond JC, et al (Univ of Iowa Carver College of Medicine; Brigham and Women's Hosp, Boston, MA; Univ of California, San Diego)
Anesth Analg 113:969-971, 2011

Background.—Anesthetic neurotoxicity is a topic that is being widely discussed without much solid evidence other than indications noted in animal studies. It is difficult to design prospective, randomized controlled trials (RCTs) that can determine if anesthetic neurotoxicity occurs in children and what adverse effects it produces. Researchers currently lack sufficient knowledge about possible confounding issues. An administrative database of siblings was used to determine if anesthesia and surgery in the child's first 3 years of life produce subsequent behavioral or developmental disorders.

Methods.—From a Medicaid database, 5824 sibling pairs were identified. Three hundred four had surgery before age 3 years, and their outcomes were compared with those of 10,146 children who did not have surgery.

Results.—Of the 304 children having surgery, 24.7% had a diagnosis of a developmental or behavioral disorder, whereas 8.8% of the comparison group had these diagnoses. After adjusting for other perinatal disorders that could have altered outcome, the hazard ratio for having a developmental or behavioral diagnosis and anesthesia and surgery was 1.7. However, the difference between groups disappeared when the analysis considered only children who had a single procedure. When the analysis was limited to 138 matched twin pairs, the children having surgery had no greater risk of a diagnosis of developmental or behavioral problems than those not having surgery.

Conclusions.—The best-controlled studies have not supported the concept that anesthesia negatively impacts the neurodevelopmental status of infants. The data indicate that the association does not prove causation. It is true that children who have multiple surgeries are more likely to have serious underlying medical disorders than other children, and these disorders are likely to influence development and behavior. Parents who fear that their child's well-being will be threatened by the use of general anesthesia should be reassured that to date, no evidence justifies their fear. There is currently no reason to change medical, surgical, or anesthetic practice in infants. Rigorous, appropriately designed studies will be needed to prove that neurotoxicity exists. Until the results of a multitude of such investigations are available, medical practitioners should exercise restraint and caution in publicly sharing interim findings.

▶ This editorial is informative and important for all anesthesiologists involved in the perioperative care of children. In reviewing the available data and its strengths and limitations related to neurotoxicity, they draw several conclusions. First, the neurotoxicity of anesthetics in infants, while clearly demonstrated in the laboratory setting, has not been conclusively demonstrated in clinical studies.[1] In particular, they point out that the best evidence available suggests that a single anesthetic in an otherwise healthy child under the age of 3 does not predispose to neurologic deficits or developmental delays. The impact of anesthetics versus the disease, versus other factors, cannot be defined at this point. They wisely conclude that recommendations to delay needed surgery due to as yet undefined risks of anesthesia are unfounded at this time.

S. Black, MD

Reference

1. DiMaggio C, Sun LS, Li G. Early childhood exposure to anesthesia and risk of developmental and behavioral disorders in a sibling birth cohort. *Anesth Analg.* 2011;113:1143-1151.

Beyond Opioid Patient-Controlled Analgesia: A Systematic Review of Analgesia After Major Spine Surgery

Sharma S, Balireddy RK, Vorenkamp KE, et al (Northwestern Univ, Chicago, IL; Univ of Virginia, Charlottesville)
Reg Anesth Pain Med 37:79-98, 2012

Postoperative pain control in patients undergoing spine surgery remains a challenge for the anesthesiologist. In addition to incisional pain, these patients experience pain arising from deeper tissues such as bones, ligaments, muscles, intervertebral disks, facet joints, and damaged nerve roots. The pain from these structures may be more severe and can lead to neural sensitization and release of mediators both peripherally and centrally. The problem is compounded by the fact that many of these patients are either opioid dependent or opioid tolerant, making them less responsive to the most commonly used therapy for postoperative pain (opioid-based intermittent or patient-controlled analgesia). The purpose of this review was to compare all published treatment options available that go beyond intravenous opiates and attempt to find the best possible treatment modality.

▶ This excellent article compares multiple modalities for management of postoperative pain after spine surgery. Patients undergoing spine surgery frequently have substantial postoperative pain and often report inadequate pain relief. As the authors point out, the etiology of this problem is likely multifactorial, including the nature of the surgery itself, which may be more painful than we realize, the multiple tissue types traumatized, and the frequent opioid dependence of the patients preoperatively. Unfortunately, few individual maneuvers have consistently been shown to be effective. With the exception of intraoperative ketamine, use of nonsteroidal anti-inflammatory drugs, and epidural techniques, no other single interventions are shown to be effective consistently. The authors recommend studies utilizing multiple modalities, which may prove effective in tackling the challenging problem of pain control after spine surgery.

S. Black, MD

Comparison of the C-MAC®, Airtraq®, and Macintosh laryngoscopes in patients undergoing tracheal intubation with cervical spine immobilization
McElwain J, Laffey JG (Galway Univ Hosps, Ireland)
Br J Anaesth 107:258-264, 2011

Background.—We aimed at comparing the performance of the C-MAC®, Airtraq®, and Macintosh laryngoscopes when performing tracheal intubation in patients undergoing neck immobilization using manual inline axial cervical spine stabilization.

Methods.—Ninety consenting patients presenting for surgery requiring tracheal intubation were randomly assigned to undergo intubation using a C-MAC® ($n=30$), Airtraq® ($n=29$), or Macintosh ($n=31$) laryngoscope. All patients were intubated by one anaesthetist experienced in the use of each laryngoscope.

Results.—The Airtraq® laryngoscope performed best in these patients, reducing the Intubation Difficulty Scale score, improving the Cormack and Lehane glottic view, and reducing the need for optimization manoeuvres, compared with both the Macintosh and the C-MAC®. The C-MAC® and Macintosh laryngoscopes performed similarly. There were no differences in success rates or haemodynamic profiles post-intubation between any of the devices tested.

Conclusions.—The Airtraq® laryngoscope performed better than the C-MAC® and Macintosh laryngoscopes in patients undergoing cervical immobilization (Figs 1 and 2).

► Manual in-line stabilization is an effective maneuver to decrease motion of the cervical spine during airway management and is commonly used to protect patients with known or suspected cervical spine instability from cervical cord injury during intubation. However, manual in-line stabilization has also been shown to increase difficulty of intubation. This prospective trial compares the Macintosh, C-MAC, and Airtraq laryngoscopes (Fig 1) in intubation difficulty during manual in-line stabilization. The Airtraq was most effective in decreasing the difficulty of intubation. Fig 2 shows the intubation difficulty score (described in the Appendix in the original article). All measures of intubation difficulty were improved with the Airtraq compared with the other devices during manual in-line stabilization (Fig 3 and Table 2 in the original article).

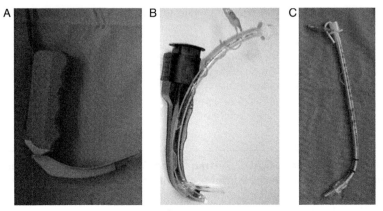

FIGURE 1.—(A) Photograph of the C-MAC® laryngoscope. The cable is connected to a display unit. (B) Photograph of the Airtraq® laryngoscope. The TT is preloaded into the chamber of the device. (C) Photograph of the TT in the hockey stick configuration used for tracheal intubation with the C-MAC®. (Reprinted from McElwain J, Laffey JG. Comparison of the C-MAC®, Airtraq®, and Macintosh laryngoscopes in patients undergoing tracheal intubation with cervical spine immobilization. *Br J Anaesth*. 2011;107:258-264, by permission of The Board of Management and Trustees of the British Journal of Anaesthesia, Oxford University Press.)

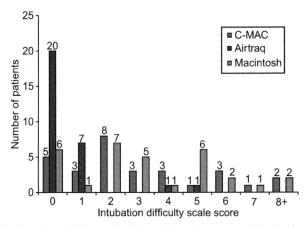

FIGURE 2.—Comparison of IDS score distributions with each laryngoscope. Number of patients is shown above each bar. The IDS scores were lowest with the Airtraq® compared with both Macintosh and C-MAC® laryngoscopes. $P<0.001$ between groups, Kruskal–Wallis ANOVA on ranks. (Reprinted from McElwain J, Laffey JG. Comparison of the C-MAC®, Airtraq®, and Macintosh laryngoscopes in patients undergoing tracheal intubation with cervical spine immobilization. *Br J Anaesth*. 2011;107:258-264, by permission of The Board of Management and Trustees of the British Journal of Anaesthesia, Oxford University Press.)

However, it is most important to use a tool with which the anesthesiologist is familiar during management of patients with potential unstable cervical spine.

S. Black, MD

Continuous Noninvasive Hemoglobin Monitoring During Complex Spine Surgery

Berkow L, Rotolo S, Mirski E (Johns Hopkins School of Medicine, Baltimore, MD)
Anesth Analg 113:1396-1402, 2011

Background.—Monitoring hemoglobin levels in the operating room currently requires repeated blood draws, several steps, and a variable time delay to receive results. Consequently, blood transfusion management decisions may be delayed or made before hemoglobin results become available. The ability to measure hemoglobin continuously and noninvasively may enable a more rapid assessment of a patient's condition and more appropriate blood management. A new technology, Pulse CO-Oximetry, provides a continuous, noninvasive estimate of hemoglobin concentration (SpHb) from a sensor placed on the finger. We evaluated the accuracy of SpHb compared with laboratory CO-Oximetry measurements of total hemoglobin (tHb) during complex spine procedures in patients at high risk for blood loss.

Methods.—Patients eligible for the study were undergoing complex spine surgery with planned invasive arterial or central venous monitoring and hourly blood draws for hemoglobin measurement. During each surgery, blood samples were obtained hourly (or more often if clinically indicated) and analyzed by the central laboratory with CO-Oximetry, a standard method of hemoglobin measurement in many hospitals. The tHb measurements were compared with SpHb obtained at the time of the blood draw.

Results.—Twenty-nine patients were included in the study. The tHb values ranged from 6.9 to 13.9 g/dL, and the SpHb values ranged from 6.9 to 13.4 g/dL. A total of 186 data pairs (tHb/SpHb) were analyzed; after removal of SpHb readings with low signal quality, the bias (defined as the difference between SpHb and tHb) and precision (defined as 1 SD of the bias) were -0.1 g/dL $\pm$ 1.0 g/dL for the remaining 130 data pairs. Bland-Altman analysis showed good agreement of SpHb to tHb values

TABLE 1.—Comparison of Hemoglobin Concentration (SpHb) to Total Hemoglobin (tHb) Values; Mean Percent Error and Number of Points Within a Bias Range, by tHb Range

tHb Range (g/dL)	n (%)	Mean % Error	Bias < ±1.0 g/dL, n (%)	Bias < ±1.5 g/dL, n (%)
A. All SpHb—tHb data pairs ($n = 186$)				
<10.0	38 (20.4)	19.01	26 (68.4)	36 (94.7)
10.0–11.9	114 (61.3)	19.89	69 (60.5)	86 (75.4)
12.0–13.9	34 (18.3)	12.37	15 (44.1)	31 (91.1)
6.9–13.9	186 (100)	17.90	110 (59.1)	153 (82.3)
B. SpHb—tHb data pairs with >50% SIQ (signal-quality indicator) ($n = 130$)				
<10.0	18 (13.9)	11.70	14 (77.8)	17 (94.4)
10.0–11.9	83 (63.8)	17.28	59 (71.1)	70 (84.1)
12.0–13.9	29 (22.3)	10.22	15 (51.7)	27 (93.1)
6.9–13.9	130 (100)	16.97	88 (67.7)	114 (87.7)

Mean % error = (SD of bias SpHb − tHb) (1.96)/mean tHb of range. Bias = SpHb − tHb.

TABLE 2.—Trending of Hemoglobin Concentration (SpHb): Comparison of Changes in SpHb with Changes in Total Hemoglobin (tHb)[a]

tHb Δ (g/dL)	n	<−1.5	−1.5 to −1.1	−1.0 to −0.6	−0.5 to 0	0−0.5	0.6−1.0	1.1−1.5	>1.5
<−1.5	6	1	1	3	1	0	0	0	0
<−1.0	12	1	1	7	3	0	0	0	0
>1.0	10	0	0	0	0	3	3	2	2
>1.5	5	0	0	0	0	1	1	1	2

[a]For each specific time that the laboratory value of tHb changed by at least 1 g/dL (either increasing or decreasing) between consecutive samples, the change in SpHb was calculated for the same consecutive samples and then categorized by magnitude of change in 0.5 g/dL increments.

over the range of values; limits of agreement were −2.0 to 1.8 g/dL. The absolute bias and precision were 0.8 ± 0.6 g/dL.

Conclusions.—Continuous, noninvasive hemoglobin measurement via Pulse CO-Oximetry demonstrated clinically acceptable accuracy of hemoglobin measurement within 1.5 g/dL compared with a standard laboratory reference device when used during complex spine surgery. This technology may provide more timely information on hemoglobin status than intermittent blood sample analysis and thus has the potential to improve blood management during surgery (Tables 1 and 2).

▶ In this prospective trial of 29 patients undergoing spine surgery comparing conventional hemoglobin measurements with continuous noninvasive measurements, the authors concluded that the noninvasive device provided adequate accuracy. The primary results are displayed in Tables 1 and 2. It should be noted that the difference between hemoglobin measurements exceeds 1 g/dL in 41% of samples and 1.5 g/dL in 18% of samples. This was more common with hemoglobin levels less than 10 and in the presence of low-quality signals. Also, decreases in hemoglobin were detected with greater sensitivity by conventional blood draw measurements than the noninvasive device. Taking into account these limitations, noninvasive hemoglobin measurements will likely prove to be valuable in the management of cases in which relatively high blood loss is expected.

S. Black, MD

Controversy of non-steroidal anti-inflammatory drugs and intracranial surgery: et ne nos inducas in tentationem?
Kelly KP, Janssens MC, Ross J, et al (Western General Hosp, Edinburgh, UK; Royal Infirmary of Edinburgh, UK)
Br J Anaesth 107:302-305, 2011

Background.—Unresolved issues attend the use of nonsteroidal anti-inflammatory drugs (NSAIDs) in patients having intracranial surgery.

Developing a rational approach to NSAID use would help neurosurgeons manage patients' risk and pain more effectively.

NSAID Analgesia.—NSAIDs exert analgesic properties by inhibiting arachidonic acid-n-derived prostaglandins (PGs) generated via the cyclooxygenase (COX) pathway. Anti-inflammatory PGs are considered COX-1 forms, and inducible pro-inflammatory PGs are COX-2 forms. Arachidonic acid products also affect hemostasis, exerting either prothrombotic or antithrombotic effects. After vascular injury, endothelial cells are damaged and platelets adhere to the damaged vessel walls. PGI_2 synthesis by injured endothelial cells is reduced. Aspirin covalently and irreversibly binds to platelet COX, the activity of which cannot be recovered until new platelets are produced by the bone marrow. Platelet cohorts are completely replaced about every 10 days. Depending on the risks, aspirin use is usually stopped between 7 and 14 days before surgery, allowing all platelets exposed to aspirin to be replaced. Non-aspirin NSAIDs reversibly inhibit COX, but the duration and extent of this action vary depending on the agent involved. Single doses of piroxicam prolong platelet aggregation for 3 days, single doses of naproxen, diclofenac, or indomethacin last about 2 days, and ibuprofen lasts about 1 day. Chronic administration allows products to accumulate in adipose tissue and can further prolong the return of normal platelet function.

Dosage Recommendations.—Generally it is recommended that non-aspirin NSAIDs be stopped before surgery when hemostasis is critical or patients have a preexisting coagulopathy. However, the individual patient, the specific NSAID, and the procedure being done must be considered a unique combination. When doubt exists, some clinicians omit non-aspirin NSAIDs for 2 weeks. A concern after craniotomy is the development of hematoma. Some studies show that 88% of postoperative hematomas develop in 6 hours, so clinicians justify the postoperative use of NSAIDs after 6 hours. However, the distribution of cases was actually dichotomous, falling before 6 hours or after 24 hours, so any NSAID administered in the interim could contribute to hematoma development. In addition, COX-2 inhibitors and even some non-selective NSAIDs actually both inhibit platelet function and promote thrombosis, depending on the patient and other interactive mechanisms. Some research even indicates that NSAIDs are not needed after craniotomy, with sufficient pain control obtained using dexamethasone. Subjecting all patients to parecoxib, for example, may expose them to a higher risk of adverse events without gaining an advantage in terms of pain control.

Conclusions.—There is concern about the link between NSAIDs and hemostasis when intracranial procedures are done. Some evidence indicates patients may not even need these agents and should not be exposed to their adverse effects. Current evidence supports the avoidance of NSAIDs in close proximity to the performance of a craniotomy and waiting at least 24 hours postoperatively to employ them and then only if other measures have not produced adequate analgesia.

▶ In this editorial, the authors point out the poorly defined risks of nonaspirin nonsteroidal anti-inflammatory agents used routinely after craniotomy. Although use of these agents has not been consistently associated with a substantial increase in volume of estimated blood loss, the authors note that small increases in postoperative bleeding after craniotomy may well be associated with new neurologic deficits. Pain relief after craniotomy is often not well addressed.

S. Black, MD

Decompressive Craniectomy and Early Cranioplasty for the Management of Severe Head Injury: A Prospective Multicenter Study on 147 Patients
Chibbaro S, Di Rocco F, Mirone G, et al (Lariboisiére Univ Hosp, Paris, France; Necker Univ Hosp, Paris, France; Naples Univ Hosp, Italy; et al)
World Neurosurg 75:558-562, 2011

Objective.—In emergency care of patients with severe blunt head injury, uncontrollable high intracranial pressure is one of major causes of morbidity and mortality. The purpose of this study was to evaluate the efficacy of aggressive surgical treatment in managing uncontrollable elevated intracranial pressure coupled with early skull reconstruction.

Methods.—This was a prospective study on a series of 147 consecutive patients, managed according to the same protocol by five different neurosurgical units, for severe head injuries (Glasgow coma scale score ≤8/15 and high intracranial pressure >25 mm Hg) during a five-year period. All patients received a wide decompressive craniectomy and duroplasty in the acute phase, and a cranioplasty was also performed within 12 weeks (median 6 weeks, range 4—12 weeks).

Results.—The emergency decompressive surgery was performed within 28 hours (median 16 hours, range 6—28 hours) after sustaining the head injury. The median preoperative Glasgow coma scale score was 6/15 (range 3—8/15). At a mean follow-up of 26 months (range 14—74 months) 14 patients were lost to long-term follow-up, leaving only 133 patients available for the study. The outcome was favorable in 89 (67%, Glasgow outcome score 4 or 5), it was not favorable in 25 (19%, Glasgow outcome score 2 and 3), and 19 patients (14%) died. A younger age (<50 years) and earlier operation (within 9 hours from trauma) had a significant effect on positive outcomes (*P* < 0.0001 and *P* < 0.03, respectively).

Conclusions.—A prompt aggressive surgery, including a wide decompressive craniectomy coupled with early cranioplasty, could be an effective treatment method to improve the outcome after a severe closed head injury reducing, perhaps, many of the complications related to decompressive craniectomy (Fig 1, Table 2).

▶ Traumatic brain injury (TBI) is one of the common causes of death in the young population and carries high morbidity and mortality rates. Those who survive have considerable disability, which makes it very difficult to integrate them back into the society. This creates a very high economic burden on the society. Brain swelling caused by TBI increases the intracranial pressure, which reduces cerebral perfusion pressure leading to brain ischemia. Increases

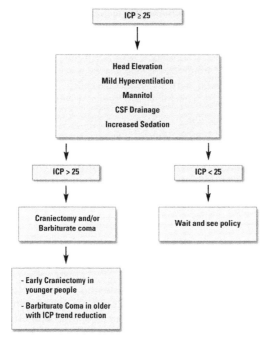

FIGURE 1.—Algorithm for Patient's Management Implemented in All Five Centers. (Reprinted from Chibbaro S, Di Rocco F, Mirone G, et al. Decompressive craniectomy and early cranioplasty for the management of severe head injury: a prospective multicenter study on 147 patients. *World Neurosurg.* 2011;75:558-562, with permission from Elsevier.)

TABLE 2.—Review of Most Recent Literature on Decompressive Craniectomy for Traumatic Brain Injury

Author, Year	No. of Patients	Mean Delay to Cranioplasty	Good Outcome (GOS 4-5)	Mortality Rate	Complication Rate
Polin et al. 1997 (34)	35	NA	37%	23%	NA
Kunze et al. 1998 (18)	28	NA	56%	11%	NA
Munch et al. 2000 (31)	49	NA	41%	NA	NA
Guerra et al. 1999 (10)	57	NA	58%	19%	NA
Timofeev et al. 2006 (43)	49	NA	61%	18%	NA
Olivecrona et al. 2007 (33)	21	NA	71%	14%	NA
Williams et al. 2009 (44)	171	NA	56%	22%	NA
Honeybul et al. 2010 (13)	147	NA	39.5%	18.4%	25%
Present study	147	6 weeks	67%	23%	23%

NA, not applicable; GOS, Glasgow outcome score.
Editor's Note: Please refer to original journal article for full references.

in intracranial pressure are traditionally treated with several modalities, including hyperosmolar therapy, cerebrospinal fluid drainage, barbiturate coma, and short-term hyperventilation. This study examined the impact of decompressive craniectomy and early cranioplasty in TBI with intractable intracranial hypertension. Previous studies have reported a complication rate of 14%—25% and mortality range between 14% and 90%. Unlike the previous studies, this study showed good outcome in younger (mean age, 36 years) patents with a Glasgow Coma Score of 4 and 5 compared with patients with a mean age of 56 years. In addition, those who underwent early surgery (within 9 hours of injury) had a better outcome. Furthermore, complications associated with decompressive craniectomy were fewer compared with the previous series. This is attributed to the application of early cranioplasty following hemicraniectomy.

M. Mathru, MD

Effect of intravenous parecoxib on post-craniotomy pain

Williams DL, Pemberton E, Leslie K (Royal Melbourne Hosp, Parkville, Victoria, Australia)
Br J Anaesth 107:398-403, 2011

Background.—Pain management in craniotomy patients is challenging, with mild-to-moderate pain intensity, moderate-to-high risk of postoperative nausea and vomiting (PONV), and potentially catastrophic consequences of analgesic-related side-effects. The aim of this study was to determine whether i.v. parecoxib administered at dural closure during craniotomy decreased total morphine consumption and morphine-related side-effects compared with placebo.

Methods.—One hundred adult patients presenting for supratentorial craniotomy under propofol/remifentanil anaesthesia were randomized to receive parecoxib, 40 mg i.v., or placebo in a double-blind manner. All patients received local anaesthetic scalp infiltration, regular i.v. paracetamol, nurse-administered morphine in the post-anaesthesia care unit (PACU) until verbal analogue pain scores were ≤4/10 and patient-controlled morphine thereafter. Morphine consumption, pain intensity, and analgesia-related side-effects were recorded during the first 24 h after operation.

Results.—Ninety-six patients (49 control and 47 parecoxib) were included in the analyses. Fifty-nine (61) patients received morphine in the PACU and only one patient (control) did not receive any morphine in the postoperative period. There were no significant differences between the two groups in morphine consumption [20 (range: 0—102) *vs* 16 (range: 1—92) mg; $P=$ 0.38], pain intensity [excellent/very good pain relief in 78% of parecoxib patients; 74% of control patients ($P=0.72$)] or analgesia-related side-effects (PONV in 51% of parecoxib patients; 56 of control patients; $P=0.55$) in the first 24 h after operation. No major morbidity was recorded.

Conclusions.—Our study demonstrated no clinical benefit to adding i.v. parecoxib to local anaesthetic scalp infiltration, i.v. paracetamol, and patient-controlled i.v. morphine after supratentorial craniotomy.

Trial Registration.—ClinicalTrials.gov registry NCT00455117; Australian Clinical Trials Registry ACTRN12605000600640 (Fig 2, Tables 2 and 3).

▶ Management of postoperative pain after craniotomy has received less attention than pain management after other surgical procedures. Some feel that little

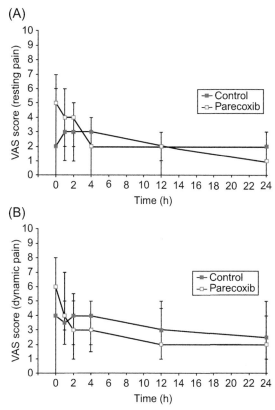

FIGURE 2.—VAS score for resting pain (A) and dynamic pain (B) in patients receiving parecoxib and placebo. Data are presented as median (inter-quartile range). (Reprinted from Williams DL, Pemberton E, Leslie K. Effect of intravenous parecoxib on post-craniotomy pain. *Br J Anaesth*. 2011;107:398-403, with permission from The Author.)

TABLE 2.—Intraoperative and Postoperative Data. Data are Expressed as Median (Range) or Number (%). PACU, Post-Anaesthesia Care Unit; PCA, Patient-Controlled Analgesia

Characteristic	Control	Parecoxib	*P*-Value
Induction, wound closure (min)	195 (97–614)	188 (73–520)	0.62
Wound closure, eyes open (min)	15 (0–80)	15 (0–65)	0.72
Wound closure, PACU discharge (min)	100 (67–247)	90 (40–162)	0.64
Dexamethasone administered	42 (86)	41 (87)	0.87
Dexamethasone dose (mg)	12 (4–20)	8 (4–20)	0.03
Bispectral index monitoring used	24 (49)	20 (43)	0.53
Morphine administered in PACU	26 (53)	33 (70)	0.08
Morphine administration in PACU (mg)	5 (1–14)	6 (1–14)	0.88
Morphine administration via PCA (mg)	18 (0–97)	11 (0–86)	0.32
Morphine total (mg)	20 (0–102)	16 (1–92)	0.38
Postoperative nausea and/or vomiting	28 (56)	24 (51)	0.55
Excellent or very good pain relief	38 (78)	35 (74)	0.72

TABLE 3.—Postoperative Characteristics. Results are Presented as Median (Inter-Quartile Range) or Mean (SD)

		0 h	1 h	2 h	4 h	12 h	24 h	P-Value
PONV score	Control	—	1 (1–1)	1 (1–2)	1 (1–2)	1 (1–1)	1 (1–1)	1.0*
	Parecoxib	—	1 (1–1)	1 (1–2)	1 (1–2)	1 (1–1)	1 (1–1)	
Sedation score	Control	2 (0–2)	0 (0–2)	0 (0–2)	0 (0–2)	0 (0–2)	0 (0–0)	1.0*
	Parecoxib	2 (2–4)	1 (0–2)	0 (0–2)	0 (0–2)	0 (0–2)	0 (0–0)	
Systolic arterial pressure (mm Hg)	Control	145 (24)	139 (22)	127 (16)	125 (15)	121 (14)	122 (17)	Between groups 0.26; within groups <0.0001**
	Parecoxib	139 (20)	133 (17)	126 (14)	122 (15)	122 (14)	121 (15)	
Heart rate (beats min^{-1})	Control	76 (16)	72 (14)	78 (16)	76 (17)	72 (17)	76 (13)	Between groups 0.50; within groups 0.0003**
	Parecoxib	74 (17)	70 (16)	75 (16)	73 (17)	72 (14)	74 (15)	
Ventilatory frequency (bpm)	Control	15 (3)	15 (2)	15 (3)	15 (2)	16 (2)	16 (2)	Between groups 0.06; within groups 0.002**
	Parecoxib	15 (3)	15 (2)	16 (2)	16 (3)	16 (2)	16 (2)	

*Friedman Test.
**Repeated-Measures Analysis of Variance. PONV, Postoperative Nausea and Vomiting; PONV was Rated by Patients as: 0, Absent; 1, Nausea not Requiring Treatment; 2, Nausea Requiring Treatment; and 3, Vomiting. Sedation was Rated by Attending Nurses as: 1, Awake and Alert; 2, Easy to Rouse with Verbal Commands; 3, Drowsy, Roused only by Touch; 4, Somnolent, Roused Only by Pain

pain occurs after craniotomy. Concern over respiratory depression in neurosurgical patients receiving narcotics limits their use by many surgeons. In this prospective trial, addition of parecoxib to scalp infiltration after craniotomy had no impact on postoperative pain, requirement for narcotics, or complications (Tables 2 and 3, Fig 2). Perhaps the lack of difference in pain scores or requirement for narcotics has to do with the high quality of pain management from the local anesthetic scalp infiltration.

S. Black, MD

Erythropoietin Administration Modulates Pulmonary Nrf2 Signaling Pathway After Traumatic Brain Injury in Mice

Jin W, Wu J, Wang H, et al (Med School of Nanjing Univ, China)
J Trauma 71:680-686, 2011

Background.—In our previous studies, antioxidant transcription factor, nuclear factor erythroid 2-related factor 2 (Nrf2) signaling pathway has been shown to play an important role in protecting traumatic brain injury (TBI)-induced acute lung injury (ALI). This study was designed to explore whether recombinant human erythropoietin (rhEPO) administration modulates pulmonary Nrf2 signaling pathway in a murine TBI model.

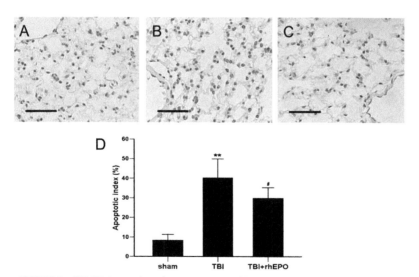

FIGURE 3.—TUNEL immunohistochemistry staining of lung in sham group, TBI group, and TBI + rhEPO group (n = 6). (A) Sham group mice showing few TUNEL positive cells (*stained brown*); (B) TBI group mice showing more TUNEL positive cells; (C) TBI + rhEPO group mice showing less TUNEL positive cells than TBI group; and (D) the rhEPO treatment significantly decreased the AI in the lung tissue after TBI. **p < 0.01 versus sham group and #*p* < 0.05 versus TBI group. Scale bars, 50 μm. For interpretation of the references to color in this figure legend, the reader is referred to web version of this article. (Reprinted from Jin W, Wu J, Wang H, et al. Erythropoietin administration modulates pulmonary Nrf2 signaling pathway after traumatic brain injury in mice. *J Trauma.* 2011;71:680-686, with permission from Lippincott Williams & Wilkins.)

Methods.—Closed head injury was made by Hall's weight-dropping method. The rhEPO was administered at a dose of 5,000 IU/kg 30 minutes after TBI. Pulmonary capillary permeability, wet or dry weight ratio, apoptosis, Nrf2 and its downstream cytoprotective enzymes including NAD(P)H:quinone oxidoreductase 1, and glutathione S-transferase were investigated at 24 hours after TBI.

Results.—We found that treatment with rhEPO markedly ameliorated TBI-induced ALI, as characterized by decreased pulmonary capillary permeability, wet or dry weight ratio, and alveolar cells apoptosis. Administration of rhEPO also significantly upregulated the mRNA expressions and activities of Nrf2 signaling pathway-related agents, including Nrf2, NAD(P)H: quinone oxidoreductase 1, and glutathione S-transferase.

Conclusions.—The results of this study suggest that post-TBI rhEPO administration may induce Nrf2-mediated cytoprotective response in the lung, and this may be a mechanism whereby rhEPO reduces TBI-induced ALI (Figs 3 and 5).

▶ Acute lung injury (ALI) often accompanies traumatic brain injury (TBI). The presence of ALI in the presence TBI impairs brain oxygenation and aggravates neurogenic injury. Several lines of experimental evidence indicate that oxidative stress and inflammatory responses are involved in the pathogenesis of TBI-induced

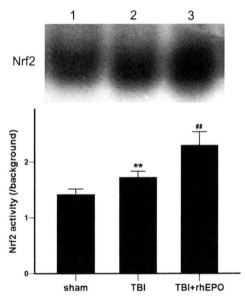

FIGURE 5.—Nrf2 activity in the lung samples in sham group, TBI group, and TBI + rhEPO group (n = 6). EMSA autoradiography of Nrf2 DNA binding is shown on top of the graph and the order of individual bands corresponds to that of graph bars. *Lane 1*, sham group; *Lane 2*, TBI group; and *Lane 3*, TBI + rhEPO group. The rhEPO treatment significantly promoted the Nrf2 activation in the lung tissue after TBI. $**p < 0.01$ versus sham group and $\#\#p < 0.01$ versus TBI group. (Reprinted from Jin W, Wu J, Wang H, et al. Erythropoietin administration modulates pulmonary Nrf2 signaling pathway after traumatic brain injury in mice. *J Trauma.* 2011;71:680-686, with permission from Lippincott Williams & Wilkins.)

ALI. Evidence also suggests that oxidative stress can modulate the inflammatory responses during tissue injury through activation of transcription factor erythroid 2 related factor (Nrf2). Nrf2 upregulation induces the expression and upregulation of downstream cytoprotective enzymes, such as NADPH and glutathione transferase, that attenuate tissue injury. Experimental and clinical studies suggest that erythropoietin (EPO) has pleiotropic actions beside the stimulation of erythroid precursors. Previous studies have found protective effects of EPO in experimental models of ischemia-reperfusion—induced lung injury and in necrotizing pancreatitis. This study examined whether EPO promotes the TBI-induced activation of Nrf2 signaling pathway in the lung in TBI model. The study convincingly demonstrates that the pulmonary Nrf2 signaling pathway was significantly activated after TBI and could be promoted when treated with rhEPO. This is supported by their observation that EPO induced decreases in pulmonary capillary permeability, wet or dry weight ratio, and alveolar cell apoptosis. Clinical studies are needed to confirm their observation.

M. Mathru, MD

Evoked Potential Monitoring Identifies Possible Neurological Injury During Positioning for Craniotomy

Anastasian ZH, Ramnath B, Komotar RJ, et al (Columbia Univ, NY)
Anesth Analg 109:817-821, 2009

Somatosensory-evoked potential (SSEP) monitoring is commonly used to detect changes in nerve conduction and prevent impending nerve injury. We present a case series of two patients who had SSEP monitoring for their surgical craniotomy procedure, and who, upon positioning supine with their head tilted $30°-45°$, developed unilateral upper extremity SSEP changes. These SSEP changes were reversed when the patients were repositioned. These cases indicate the clinical usefulness of monitoring SSEPs while positioning the patient and adjusting position accordingly to prevent injury (Fig 1).

▶ This case report illustrates 2 important points. First, the positions our patients are placed in to facilitate surgical exposure have the potential to cause permanent injury. Results from closed claims analysis support this point. Many of the injuries are position-related peripheral nerve injuries. It is incumbent on us as anesthesiologists to understand position-related risks and carefully examine our patients as they are being positioned for surgery. Clearly, the surgeons who direct the positioning have a major component of this responsibility, but we, too, must participate actively in the positioning process. Second, neurologic monitoring should be attended to. Fig 1 shows a change that occurred at an unusual time in the procedure and that occurred at an unexpected point in the pathway. Responding to this change likely saved these patients at least temporary if not permanent neurologic injury. Too often, we are tempted to

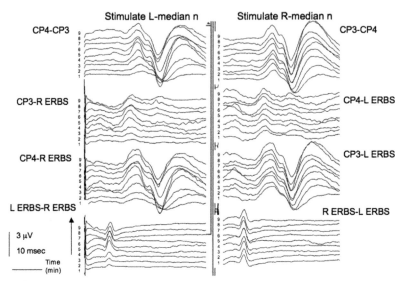

FIGURE 1.—Somatosensory-evoked potential (SEEP) changes in the left median nerve in Case 1. SSEPs from bilateral median nerves were recorded using needle electrodes placed at Erb's point over the brachial plexus, for assessing peripheral conduction, and on the scalp at CP3 and CP4 locations, for assessing central conduction. Time in minutes is recorded on the y axis. From the start of the recordings (time = 1 min), there is a unilateral decrease in the amplitude of the left median nerve recordings compared with that of the right median nerve. This difference exists at both peripheral (Erb's) and central (CP3 and CP4) recordings, suggesting a peripheral mechanism. With repositioning of the shoulder, the amplitude increases on the left side with time in central and peripheral recordings, approaching the amplitude on the right side. (Reprinted from Anastasian ZH, Ramnath B, Komotar RJ, et al. Evoked potential monitoring identifies possible neurological injury during positioning for craniotomy. *Anesth Analg.* 2009;109:817-821, with permission from International Anesthesia Research Society.)

ignore a monitor we do not use frequently that gives data inconsistent with what we expect.

S. Black, MD

Hyperglycemia During Craniotomy for Adult Traumatic Brain Injury

Pecha T, Sharma D, Hoffman NG, et al (Univ of Washington, Seattle; Univ of Washington School of Medicine, Seattle)
Anesth Analg 113:336-342, 2011

Background.—Hyperglycemia after traumatic brain injury (TBI) is associated with poor outcome, but previous studies have not addressed intraoperative hyperglycemia in adult TBI. In this study, we examined glucose value variability and risk factors for hyperglycemia during craniotomy in adults with TBI.

Methods.—A retrospective cohort study of patients ≥18 years who underwent urgent or emergent craniotomy for TBI at Harborview Medical Center (level 1 adult and pediatric trauma center) between October 2007 and May 2010 was performed. Preoperative (within 24 hours of anesthesia start) and intraoperative (during anesthesia) glucose values for each patient were retrieved. The prevalence of intraoperative hyperglycemia (glucose ≥200 mg/dL), hypoglycemia (glucose <60 mg/dL), and glycemic trends was determined. Generalized Estimating Equations was used to determine the independent predictors of intraoperative hyperglycemia. Data are presented as adjusted odds ratio (AOR) (95% confidence interval [CI]), and $P < 0.05$ reflects significance.

Results.—Intraoperative hyperglycemia was common (26 [15%]) and intraoperative hypoglycemia was not observed. *Independent risk factors* of intraoperative hyperglycemia were age ≥65 years (AOR 3.9 [95% CI: 1.4−10.3]; $P = 0.007$), Glasgow Coma Scale score <9 (AOR 4.9 [95% CI: 1.6−15.1]; $P = 0.006$), preoperative hyperglycemia (AOR 4.4 [95% CI: 1.7−11.6]; $P = 0.003$), and subdural hematoma (AOR 5.6 [95% CI: 1.4−22.2]; $P = 0.02$). Mean intraoperative glucose was highest in severe TBI patients ($P = 0.02$). There was both between-patient (79.5% variance; $P < 0.001$) and within-patient (20.5% variance; $P < 0.001$) intraoperative glucose value variability. Patients with intraoperative hyperglycemia had higher in-hospital mortality (8 [31%] vs 20 [13%]; $P < 0.02$).

Conclusion.—Intraoperative hyperglycemia was common in adults undergoing urgent/emergent craniotomy for TBI and was predicted by severe TBI, the presence of subdural hematoma, preoperative hyperglycemia, and

TABLE 2.—Univariate Factors Associated with Intraoperative Hyperglycemia in 176 Adult Patients with Traumatic Brain Injury

Variable	Hyperglycemia (any Glucose ≥200 mg/dL) ($n = 26$)	No Hyperglycemia (all Glucose <200 mg/dL) ($n = 150$)	P Value
Age, mean ± SD (range)	57 ± 19 (18−86)	50 ± 20 (18−93)	0.09
Age ≥40 y ($n = 117$)	19	98	0.17
Age ≥65 y ($n = 49$)	16	33	<0.0001
Male gender ($n = 129$)	16	113	0.26
Admission GCS score ≤8 ($n = 85$)	20	65	0.002
Isolated SDH ($n = 111$)	22	89	0.005
Any SDH ($n = 136$)	24	112	0.02
Isolated EDH ($n = 26$)	1	25	0.10
Isolated ICH ($n = 9$)	0	9	0.21
Multiple lesions ($n = 23$)	2	21	0.42
In-hospital mortality ($n = 28$)	8	20	0.02
Mannitol ($n = 68$)	9	59	0.75
Median anesthesia duration (min)	201 (130−317)	203 (93−437)	0.95
Anesthetic agent			
Isoflurane ($n = 55$)	8	47	0.88
Sevoflurane ($n = 114$)	16	98	0.77
Desflurane ($n = 3$)	0	3	0.48
Propofol ($n = 4$)	1	4	0.55
Preoperative hyperglycemia ($n = 31$)	11	20	<0.0001
Median discharge GCS score	13 (5−15)	15 (6−15)	0.09

GCS = Glasgow Coma Scale; SDH = subdural hematoma; EDH = extradural hematoma; ICH = intracranial hemorrhage.

TABLE 3.—Independent Predictors of Intraoperative Hyperglycemia

Risk Factors	Adjusted Odds Ratio (95% CI)	P Value
Age ≥65 y	3.9 (1.4−10.3)	0.007
Admission GCS score ≤9	4.9 (1.6−15.1)	0.006
Preoperative hyperglycemia	4.4 (1.7−11.6)	0.003
Isolated SDH	5.6 (1.4−22.2)	0.02

Data from 176 of 185 adults (9 patients with no intraoperative glucose values). Data are adjusted for age and gender. The maximum percentage of patients per anesthesiologist was 9%. Because of the large number of anesthesiologists, we were not able to enter anesthesiologist in the model of glucose check timing. However, the anesthesiologists were linked to each patient and data reflect the effect of these predictors on the combination of patient and anesthesiologist.

CI = confidence interval; GCS = Glasgow Coma Scale; SDH = subdural hematoma.

age ≥65 years. However, there was significant variability in intraoperative glucose values (Tables 2 and 3).

▶ Data for almost 200 head trauma patients requiring surgery emergently were reviewed to determine incidence of and predictors for intraoperative hyperglycemia. Intraoperative hyperglycemia was relatively common, occurring in 15% of patients. No patients experienced hypoglycemia. In addition, there was significant within-patient variability. These observations suggest that close monitoring and treatment of hyperglycemia are warranted and safe with little risk for hypoglycemia. The study was too small to define whether insulin treatment of intraoperative hyperglycemia improved outcome. Predictors of intraoperative hyperglycemia (Tables 2 and 3) include preoperative hyperglycemia, age over 65, severe head injury, and subdural hematoma. Patients with hyperglycemia intraoperatively had a worse outcome, which could be related to the hyperglycemia. However, equally likely is the fact that they are older and more severely injured.

S. Black, MD

Immune Cell Populations Decrease During Craniotomy Under General Anesthesia
Liu S, Wang B, Li S, et al (Beijing Tiantan Hosp, China)
Anesth Analg 113:572-577, 2011

Background.—Postoperative infections are common and potentially fatal complications in neurosurgical intensive care medicine. An impairment of immune function after central nervous system surgery is associated with higher risk of infection and postoperative complications. The aim of our study was to investigate how the immune cell population changes during the anesthesia process in patients undergoing craniotomy surgery.

Methods.—Patients undergoing craniotomy who had an inhaled general anesthetic were studied. Blood samples were collected before anesthesia and 30, 45, 60, 120, and 240 minutes after anesthesia began. Blood counts for neutrophils, monocytes, and lymphocytes were determined along with lymphocyte subpopulations (T cells, inducer and helper T cells, suppressor and cytotoxic T cells, natural killer cells, and B cells). Plasma concentrations of interleukin (IL)−2, IL-4, IL-6, and IL-10 were also measured along with tumor necrosis factor-α and interferon-γ. Data were analyzed by SPSS 13.0 software using repeated-measures analysis of variance followed by a Bonferroni correction.

Results.—Eighteen patients were enrolled in this study. In the comparison of the immune cell counts during neuroanesthesia, we found that at 30 minutes after anesthesia induction, neutrophils, monocytes, and lymphocytes decreased 18% (95% confidence interval [CI]: 11.0%−24.6%), 34% (95% CI: 16.2%−51.1%), and 39% (95% CI: 29.0%−48.9%) compared with their levels before anesthesia. At extubation the neutrophils returned to the base level. It also showed that natural killer cells decreased significantly during anesthesia. The concentration of cytokines in peripheral blood did not change significantly.

Conclusion.—Our results showed that anesthesia and surgery upset the balance of the immune system during craniotomy, and a significant decrease in immune cell populations emerged after induction under general anesthesia (Figs 1 and 2, Tables 2 and 3).

▶ This prospective trial in 18 patients undergoing craniotomy for mass resection investigates changes in immune cells with induction of anesthesia through completion of the procedure. It is interesting to note that while anesthesia and

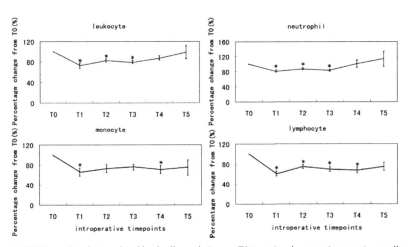

FIGURE 1.—Circulating white blood cell populations at T0 (entering the operating room), as well as 30 minutes after anesthesia induction (T1), 45 minutes after anesthesia induction (T2), 60 minutes (craniotomy start, T3), 120 minutes (tumor resection, T4), and 240 minutes (before extubation, T5) after anesthesia began. The T0 group was taken as control. *$P < 0.05$ in comparison with T0 group. Mean and standard deviation (SD) values are shown. (Reprinted from Liu S, Wang B, Li S, et al. Immune cell populations decrease during craniotomy under general anesthesia. *Anesth Analg.* 2011;113:572-577, with permission from International Anesthesia Research Society.)

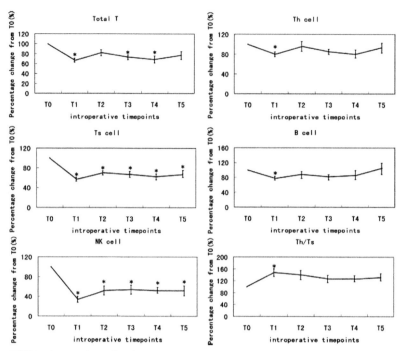

FIGURE 2.—Circulating lymphocyte subsets at T0 (entering the operating room), as well as 30 minutes after anesthesia induction (T1), 45 minutes after anesthesia induction (T2), 60 minutes (craniotomy start, T3), 120 minutes (tumor resection, T4), and 240 minutes (before extubation, T5) after anesthesia began. Lymphocyte subsets were analyzed by flow cytometry. The T0 group was taken as control. *$P < 0.05$ in comparison with T0 group. Mean and standard deviation (SD) values are shown. (Reprinted from Liu S, Wang B, Li S, et al. Immune cell populations decrease during craniotomy under general anesthesia. *Anesth Analg.* 2011;113:572-577, with permission from International Anesthesia Research Society.)

surgery lead to alternations in immune cell numbers, the most profound changes occur with the induction of anesthesia, and, for many cell types, numbers return to or near baseline levels at the end of the procedure (Tables 2 and 3 and Figs 1 and 2). These data suggest that the perioperative period is associated with significant changes in immune system balance. The authors postulate this may in part be due to the blunting of the stress response by general anesthesia and the proinflammatory response to surgical trespass. The impact of the anesthetic agent immune modulation on risk for perioperative infections is at yet undefined. Likewise, effects of different anesthetic agents and techniques have not been studied. This is important for further research. If it is demonstrated that the anesthetic agents and techniques that can be identified have minimum negative impact on the patient's immune system and that these agents are associated with a lower risk of perioperative infection, potential for great benefit to our patients exist. Many factors currently influence our choice of agents for individual patients. Impact of the agent on the immune

TABLE 2.—Blood Cell Populations During Surgery

	T0 Mean ± SD	T1 Mean ± SD	P	T2 Mean ± SD	P	T3 Mean ± SD	P	T4 Mean ± SD	P	T5 Mean ± SD	P
Leukocyte (1 nL^{-1})	6.82 ± 0.75	4.90 ± 0.68	0.022	5.64 ± 0.67	0.007	5.39 ± 0.65	0.009	5.99 ± 0.73	0.127	6.46 ± 0.87	>0.99
Neutrophil (1 nL^{-1})	4.35 ± 0.58	3.51 ± 0.46	0.021	3.78 ± 0.51	0.105	3.62 ± 0.50	0.05	4.34 ± 0.69	>0.99	4.66 ± 0.78	>0.99
Monocyte (1 nL^{-1})	0.50 ± 0.06	0.31 ± 0.05	0.022	0.34 ± 0.04	0.083	0.35 ± 0.04	0.122	0.32 ± 0.05	0.139	0.32 ± 0.05	0.482
Lymphocyte (1 nL^{-1})	1.92 ± 0.23	1.18 ± 0.18	0.003	1.45 ± 0.19	0.002	1.36 ± 0.20	0.001	1.27 ± 0.17	0.015	1.42 ± 0.22	0.124
Total T (1 nL^{-1})	1.31 ± 0.16	0.86 ± 0.12	0.011	1.05 ± 0.15	0.09	0.95 ± 0.15	0.013	0.87 ± 0.12	0.027	0.98 ± 0.16	0.294
Th cell (1 nL^{-1})	0.65 ± 0.10	0.49 ± 0.06	0.561	0.60 ± 0.10	>0.99	0.55 ± 0.10	0.316	0.51 ± 0.08	0.435	0.59 ± 0.11	>0.99
Ts cell (1 nL^{-1})	0.57 ± 0.09	0.35 ± 0.07	<0.001	0.40 ± 0.07	0.007	0.38 ± 0.07	0.07	0.33 ± 0.05	0.053	0.37 ± 0.07	0.209
B cell (1 nL^{-1})	0.27 ± 0.05	0.20 ± 0.03	0.113	0.23 ± 0.04	0.705	0.22 ± 0.04	0.565	0.23 ± 0.04	>0.99	0.27 ± 0.05	>0.99
NK cell (1 nL^{-1})	0.33 ± 0.04	0.10 ± 0.02	0.003	0.16 ± 0.04	0.012	0.19 ± 0.05	0.041	0.16 ± 0.02	0.004	0.17 ± 0.05	0.077
Th/Ts	1.44 ± 0.15	2.03 ± 0.21	0.122	1.94 ± 0.24	0.44	1.76 ± 0.20	>0.99	1.76 ± 0.17	0.468	1.82 ± 0.18	0.809

Values are expressed as mean values ± SD.
T0 = before anesthesia; T1 = 30 minutes after anesthesia induction; T2 = 45 minutes after anesthesia induction; T3 = craniotomy start (60 minutes after anesthesia began); T4 = tumor resection (120 minutes after anesthesia began); T5 = before extubation (240 minutes after anesthesia began); NK = natural killer; Th = inducer and helper T cells; Ts = suppressor and cytotoxic T cells.
Listed P values compared with T0 group have been Bonferroni corrected.

TABLE 3.—Cytokine Concentrations During Surgery

	T0 Mean ± SD	T1 Mean ± SD	P	T2 Mean ± SD	P	T3 Mean ± SD	P	T4 Mean ± SD	P	T5 Mean ± SD	P
IFN-γ (pg·mL^{-1})	5.44 ± 0.29	5.64 ± 0.27	>0.99	5.74 ± 0.26	>0.99	5.28 ± 0.40	>0.99	6.02 ± 0.89	>0.99	5.38 ± 0.33	>0.99
TNF-α (pg·mL^{-1})	2.80 ± 0.09	2.98 ± 0.15	>0.99	2.91 ± 0.06	>0.99	2.84 ± 0.13	>0.99	2.94 ± 0.29	>0.99	2.86 ± 0.11	>0.99
IL-10 (pg·mL^{-1})	5.78 ± 1.18	5.41 ± 1.13	0.305	5.60 ± 1.19	>0.99	5.82 ± 1.70	>0.99	6.90 ± 1.21	>0.99	6.34 ± 1.25	>0.99
IL-6 (pg·mL^{-1})	6.38 ± 2.41	3.91 ± 0.18	>0.99	3.83 ± 0.18	>0.99	3.90 ± 0.13	>0.99	4.65 ± 0.23	>0.99	7.46 ± 0.55	>0.99
IL-4 (pg·mL^{-1})	5.15 ± 0.28	5.32 ± 0.10	>0.99	5.43 ± 0.12	>0.99	5.44 ± 0.15	>0.99	5.48 ± 0.19	>0.99	5.22 ± 0.12	>0.99
IL-2 (pg·mL^{-1})	5.91 ± 0.38	6.48 ± 0.10	>0.99	6.51 ± 0.12	>0.99	6.43 ± 0.11	>0.99	6.57 ± 0.29	>0.99	6.17 ± 0.12	>0.99

Values are expressed as mean values ± SD.

T0 = before anesthesia; T1 = 30 minutes after anesthesia induction; T2 = 45 minutes after anesthesia induction; T3 = craniotomy start (60 minutes after anesthesia began); T4 = tumor resection (120 minutes after anesthesia began); T5 = before extubation (240 minutes after anesthesia began); IFN = interferon; TNF = tumor necrosis factor; IL = interleukin.

Listed P values compared with T0 group have been Bonferroni corrected.

system would be another important variable to consider as we tailor our approach for each patient.

S. Black, MD

Local Brain Temperature Reduction Through Intranasal Cooling With the RhinoChill Device: Preliminary Safety Data in Brain-Injured Patients

Abou-Chebl A, Sung G, Barbut D, et al (Univ of Louisville School of Medicine, KY; Univ of Southern California, Los Angeles, CA; BeneChill Inc, San Diego, CA)

Stroke 42:2164-2169, 2011

Background and Purpose.—Hypothermia is neuroprotectant but currently available cooling methods are laborious, invasive, and require whole-body cooling. There is a need for less invasive cooling of the brain. This study was conducted to assess the safety and efficacy of temperature reduction of the RhinoChill transnasal cooling device.

Methods.—We conducted a prospective single-arm safety and feasibility study of intubated patients for whom temperature reduction was indicated. After rhinoscopy, the device was activated for 1 hour. Brain, tympanic, and core temperatures along with vital signs and laboratory studies were recorded. All general and device-related adverse events were collected for the entire hypothermia treatment.

Results.—A total of 15 patients (mean age, 50.3 ± 17.1 years) were enrolled. Brain injury was caused by intracerebral hemorrhage, trauma, and ischemic stroke in equal numbers. Hypothermia was induced for fever control in 9 patients and for neuroprotection/intracranial pressure control in 6. Core temperature, brain temperature, and tympanic temperature were reduced an average of 1.1 ± 0.6°C (range, 0.3 to 2.1°C), 1.4 ± 0.4°C (range, 0.8 to 5.1°C), and 2.2 ± 2°C (range, 0.5 to 6.5°C), respectively. Only 2 patients did not achieve the goal of ≥1°C decrease in temperature. Brain temperature, tympanic temperature, and core temperature reductions were similar between the afebrile and febrile patients. There were no unanticipated adverse events and only 1 anticipated adverse event: hypertension in 1 subject that led to discontinuation of cooling after 30 minutes. There were no nasal complications.

Conclusions.—Intranasal cooling with the RhinoChill device appears safe and effectively lowers brain and core temperatures. Further study is warranted to assess the efficacy of hypothermia through intranasal cooling for brain-injured patients (Figs 1 and 2, Table 2).

▶ Hypothermia is a well-established treatment adjunct for brain protection in brain injury focal and global ischemia. Here the authors describe a novel, brain-specific cooling device known as Rhinochill device (RCD, BENECHILL, San Diego, CA). The device consists of 2 nasal catheters that spray a proprietary perfluorocarbon-oxygen mixture into the nasopharynx for cooling. It takes advantage of the nasal pathways (ie, the conchal folds and turbinates) that

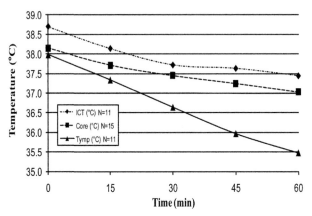

FIGURE 1.—Mean temperature reductions during the 1-hour RhinoChill induction. ICT indicates intracranial temperature. (Reprinted from Abou-Chebl A, Sung G, Barbut D, et al. Local brain temperature reduction through intranasal cooling with the rhinochill device: preliminary safety data in brain-injured patients. *Stroke.* 2011;42:2164-2169, with permission from American Heart Association, Inc.)

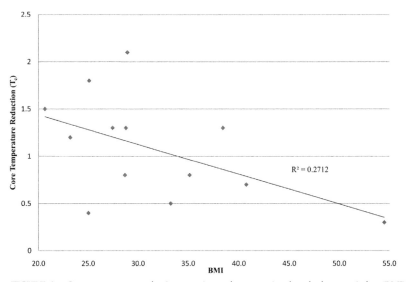

FIGURE 2.—Core temperature reduction was inversely proportional to body mass index (BMI). (Reprinted from Abou-Chebl A, Sung G, Barbut D, et al. Local brain temperature reduction through intranasal cooling with the rhinochill device: preliminary safety data in brain-injured patients. *Stroke.* 2011;42:2164-2169, with permission from American Heart Association, Inc.)

provide a large diffuse surface area in close proximity to cerebral circulation. Cooling in the nasopharynx offers brain-specific cooling through conductive mechanisms and indirect hematogenous mechanisms preferentially cooling the brain before the body. Future studies should explore the efficacy of this device in inducing hypothermia and controlling rewarming in a larger pool of

TABLE 2.—Rhinoscopy Findings

Patient No.	Baseline	1 H After RhinoChill	24 H After RhinoChill	24 H Postcooling
1-1	Normal	Erythema, minimal	Normal	Normal
1-2	Normal	Abrasion & erythema bilaterally	Erythema, mild, left nare	Normal
1-3	Normal	Mucus discharge	Minimal bloody discharge, left nare	Normal
2-1	Not performed	Normal	Not available	Not available
2-2	Normal	Normal	Not available	Not available
2-3	Minor abrasion, left nare	Normal	Normal	Normal
2-4	Minor abrasion, left concha	No change	Normal	Normal
3-1	Mild erythema, small hemorrhage, left nare	Erythema, minimal	Mild to moderate white discharge bilaterally	Not available
3-2	Erythema bilaterally, clear-white discharge, ulcer on columella	Unchanged with erythema right >left, ulcer on columella	Erythema bilaterally	Mild improvement
3-3	Normal	Erythema, medial left nare	Normal	No change
3-4	Erythema, minimal to moderate bilaterally, minimal blood left nare	No change	No change	Erythema, minimal, right nare
3-5	Mild clear discharge bilaterally	Normal mucosa bilaterally	Normal mucosa bilaterally; slight clear-white discharge	Not applicable
3-6	Bloody yellow secretions bilaterally	Erythema, mild, bilaterally	Erythema, mild, bilaterally	Erythema, mild
3-7	Erythema, mild, upper left turbinate and right nare	Erythema, mild, bilaterally with clear drainage	Small white plaque, left nare, mild erythema bilaterally	Erythema, minimal, bilaterally
3-8	Erythema, mild, turbinates bilaterally	Clear drainage bilaterally, slight increased erythema left nare, mild erythema right nare	Erythema, moderate, right turbinate	Erythema, mild, right nare

patients, because this has broad potential applications in patients with brain-injury cardiac arrest and large hemispheric infarcts.

M. Mathru, MD

Risk Factors Associated with Ischemic Optic Neuropathy after Spinal Fusion Surgery

The Postoperative Visual Loss Study Group (Univ of Washington School of Medicine, Seattle; Univ of Chicago, IL; Univ of Iowa Carver College of Medicine; et al)
Anesthesiology 116:15-24, 2012

Background.—Perioperative visual loss, a rare but dreaded complication of spinal fusion surgery, is most commonly caused by ischemic optic neuropathy (ION). The authors sought to determine risk factors for ION in this setting.

Methods.—Using a multicenter case-control design, the authors compared 80 adult patients with ION from the American Society of Anesthesiologists Postoperative Visual Loss Registry with 315 adult control subjects without ION after spinal fusion surgery, randomly selected from 17 institutions, and matched by year of surgery. Preexisting medical conditions and perioperative factors were compared between patients and control subjects using stepwise multivariate analysis to assess factors that might predict ION.

Results.—After multivariate analysis, risk factors for ION after spinal fusion surgery included male sex (odds ratio [OR] 2.53, 95% CI 1.35–4.91, $P = 0.005$), obesity (OR 2.83, 95% CI 1.52–5.39, $P = 0.001$), Wilson frame use (OR 4.30, 95% CI 2.13–8.75, $P < 0.001$), anesthesia duration (OR per 1 h = 1.39, 95% CI 1.22–1.58, $P < 0.001$), estimated blood loss (OR per 1 l = 1.34, 95% CI 1.13–1.61, $P = 0.001$), and colloid as percent of non-blood replacement (OR per 5% = 0.67, 95% CI 0.52–0.82, $P < 0.001$). After cross-validation, area under the curve = 0.85, sensitivity = 0.79, and specificity = 0.82.

Conclusions.—This is the first study to assess ION risk factors in a large, multicenter case-control fashion with detailed perioperative data. Obesity, male sex, Wilson frame use, longer anesthetic duration, greater estimated blood loss, and decreased percent colloid administration were significantly and independently associated with ION after spinal fusion surgery (Tables 3 and 4).

▶ Ischemic optic neuropathy is a rare but devastating complication most commonly associated with prone spine surgery. Due to the rarity of the complication, determination of etiology, risk factors, and preventative maneuvers have proven to be difficult. This is a case-control study using cases reported to the American Society of Anesthesiologists Postoperative Vision Loss Registry and matched controls from multiple institutions performing large numbers of spine procedures. From this work, several risk factors are identified: male sex, obesity, use of the Wilson frame, duration, blood loss, and lower percentage use of colloid

TABLE 3.—Multivariate Regression Analysis*

	Stage 1 Model Preexisting Conditions		Stage 2 Model Predetermined Procedural Factors		Stage 3 Model Potentially Modifiable Intraoperative Procedural Factors		Stage 4 Model Potentially Modifiable Intraoperative Management Factors	
	OR (95% CI)	P Value	OR (95% CI)	P Value	OR (95% CI)	P Value	OR (95% CI)	P Value
Male	2.80 (1.66–4.85)	<0.001	2.49 (1.46–4.37)	0.001	2.72 (1.47–5.18)	0.002	2.53 (1.35–4.91)	0.005
Obesity	2.38 (1.43–3.99)	<0.001	2.07 (1.22–3.53)	0.007	2.35 (1.30–4.32)	0.005	2.83 (1.52–5.39)	0.001
Wilson	—	—	3.40 (1.90–6.06)	<0.001	4.87 (2.48–9.68)	<0.001	4.30 (2.13–8.75)	<0.001
Anesthesia duration (hr), OR per 1 h	—	—	—	—	1.32 (1.18–1.50)	<0.001	1.39 (1.22–1.58)	<0.001
Estimated blood loss (l), OR per 1 l	—	—	—	—	1.31 (1.12–1.54)	<0.001	1.34 (1.13–1.61)	0.001
Colloid as % of nonblood replacement, OR per 5%	—	—	—	—	—	—	0.67 (0.52–0.82)	<0.001
AUC (all data/cross-validation)	0.64/0.60	—	0.71/0.71	—	0.85/0.83	—	0.87/0.85	—
Sensitivity† (all data/crossvalidation)	0.69/0.36	—	0.55/0.63	—	0.85/0.88	—	0.81/0.79	—
Specificity† (all data/crossvalidation)	0.54/0.86	—	0.80/0.73	—	0.73/0.65	—	0.82/0.80	—

AUC = area under the curve; OR = odds ratio.

*Only variables with $P < 0.2$ in the univariate analysis (table 1 in original article) were considered. Selection criterion: $P < 0.05$. At the end of each stage, interactions were tested for variables in the model and were added if $P < 0.01$ (no interactions in this model had P values < 0.01). The same model was derived using backward elimination ($P < 0.05$ for exclusion). The following variables were considered: stage 1: sex, obesity, diabetes, hypertension, atherosclerosis, clinic systolic blood pressure, clinic mean arterial blood pressure; stage 2: Wilson frame; stage 3: anesthesia duration and estimated blood loss, stage 4: lowest intraoperative hematocrit, systolic or mean arterial blood pressure ≥40% below baseline 30 min, and colloid as percent of nonblood replacement. Because of the high correlation with anesthesia duration, estimated blood loss, total volume replacement and total nonblood replacement variables (table 2 in original article), colloid as percent of nonblood replacement was chosen as the volume variable considered in stage 4 of the multivariate analysis (see Discussion). Alternative multivariate models including total nonblood replacement in stage 4 are shown in Supplemental Digital Content 1, tables describing these models, http://links.lww.com/ALN/A793.

†This combination of sensitivity and specificity optimizes the sum of the two. Other combinations can be calculated with trade-offs between better/worse sensitivity combined with worse/better specificity, respectively.

TABLE 4.—Risk Prediction for ION after Major Spine Surgery: Effect of Changes in Variables on ION Risk

Sex	Obesity	Wilson Frame	Anesthesia (h)	EBL (l)	Colloid (%)*	Absolute Risk of ION per 10,000 Procedures[†] (Based on 0.017% Overall Rate)	Absolute Risk of ION per 10,000 Procedures[†] (Based on 0.1% Overall Rate)	Relative Risk[‡]
Female	**No**	**No**	**5**	**1**	**10**	**0.08**	**0.45**	**1.00**[§]
Female	Yes	No	5	1	10	0.22	1.27	2.83
Female	No	Yes	5	1	10	0.33	1.93	4.30
Female	No	No	7.5	1	10	0.17	1.01	2.26
Female	No	No	10	1	10	0.39	2.30	5.12
Female	No	No	5	2	10	0.10	0.60	1.34
Female	No	No	5	3	10	0.14	0.80	1.78
Female	No	No	5	1	0	0.17	1.00	2.24
Female	**Yes**	**Yes**	**10**	**3**	**0**	**18.98**	**111.67**	**249.27**
Male	No	No	5	1	10	0.19	1.14	2.53
Male	Yes	No	5	1	10	0.55	3.21	7.17
Male	No	Yes	5	1	10	0.83	4.89	10.91
Male	No	No	7.5	1	10	0.44	2.57	5.74
Male	No	No	10	1	10	0.99	5.82	12.98
Male	No	No	5	2	10	0.26	1.52	3.39
Male	No	No	5	3	10	0.34	2.03	4.52
Male	No	No	5	1	0	0.43	2.54	5.67
Male	**Yes**	**Yes**	**10**	**3**	**0**	**48.11**	**283.00**	**631.73**

Variables in bold and shaded areas indicate changes in risk factors from the female reference patient with the lowest risk variables in this table (bold, first line), to demonstrate the effect on the range of absolute and relative risks of ION using examples of common clinical scenarios. For example, a male patient has an increased relative risk = 2.53 for ION compared with the reference female patient, with an absolute risk range of 0.19−1.14 per 10,000 procedures; an obese female patient has an increased relative risk=2.83 for ION compared with the reference nonobese female patient, with an absolute risk range of 0.22−1.27 per 10,000 procedures; a female patient placed on a Wilson frame has an increased relative risk=4.30 for ION compared with the reference female patient (non-Wilson frame), with an absolute risk range of 0.33−1.93 per 10,000 procedures; etc. The highest risk variables for females and males are shown in the last row of each sex group. In this table, the clinical scenario with the highest risk variables for males (obese, Wilson frame use, 10-h duration, 3 l EBL, no colloid in the total nonblood replacement) has a 631-fold increased risk of ION compared with the clinical scenario with the lowest risk variables for females (nonobese, no Wilson frame use, 5-h duration, 1 l EBL, and 10% colloid of total nonblood replacement).

EBL = estimated blood loss; ION = ischemic optic neuropathy.

Editor's Note: Please refer to original journal article for full references.

*Colloid as % of total non-blood replacement, where total non-blood replacement = (crystalloid + albumin + hetastarch).
[†]Range of low and high absolute risks of ION based on the literature from multicenter studies or national databases.[5−7]
[‡]Relative risk of ION compared with the lowest risk set of patient variables in this table: first row (bold, no shading), reference value = 1·0.
[§]Reference category for relative risk: female, non-obese, non-Wilson frame, 5 h anesthesia duration, 1 l EBL, and 10% colloid of non-blood replacement administered, first row (bold, no shading).

as a portion of nonblood infusions (Table 3). Most of these predictors of risk do not offer opportunities for prevention but do provide evidence to guide discussions of risk (Table 4). This article helps guide our care, in particular, helping patients make informed decisions.

S. Black, MD

The Success of Emergency Endotracheal Intubation in Trauma Patients: A 10-Year Experience at a Major Adult Trauma Referral Center

Stephens CT, Kahntroff S, Dutton RP (Univ of Maryland School of Medicine, Baltimore)
Anesth Analg 109:866-872, 2009

Background.—Emergency airway management is a required skill for many anesthesiologists. We studied 10 yr of experience at a Level 1 trauma center to determine the outcomes of tracheal intubation attempts within the first 24 h of admission.

Methods.—We examined Trauma Registry, quality management, and billing system records from July 1996 to June 2006 to determine the number of patients requiring intubation within 1 h of hospital arrival and to estimate the number requiring intubation with the first 24 h. We reviewed the medical record of each patient in either cohort who underwent a surgical airway access procedure (tracheotomy or cricothyrotomy) to determine the presenting characteristics of the patients and the reason they could not be orally or nasally intubated.

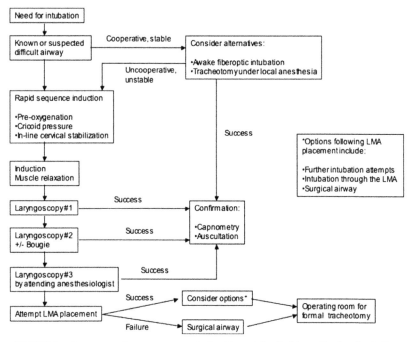

FIGURE 1.—Emergency airway management algorithm at the R Adams Cowley Shock Trauma Center. It is assumed that an airway is absolutely required and that patients cannot be reawakened electively. LMA = laryngeal mask airway. (Reprinted from Stephens CT, Kahntroff S, Dutton RP. The success of emergency endotracheal intubation in trauma patients: a 10-year experience at a major adult trauma referral center. *Anesth Analg.* 2009;109:866-872, with permission from International Anesthesia Research Society.)

Results.—All intubation attempts were supervised by an anesthesiologist experienced in trauma patient care. Rapid sequence intubation with direct laryngoscopy was the standard approach throughout the study period. During the first hour after admission, 6088 patients required intubation, of whom 21 (0.3%) received a surgical airway. During the first 24 h, 10 more patients, for a total of 31, received a surgical airway, during approximately 32,000 attempts (0.1%). Unanticipated difficult upper airway anatomy was the leading reason for a surgical airway. Four of the 31 patients died of their injuries but none as the result of failed intubation.

Conclusions.—In the hands of experienced anesthesiologists, rapid sequence intubation followed by direct laryngoscopy is a remarkably effective

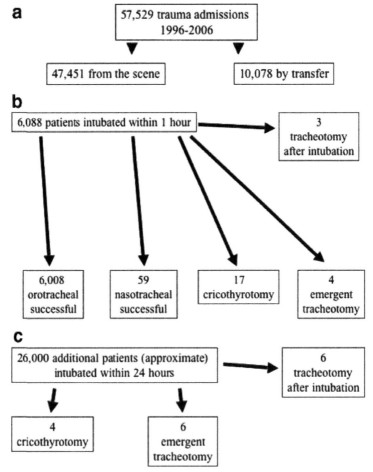

FIGURE 2.—a–c, Trauma admission and outcomes of urgent and emergency airway management. (Reprinted from Stephens CT, Kahntroff S, Dutton RP. The success of emergency endotracheal intubation in trauma patients: a 10-year experience at a major adult trauma referral center. *Anesth Analg.* 2009;109: 866-872, with permission from International Anesthesia Research Society.)

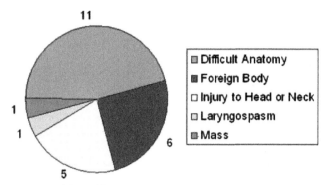

FIGURE 3.—Causes of the need for surgical airway access. (Reprinted from Stephens CT, Kahntroff S, Dutton RP. The success of emergency endotracheal intubation in trauma patients: a 10-year experience at a major adult trauma referral center. *Anesth Analg.* 2009;109:866-872, with permission from International Anesthesia Research Society.)

approach to emergency airway management. An algorithm designed around this approach can achieve very high levels of success (Figs 1-3).

▶ This large retrospective study reports on success rates and complications in trauma patients requiring intubation within the first hour and first 24 hours of admission (Fig 2). Just over 6000 patients were intubated within 1 hour during the 10 years reviewed. Of those, only 21 required a surgical airway. More than 30 000 patients were intubated within 24 hours with only 0.1% requiring a surgical airway. Morbidity related to airway management was identified in only 1 patient. There was no mortality related to failed intubations. In this center, airway management is supervised by anesthesiologists and follows an algorithm based on the American Society of Anesthesiologists difficult airway algorithm (Fig 1). Fig 3 shows causes of difficulty in airway management that led to a surgical airway. Of note, head and neck injury was a relatively common factor. In addition, as the authors note in the introduction, the rate of need for surgical airway is less than that reported recently from centers in which emergency medicine physicians manage the airways.

S. Black, MD

7 Critical Care Medicine

Adult Critical Care

A Description of Intraoperative Ventilator Management in Patients with Acute Lung Injury and the Use of Lung Protective Ventilation Strategies
Blum JM, Maile M, Park PK, et al (Univ of Michigan Health System, Ann Arbor)
Anesthesiology 115:75-82, 2011

Background.—The incidence of acute lung injury (ALI) in hypoxic patients undergoing surgery is currently unknown. Previous studies have identified lung protective ventilation strategies that are beneficial in the treatment of ALI. The authors sought to determine the incidence and examine the use of lung protective ventilation strategies in patients receiving anesthetics with a known history of ALI.

Methods.—The ventilation parameters that were used in all patients were reviewed, with an average preoperative $Paco_2/Fio_2$ ratio of ≤ 300 between January 1, 2005 and July 1, 2009. This dataset was then merged with a dataset of patients screened for ALI. The median tidal volume, positive end-expiratory pressure, peak inspiratory pressures, fraction inhaled oxygen, oxygen saturation, and tidal volumes were compared between groups.

Results.—A total of 1,286 patients met criteria for inclusion; 242 had a diagnosis of ALI preoperatively. Comparison of patients with ALI *versus* those without ALI found statistically yet clinically insignificant differences between the ventilation strategies between the groups in peak inspiratory pressures and positive end-expiratory pressure but no other category. The tidal volumes in cc/kg predicted body weight were approximately 8.7 in both groups. Peak inspiratory pressures were found to be 27.87 cm H_2O on average in the non-ALI group and 29.2 in the ALI group.

Conclusion.—Similar ventilation strategies are used between patients with ALI and those without ALI. These findings suggest that anesthesiologists are not using lung protective ventilation strategies when ventilating patients with low $Paco_2/Fio_2$ ratios and ALI, and instead are treating

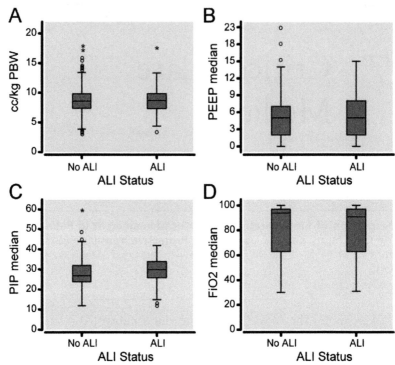

FIGURE 2.—(A–D) Distribution of ventilator settings by ALI status. (A) cc of ventilation per kg PBW by ALI status. *Solid lines* represent median values, *boxes* represent the interquartile range, *T bars* represent 95% of total sample, O represent outliers (1.5–3 X box length), * represent extreme outliers (more than 3 X box length). (B) Median positive end-expiratory pressure (PEEP) by ALI status. *Solid lines* represent median values, *boxes* represent the interquartile range, *T bars* represent 95% of total sample, O represent outliers (1.5–3 X box length), * represent extreme outliers (more than 3 X box length). (C) Median PIP by ALI status. *Solid lines* represent median values, *boxes* represent the interquartile range, *T bars* represent 95% of total sample, O represent outliers (1.5–3 X box length), * represent extreme outliers (more than three times box length). (D) Median FiO_2 by ALI status. *Solid lines* represent median values, *boxes* represent the interquartile range, *T bars* represent 95% of total sample, O represent outliers (1.5–3 X box length), * represents extreme outliers (more than 3 X box length). ALI = acute lung injury; FiO_2 = fraction inspired oxygen; PBW = predicted body weight; PEEP = positive end expiratory pressure; PIP = peak inspiratory pressure. (Reprinted from Blum JM, Maile M, Park PK, et al. A description of intraoperative ventilator management in patients with acute lung injury and the use of lung protective ventilation strategies. *Anesthesiology.* 2011;115:75-82, with permission from the American Society of Anesthesiologists, Inc.)

hypoxia and ALI with higher concentrations of oxygen and peak pressures (Figs 2, Tables 4 and 5).

▶ Protective ventilatory strategy is the standard of practice in the management of acute respiratory distress syndrome (ARDS) patients. There is considerable evidence suggesting that acute lung injury (ALI) outcomes are improved if patients are treated using lung protective ventilatory strategies (LPVS) while they are in the intensive care unit (ICU). In this retrospective review, 20% of patients who meet the criteria for ALI ($PaCO_2/FiO_2$ ratio < 300) were treated intraoperatively in the usual manner, such as increasing FiO_2, tolerating high

TABLE 4.—Preoperative and Intraoperative Ventilator Settings for All Patients

	N	Preoperative Mean	SD	Intraoperative Mean	SD	P Value
F$_{IO_2}$	719	52.13	21.56	81.61	20.14	<.001
PIP	668	26.41	5.99	28.18	6.16	<.001
V$_t$	703	551.74	119.46	564.06	124.66	.009
cc/kg PBW	703	8.41	1.71	8.64	1.99	.002
PEEP	695	6.61	2.45	5.20	3.71	<.001

A comparison of preoperative and intraoperative ventilator settings for all patients using the paired Student *t* test or Wilcoxon signed-rank test.

F$_{IO_2}$ = fraction inspired oxygen; PBW = predicted body weight; PEEP = positive end expiratory pressure; PIP = peak inspiratory pressure; V$_T$ = tidal volume.

TABLE 5.—Preoperative and Intraoperative Ventilator Settings for Patients with Preoperative ALI

	N	Preoperative Mean	SD	Intraoperative Mean	SD	P Value
F$_{IO_2}$	149	47.99	15.06	82.38	18.63	<.001
PIP	138	27.83	6.47	30.17	6.19	<.001
V$_T$	144	535.53	131.25	556.31	146.28	.092
cc/kg PBW	144	8.25	1.97	8.58	2.18	.098
PEEP	140	6.82	2.39	5.86	3.72	<.001

A comparison of preoperative and intraoperative ventilator settings for ALI patients using the paired Student *t* test or Wilcoxon signed-rank test.

ALI = acute lung injury; F$_{IO_2}$ = fraction of inspired oxygen; PBW = predicted body weight; PEEP = positive end expiratory pressure; PIP = peak inspiratory pressure; V$_T$ = tidal volume.

positive-end expiratory pressure (PEEP), and prescribing lower amount of PEEP than prescribed by the ARDS network group, and they tend to use pre-existing ventilator settings that are similar to those found in the ICU. This study convincingly shows that anesthesiologists are favoring increased oxygen-ation over a proven modality in the treatment of ALI. This is shown by increased intraoperative Pao$_2$ compared with the preoperative Pao$_2$. This reluctance of the anesthesiologist to follow ARDS net protocol may be based on the premise that LPVS would be harmful because of potentially increased cytokines from increased PEEP and potential hypercapnia in patients who do not have ALI. However, it has been shown that LPVS does not increase biologic markers of lung injury in normal lung. Future prospective studies should determine if the use of LPVS intraoperatively has any impact on reducing mortality of hypoxic patients who undergo surgery both with and without ALI.

M. Mathru, MD

A Randomized and Blinded Single-Center Trial Comparing the Effect of Intracranial Pressure and Intracranial Pressure Wave Amplitude-Guided Intensive Care Management on Early Clinical State and 12-Month Outcome in Patients With Aneurysmal Subarachnoid Hemorrhage

Eide PK, Bentsen G, Sorteberg AG, et al (Oslo Univ Hosp-Rikshospitalet, Norway)

Neurosurgery 69:1105-1115, 2011

Background.—In patients with aneurysmal subarachnoid hemorrhage (SAH), preliminary results indicate that the amplitude of the single intracranial pressure (ICP) wave is a better predictor of the early clinical state and 6-month outcome than the mean ICP.

Objective.—To perform a randomized and blinded single-center trial comparing the effect of mean ICP vs mean ICP wave amplitude (MWA)-guided intensive care management on early clinical state and outcome in patients with aneurysmal SAH.

Methods.—Patients were randomized to 2 different types of ICP management: maintenance of mean ICP less than 20 mm Hg and MWA less than 5 mm Hg. Early clinical state was assessed daily using the Glasgow Coma Scale. The primary efficacy variable was 12-month outcome in terms of the Rankin Stroke Score.

Results.—Ninety-seven patients were included in the study. There were no significant differences in treatment between the 2 groups apart from a larger volume of cerebrospinal fluid drained during week 1 in the MWA group. There was a tendency toward higher Glasgow Coma Scale scores in the MWA group during weeks 1 ($P=.08$) and 2 ($P=.07$). Outcome in terms of Rankin Stroke Score at 12 months was significantly better in the MWA group ($P < .05$).

Conclusion.—This randomized and blinded trial disclosed a significant better primary efficacy variable (Rankin Stroke Score after 12 months) in the MWA patient group. We suggest that proactive intensive care management with MWA-tailored cerebrospinal fluid drainage during the first week improves aneurysmal SAH outcome (Fig 3, Table 4).

▶ Nearly 30 000 patients are admitted to neurological intensive care units with the diagnosis of subarachnoid hemorrhage (SAH). Although aneurysm repair by surgical clipping or endovascular treatment plays a key role in the management of SAH patients, subsequent critical care management is critical for the outcome. Controlling intracranial pressure (ICP) and maintaining cerebral perfusion pressure levels are core elements of intensive care management. ICP control is usually accomplished by external ventricular drainage and osmotherapy. In recent years, the ICP wave-guided management is used instead of controlling mean ICP. The ICP mean wave amplitude (MWA) is related to intracranial compliance and intracranial volume-reserve capacity. The ICP wave amplitude was caused by cardiac contraction, creating a net change in intracranial volume of approximately 1 mL. In this randomized, blinded trial, the authors compared the effects of ICP and ICP pressure wave amplitude-guided management in

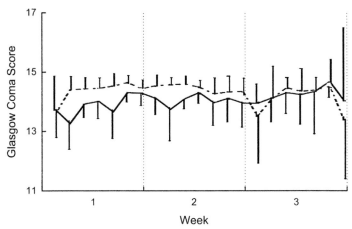

FIGURE 3.—The average daily Glasgow Coma Scale (GCS) score is plotted for weeks 1 to 3 after subarachnoid hemorrhage for the mean intracranial pressure (ICP) (solid line) and mean ICP wave amplitude (MWA) (dotted line) groups (error bars represent the 95% confidence interval). The daily GCS score was borderline significantly higher in the MWA group than the ICP group during weeks 1 ($P = .08$) and 2 ($P = .07$), but not during week 3 ($P = .9$). The change over time in GCS score was significantly different between groups ($P = .02$; mixed-model analysis). Total number of observations for the entire period: ICP group ($n = 345$), MWA group ($n = 385$). (Reprinted from Eide PK, Bentsen G, Sorteberg AG, et al. A randomized and blinded single-center trial comparing the effect of intracranial pressure and intracranial pressure wave amplitude-guided intensive care management on early clinical state and 12-month outcome in patients with aneurysmal subarachnoid hemorrhage. *Neurosurgery.* 2011;69:1105-1115, with permission from the Congress of Neurological Surgeons.)

TABLE 4.—Outcome Data 12 Months After Subarachnoid Hemorrhage[a]

	Rankin Stroke Score	ICP Group (%)	MWA Group (%)
0	No symptoms at all	5 (10.2)	15 (31.3)
1	No significant disability despite symptoms; able to carry out all usual duties and activities	20 (40.8)	9 (18.8)
2	Slight disability; unable to carry out all previous activities, but able to look after own affairs without assistance	8 (16.3)	6 (12.5)
3	Moderate disability; requiring some help, but able to walk without assistance	2 (4.1)	4 (8.3)
4	Moderately severe disability; unable to walk without assistance and unable to attend to own bodily needs without assistance	3 (6.1)	3 (6.3)
5	Severe disability; bedridden, incontinent, and requiring constant nursing care and attention	2 (4.1)	4 (8.3)
6	Dead	9 (18.4)	7 (14.6)
Total		49	48

[a]Overall difference between ICP and MWA groups: $P < .05$ (Pearson χ^2; Rankin Stroke Score categories 2 and 3 were combined, and 4 and 5 were combined because of small numbers in each cell). ICP, intracranial pressure; MWA, mean intracranial pressure wave amplitude.

patients with SAH. This study convincingly demonstrates more favorable outcomes in the MWA group compared with traditional mean ICP management. The precise mechanism behind this improved outcome in MWA is not elucidated in this study. The authors speculate that a low MWA could have contributed to rescuing functional penumbra by optimizing the conditions of the brain, promoting recovery of brain cells that may succumb under less favorable conditions. The authors should be congratulated for this excellent clinical study.

M. Mathru, MD

A randomized trial of recombinant human granulocyte-macrophage colony stimulating factor for patients with acute lung injury

Paine R III, Standiford TJ, Dechert RE, et al (Univ of Michigan Med School, Ann Arbor; et al)

Crit Care Med 40:90-97, 2012

Rationale.—Despite recent advances in critical care and ventilator management, acute lung injury and acute respiratory distress syndrome continue to cause significant morbidity and mortality. Granulocyte-macrophage colony stimulating factor may be beneficial for patients with acute respiratory distress syndrome.

Objectives.—To determine whether intravenous infusion of granulocyte-macrophage colony stimulating factor would improve clinical outcomes for patients with acute lung injury/acute respiratory distress syndrome.

Design.—A randomized, double-blind, placebo-controlled clinical trial of human recombinant granulocyte-macrophage colony stimulating factor vs. placebo. The primary outcome was days alive and breathing without mechanical ventilatory support within the first 28 days after randomization. Secondary outcomes included mortality and organ failure-free days.

Setting.—Medical and surgical intensive care units at three academic medical centers.

Patients.—One hundred thirty individuals with acute lung injury of at least 3 days duration were enrolled, out of a planned cohort of 200 subjects.

Interventions.—Patients were randomized to receive human recombinant granulocyte-macrophage colony stimulating factor (64 subjects, 250 $\mu g/M^2$) or placebo (66 subjects) by intravenous infusion daily for 14 days. Patients received mechanical ventilation using a lung-protective protocol.

Measurements and Main Results.—There was no difference in ventilator-free days between groups (10.7 ± 10.3 days placebo vs. 10.8 ± 10.5 days granulocyte-macrophage colony stimulating factor, $p = .82$). Differences in 28-day mortality (23% in placebo vs. 17% in patients receiving granulocyte-macrophage colony stimulating factor ($p = .31$) and organ failure-free days (12.8 ± 11.3 days placebo vs. 15.7 ± 11.9 days granulocyte-macrophage colony stimulating factor, $p = .16$) were not statistically significant. There were similar numbers of serious adverse events in each group.

Conclusions.—In a randomized phase II trial, granulocyte- macrophage colony stimulating factor treatment did not increase the number of ventilator-free days in patients with acute lung injury/acute respiratory distress syndrome. A larger trial would be required to determine whether treatment with granulocyte-macrophage colony stimulating factor might

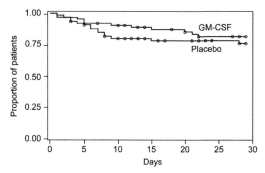

FIGURE 1.—Patient survival through day 29 after randomization. $p = .31$ using log-rank test. *GM-CSF*, granulocyte-macrophage colony stimulating factor. (Reprinted from Paine R III, Standiford TJ, Dechert RE, et al. A randomized trial of recombinant human granulocyte-macrophage colony stimulating factor for patients with acute lung injury. *Crit Care Med*. 2012;40:90-97, with permission from the Society of Critical Care Medicine and Lippincott Williams & Wilkins.)

alter important clinical outcomes, such as mortality or multiorgan failure. (ClinicalTrials.gov number, NCT00201409 [ClinicalTrials.gov]) (Fig 1).

▶ In acute lung injury protective ventilatory strategy and restrictive approach to fluid management have been shown to improve patient outcomes in large multicenter randomized trials. To date, the search for pharmacologic interventions targeted to the pathophysiology of acute respiratory distress syndrome (ARDS) have been disappointing. New therapeutic approaches are constantly being investigated by different groups to improve outcome in patients with ARDS. Granulocyte colony stimulating factor (GM-GSF) plays a pivotal role in the normal pulmonary homeostasis, including maturation of alveolar homeostasis and thus surfactant clearance and for the growth and survival of alveolar epithelial cells, which are the primary site of lung injury. In humans with lung injury, increased expression of GM-GSF in bronchoalveolar lavage fluid is correlated with increased survival, supporting the hypothesis that GM-GSF plays a critical role in the injured lung. In this randomized controlled, multicenter study, the investigators examined the efficacy of GM-GSF in patients with lung injury. The primary outcomes was days free from mechanical ventilation in the first 28 days, and secondary outcomes included 28-day mortality and duration of organ failure. Their results show no difference in ventilator-free days between patients treated with GM-GSF and those treated with placebo. Furthermore, there was no difference in the secondary end points, mortality, and organ failure-free days. The potential reasons for the failure of GM-GSF to show any beneficial effect in lung injury may include the following: preclinical data concerning the effects of GM-GSF in animal models do not reflect human biology, small sample size, and the decisions concerning the timing, dose, or route of administration.

M. Mathru, MD

A Systematic Review and Meta-Analysis on the Use of Preemptive Hemodynamic Intervention to Improve Postoperative Outcomes in Moderate and High-Risk Surgical Patients

Hamilton MA, Cecconi M, Rhodes A (St George's Healthcare NHS Trust, London, UK)

Anesth Analg 112:1392-1402, 2011

Background.—Complications from major surgery are undesirable, common, and potentially avoidable. The long-term consequences of short-term surgical complications have recently been recognized to have a profound influence on longevity and quality of life in survivors. In the past 30 years, there have been a number of studies conducted attempting to reduce surgical mortality and morbidity by deliberately and preemptively manipulating perioperative hemodynamics. Early studies had a high control-group mortality rate and were criticized for this as being unrepresentative of current practice and raised opposition to its implementation as routine care. We performed this review to update this body of literature and to examine the effect of changes in current practice and quality of care to see whether the conclusions from previous quantitative analyses of this field remain valid.

Methods.—Randomized clinical trials evaluating the use of preemptive hemodynamic intervention to improve surgical outcome were identified using multiple methods. Electronic databases (MEDLINE, EMBASE, and the Cochrane Controlled Clinical Trials register) were screened for potential trials, reference lists of identified trials were examined, and additional sources were sought from experts and industry representatives. Identified studies that fulfilled the entry criteria were examined in full and subjected to quantifiable analysis, subgroup analysis, and sensitivity analysis where possible.

Results.—There were 29 studies identified, 23 of which reported surgical complications. In total, the 29 trials involved 4805 patients with an overall mortality of 7.6%. The use of preemptive hemodynamic intervention significantly reduced mortality (pooled odds ratio [95% confidence interval] of 0.48 [0.33–0.78]; $P = 0.0002$) and surgical complications (odds ratio 0.43 [0.34–0.53]; $P < 0.0001$). Subgroup analysis showed significant reductions in mortality for studies using a pulmonary artery catheter, supranormal resuscitation targets, studies using cardiac index or oxygen delivery as goals, and the use of fluids and inotropes as opposed to fluids alone. By contrast, there was a significant reduction in morbidity for each of the 4 subgroups analyzed.

Conclusion.—The use of a preemptive strategy of hemodynamic monitoring and coupled therapy reduces surgical mortality and morbidity (Figs 4 and 5).

▶ Preemptive optimization of hemodynamics in the perioperative period to reduce postoperative complications and improve outcome has been in use for at least the past 3 decades. Previous systematic reviews and meta-analysis have demonstrated reduced morbidity and mortality with this approach. However,

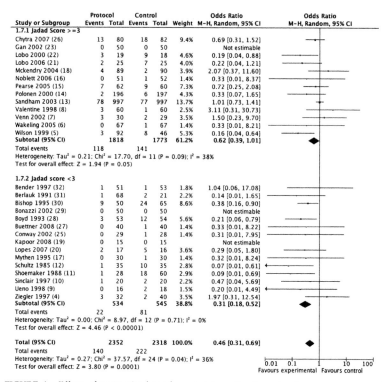

Study or Subgroup	Protocol Events	Total	Control Events	Total	Weight	Odds Ratio M-H, Random, 95% CI
1.7.1 Jadad Score >=3						
Chytra 2007 (26)	13	80	18	82	9.4%	0.69 [0.31, 1.52]
Gan 2002 (23)	0	50	0	50		Not estimable
Lobo 2000 (22)	3	19	9	18	4.6%	0.19 [0.04, 0.88]
Lobo 2006 (21)	2	25	7	25	4.0%	0.22 [0.04, 1.21]
Mckendry 2004 (18)	4	89	2	90	3.9%	2.07 [0.37, 11.60]
Noblett 2006 (16)	0	51	1	52	1.4%	0.33 [0.01, 8.37]
Pearse 2005 (15)	7	62	9	60	7.3%	0.72 [0.25, 2.08]
Polonen 2000 (14)	2	196	6	197	4.3%	0.33 [0.07, 1.65]
Sandham 2003 (13)	78	997	77	997	13.7%	1.01 [0.73, 1.41]
Valentine 1998 (8)	3	60	1	60	2.5%	3.11 [0.31, 30.73]
Venn 2002 (7)	3	30	2	29	3.5%	1.50 [0.23, 9.70]
Wakeling 2005 (6)	0	67	1	67	1.4%	0.33 [0.01, 8.21]
Wilson 1999 (5)	3	92	8	46	5.3%	0.16 [0.04, 0.64]
Subtotal (95% CI)		**1818**		**1773**	**61.2%**	**0.62 [0.39, 1.01]**
Total events	118		141			

Heterogeneity: Tau² = 0.21; Chi² = 17.70, df = 11 (P = 0.09); I² = 38%
Test for overall effect: Z = 1.94 (P = 0.05)

Study or Subgroup	Protocol Events	Total	Control Events	Total	Weight	Odds Ratio M-H, Random, 95% CI
1.7.2 Jadad score <3						
Bender 1997 (32)	1	51	1	53	1.8%	1.04 [0.06, 17.08]
Berlauk 1991 (31)	1	68	2	21	2.2%	0.14 [0.01, 1.65]
Bishop 1995 (30)	9	50	24	65	8.6%	0.38 [0.16, 0.90]
Bonazzi 2002 (29)	0	50	0	50		Not estimable
Boyd 1993 (28)	3	53	12	54	5.6%	0.21 [0.06, 0.79]
Buettner 2008 (27)	0	40	1	40	1.4%	0.33 [0.01, 8.22]
Conway 2002 (25)	0	29	1	28	1.4%	0.31 [0.01, 7.95]
Kapoor 2008 (19)	0	15	0	15		Not estimable
Lopes 2007 (20)	2	17	5	16	3.6%	0.29 [0.05, 1.80]
Mythen 1995 (17)	0	30	1	30	1.4%	0.32 [0.01, 8.24]
Schultz 1985 (12)	1	35	10	35	2.8%	0.07 [0.01, 0.61]
Shoemaker 1988 (11)	1	28	18	60	2.9%	0.09 [0.01, 0.69]
Sinclair 1997 (10)	1	20	2	20	2.2%	0.47 [0.04, 5.69]
Ueno 1998 (9)	0	16	2	18	1.5%	0.20 [0.01, 4.49]
Ziegler 1997 (4)	3	32	2	40	3.5%	1.97 [0.31, 12.54]
Subtotal (95% CI)		**534**		**545**	**38.8%**	**0.31 [0.18, 0.52]**
Total events	22		81			

Heterogeneity: Tau² = 0.00; Chi² = 8.97, df = 12 (P = 0.71); I² = 0%
Test for overall effect: Z = 4.46 (P < 0.00001)

Total (95% CI)		**2352**		**2318**	**100.0%**	**0.46 [0.31, 0.69]**
Total events	140		222			

Heterogeneity: Tau² = 0.27; Chi² = 37.57, df = 24 (P = 0.04); I² = 36%
Test for overall effect: Z = 3.80 (P = 0.0001)

0.01 0.1 1 10 100
Favours experimental   Favours control

FIGURE 4.—Effects of preemptive hemodynamic intervention in protocol group versus control on mortality rate, grouped by quality of the study as assessed by a Jadad score of more than or less than 3. M-H = Mantel-Haenszel. (Reprinted from Hamilton MA, Cecconi M, Rhodes A. A systematic review and meta-analysis on the use of preemptive hemodynamic intervention to improve postoperative outcomes in moderate and high-risk surgical patients. *Anesth Analg.* 2011;112:1392-1402, with permission from International Anesthesia Research Society.)

previous studies were done with invasive flow directed catheters to improve hemodynamics. Accordingly, there is an updated need for meta-analysis and review, because most of the current studies have used relatively noninvasive methods, such as esophageal Doppler-based systems and arterial pressure analysis. The current study was undertaken to explore whether the preemptive strategy of hemodynamic monitoring and manipulation in the perioperative period for moderate- and high-risk surgical patients can improve postoperative outcome.

The current meta-analysis convincingly demonstrates that preemptive hemodynamically targeted therapy in the perioperative period can reduce both morbidity and mortality after surgery. The study also showed that control group mortality decreased over time. This is attributed to improved overall care of patients, as well as to clinicians learning from previous studies and applying those principles in the care of lower risk groups. However, the study has a few limitations: no attempt was made to correct for the type or quantity of fluid or inotropes given; also, the meta-analysis was done in groups of patients rather than with individual patient data. Nevertheless this meta-analysis suggests that a preemptive targeted

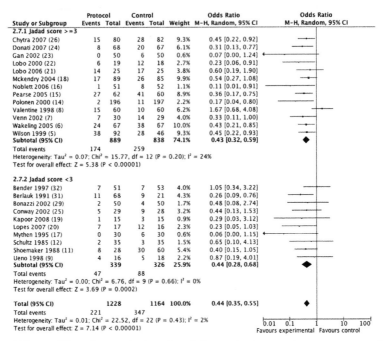

FIGURE 5.—Effects of preemptive hemodynamic intervention in protocol group versus control on complication rate, grouped by quality of the study as assessed by a Jadad score of more than or less than 3. M-H = Mantel-Haenszel. (Reprinted from Hamilton MA, Cecconi M, Rhodes A. A systematic review and meta-analysis on the use of preemptive hemodynamic intervention to improve postoperative outcomes in moderate and high-risk surgical patients. *Anesth Analg.* 2011;112:1392-1402, with permission from International Anesthesia Research Society.)

approach to the management of hemodynamics in the perioperative period may reduce morbidity and mortality for high-risk surgical patients.

M. Mathru, MD

Accuracy of a continuous noninvasive hemoglobin monitor in intensive care unit patients

Frasca D, Dahyot-Fizelier C, Catherine K, et al (Centre Hospitalier Universitaire de Poitiers, France)
Crit Care Med 39:2277-2282, 2011

Objective.—To determine whether noninvasive hemoglobin measurement by Pulse CO-Oximetry could provide clinically acceptable absolute and trend accuracy in critically ill patients, compared to other invasive methods of hemoglobin assessment available at bedside and the gold standard, the laboratory analyzer.

Design.—Prospective study.

Setting.—Surgical intensive care unit of a university teaching hospital.

Patients.—Sixty-two patients continuously monitored with Pulse CO-Oximetry (Masimo Radical-7).

Interventions.—None.

Measurements and Results.—Four hundred seventy-one blood samples were analyzed by a point-of-care device (HemoCue 301), a satellite lab CO-Oximeter (Siemens RapidPoint 405), and a laboratory hematology analyzer (Sysmex XT-2000i), which was considered the reference device. Hemoglobin values reported from the invasive methods were compared to the values reported by the Pulse CO-Oximeter at the time of blood draw. When the case-to-case variation was assessed, the bias and limits of agreement were 0.0 ± 1.0 g/dL for the Pulse CO-Oximeter, 0.3 ± 1.3 g/dL for the point-of-care device, and 0.9 ± 0.6 g/dL for the satellite lab CO-Oximeter compared to the reference method. Pulse CO-Oximetry showed similar trend accuracy as satellite lab CO-Oximetry, whereas the point-of-care device did not appear to follow the trend of the laboratory analyzer as well as the other test devices.

Conclusion.—When compared to laboratory reference values, hemoglobin measurement with Pulse CO-Oximetry has absolute accuracy and trending accuracy similar to widely used, invasive methods of hemoglobin

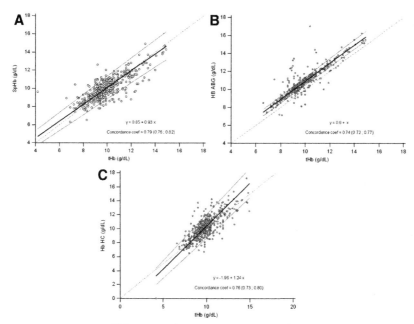

FIGURE 1.—Passing-Bablok regression for Pulse CO-Oximetry, *SpHb* (*A*), satellite lab CO-Oximeter, HbABG (*B*), and HemoCue point-of-care device, *HbHC* (*C*) vs. Laboratory Hematology Analyzer (*tHb*). *The solid line* is line of regression and the *dashed lines* represent confidence interval for regression line. *The dotted line* is line of identity. (Reprinted from Frasca D, Dahyot-Fizelier C, Catherine K, et al. Accuracy of a continuous noninvasive hemoglobin monitor in intensive care unit patients. *Crit Care Med.* 2011;39:2277-2282, with permission from the Society of Critical Care Medicine and Lippincott Williams & Wilkins.)

measurement at bedside. Hemoglobin measurement with pulse CO-Oximetry has the additional advantages of providing continuous measurements, noninvasively, which may facilitate hemoglobin monitoring in the intensive care unit (Figs 1-3).

▶ Anemia is a common occurrence in critically ill patients. Diagnosis of anemia requires a blood sample for measurement of hemoglobin. Laboratory hemoglobin analyzers utilize sodium lauryl sulphate to determine hemoglobin concentration. The recently refined Pulse CO-Oximeter provides an immediate and continuous estimation of hemoglobin concentration without the need for repeated blood sampling. In this study, the authors examined whether noninvasive hemoglobin measurement by Pulse CO-Oximetry could provide clinically acceptable accuracy in the intensive care unit setting, defined as absolute and trend accuracy comparable to common invasive methods, ie, a CO-Oximeter and a point-of-care device. The results of the study showed that the noninvasive Pulse CO-Oximeter had the best accuracy as evidenced by the highest concordance to efficient correlation and the lowest accuracy in terms of root-mean square. The satellite lab CO-Oximeter displayed the most pronounced bias (0.9 g/L), leading to constant over-estimation of hemoglobin concentration. Moreover, neither norepinephrine administration nor hyperfusion state influenced the accuracy of the noninvasive Pulse CO-Oximeter. The noninvasive measurement permits online measurement, facilitates early detection of anemia, and helps avoid the complications, expense,

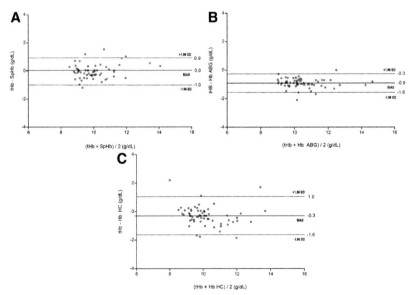

FIGURE 2.—Bland and Altman graph: Pulse CO-Oximeter, *SpHb* (*A*), satellite lab CO-Oximeter, *HbABG* (*B*), and HemoCue, *HbHC* (*C*) vs. Laboratory Hematology Analyzer, *tHb*, with the bias (*plain line*) and limits of agreement (*dotted lines*). Each point represents the bias of a single patient. (Reprinted from Frasca D, Dahyot-Fizelier C, Catherine K, et al. Accuracy of a continuous noninvasive hemoglobin monitor in intensive care unit patients. *Crit Care Med.* 2011;39:2277-2282, with permission from the Society of Critical Care Medicine and Lippincott Williams & Wilkins.)

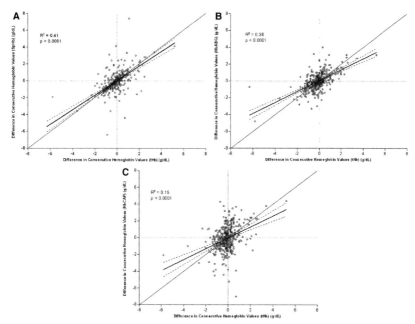

FIGURE 3.—Trend graph of hemoglobin change in consecutive measurement for Pulse CO-Oximetry, *SpHb* (A), satellite lab CO-Oximeter, *HbABG* (B), and HemoCue point-of-care device, *HbHC* (C) vs. Laboratory Hematology Analyzer (*tHb*). *The solid line* is line of regression and the *dashed lines* represent confidence interval for regression line. The plain line is line of identity. (Reprinted from Frasca D, Dahyot-Fizelier C, Catherine K, et al. Accuracy of a continuous noninvasive hemoglobin monitor in intensive care unit patients. *Crit Care Med.* 2011;39:2277-2282, with permission from the Society of Critical Care Medicine and Lippincott Williams & Wilkins.)

and discomfort associated with invasive blood draws. Despite their accuracy and convenience at very low hemoglobin levels, diagnosis and blood transfusion decisions should not be based on hemoglobin estimation with the Pulse CO-Oximeter device alone.

M. Mathru, MD

Acute kidney injury in patients with acute lung injury: Impact of fluid accumulation on classification of acute kidney injury and associated outcomes

Liu KD, for the National Institutes of Health National Heart, Lung, and Blood Institute Acute Respiratory Distress Syndrome Network (Univ of California San Francisco; et al)

Crit Care Med 39:2665-2671, 2011

Objective.—It has been suggested that fluid accumulation may delay recognition of acute kidney injury. We sought to determine the impact of fluid balance on the incidence of nondialysis requiring acute kidney injury in patients with acute lung injury and to describe associated outcomes, including mortality.

Design.—Analysis of the Fluid and Catheter Treatment Trial, a factorial randomized clinical trial of conservative vs. liberal fluid management and of management guided by a central venous vs. pulmonary artery catheter.

Setting.—Acute Respiratory Distress Syndrome Network hospitals.

Patients.—One thousand patients.

Interventions.—None.

Measurements and Main Results.—The incidence of acute kidney injury, defined as an absolute rise in creatinine of ≥ 0.3 mg/dL or a relative change of >50% over 48 hrs, was examined before and after adjustment of serum creatinine for fluid balance. The incidence of acute kidney injury before adjustment for fluid balance was greater in those managed with the conservative fluid protocol (57% vs. 51%, $p = .04$). After adjustment for fluid balance, the incidence of acute kidney injury was greater in those managed with the liberal fluid protocol (66% vs. 58%, $p = .007$). Patients who met acute kidney injury criteria after adjustment of creatinine for fluid balance (but not before) had a mortality rate that was significantly greater than those who did not meet acute kidney injury criteria both before and after adjustment for fluid balance (31% vs. 12%, $p < .001$) and those who had acute kidney injury before but not after adjustment for fluid balance (31% vs. 11%, $p = .005$). The mortality of those patients meeting acute kidney injury criteria after but not before adjustment for fluid balance was similar to patients with acute kidney injury both before and after adjustment for fluid balance (31% vs. 38%, $p = .18$).

Conclusions.—Fluid management influences serum creatinine and therefore the diagnosis of acute kidney injury using creatinine-based definitions. Patients with "unrecognized" acute kidney injury that is identified after adjusting for positive fluid balance have higher mortality rates, and patients who have acute kidney injury before but not after adjusting for fluid balance have lower mortality rates. Future studies of acute kidney injury should consider potential differences in serum creatinine caused by changes in fluid balance and the impact of these differences on diagnosis and prognosis (Table 3).

▶ Acute kidney injury (AKI) and lung injury often coexist in critically ill patients. Mortality in this population of patients increases substantially to the range of 50%–80%. Critically ill patients are often in a state of positive fluid balance. The current AKI classification system, ie, RIFLE and AKN, define AKI by using relative or absolute changes in serum creatinine without taking into account changes in positive fluid balance. In this elegantly designed study, the investigators examined the impact of positive fluid balance on more sensitive definitions of AKI. The authors hypothesized that patients who did not meet the definition of AKI using unadjusted serum creatinine values but who met criteria for AKI after adjusting creatinine for fluid balance would have poorer outcome than patients who never met AKI criteria before or after adjustment for fluid balance. The results of their study support their hypothesis: patients

TABLE 3.—Multivariable Clinical Model for Death[a]

Variable	Odds Ratio	95% Confidence Interval	p
Age[b]	1.35	1.22−1.50	<.001
Male	1.11	0.80−1.54	.53
White race	0.57	0.41−0.80	.001
Fluid conservative strategy	0.96	0.69−1.33	.81
Pulmonary artery catheter	1.02	0.74−1.41	.90
Baseline vasopressor use	1.06	0.74−1.51	.76
Baseline creatinine[c]	0.98	0.81−1.17	.81
Acute lung injury secondary to infection	1.24	0.85−1.83	.27
Acute Physiology and Chronic Health Evaluation III score[d]	1.26	1.19−1.34	<.001
No AKI before adjustment; AKI after adjustment for fluid balance (group B referent to A)	2.09	1.19−3.67	.01
AKI before adjustment; no AKI after adjustment for fluid balance (group C referent to A)	1.17	0.45−3.02	.75
AKI before AND after adjustment for fluid balance (group D referent to A)	3.16	2.04−4.87	<.001

AKI, acute kidney injury.
[a]As described in the "Methods," we controlled for age, gender, race, the trial interventions as well as other covariates that reflect the severity of acute illness, including baseline vasopressor use, the presence or absence of infection, baseline creatinine, and the Acute Physiology and Chronic Health Evaluation III score.
[b]per 10-yr increase in age.
[c]per 1-mg/dL increase in creatinine.
[d]per 10-point increase in Acute Physiology and Chronic Health Evaluation III score. Hosmer-Lemeshow goodness of fit $p = .90$.

in whom AKI was diagnosed after adjustment for fluid balance have higher mortality rates compared with patients who have AKI before but not after adjusting for fluid balance. The clinical implications of this include the following: recognizing AKI after adjustment for fluid balance indicates positive fluid balance, which carries a high mortality rate. Fluid overload per se can exacerbate AKI by tissue edema and increases in venous pressure, which can reduce the renal perfusion pressure. This needs to be addressed in future studies by using novel sensitive biomarkers of kidney injury.

M. Mathru, MD

Acute respiratory distress syndrome leads to reduced ratio of ACE/ACE2 activities and is prevented by angiotensin-(1–7) or an angiotensin II receptor antagonist

Wösten-van Asperen RM, Lutter R, Specht PA, et al (Emma Children's Hosp/ Academic Med Centre, Amsterdam, The Netherlands; Academic Med Centre, Amsterdam, The Netherlands; Erasmus Med Centre, Rotterdam, The Netherlands; et al)
J Pathol 225:618-627, 2011

Acute respiratory distress syndrome (ARDS) is a devastating clinical syndrome. Angiotensin-converting enzyme (ACE) and its effector peptide

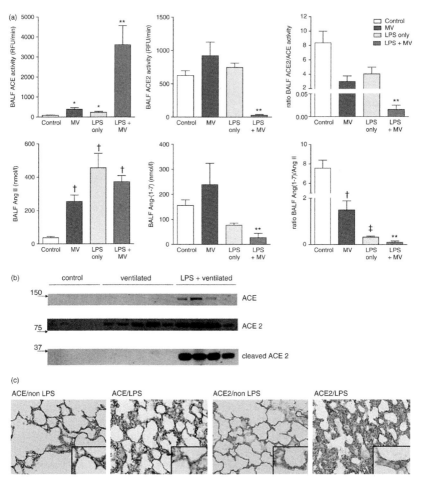

FIGURE 2.—Imbalance of the ACE/Ang II and ACE2/Ang 1−7 pathways in a rat model of ARDS. (a) BALF ACE activity, ACE2 activity and ACE2/ACE ratio, and BALF levels of Ang II and Ang-(1−7) and Ang-(1−7)/Ang II ratio in unexposed and LPS-exposed non-ventilated (spontaneously breathing) and mechanically ventilated (MV) animals. $n = 6$ per group. $*p < 0.05$ compared with control; $**p < 0.0001$ versus all other groups; $^{†}p < 0.0001$ versus control; $^{‡}p < 0.0001$ versus MV and control. (b) Western blot for ACE and ACE2 protein in equal volumes of BALF from unexposed and LPS-exposed mechanically ventilated animals. (c) Immunohistochemistry for ACE and ACE2 in lung tissue from unexposed and LPS-exposed mechanically ventilated animals. Diffuse staining was found on endothelial cells and also on epithelial cells (see inset) and infiltrating cells (macrophages, monocyte-like cells) in the alveolar walls. Representative images are shown. Original magnification 20×, inset 100×. (Reprinted from Wösten-van Asperen RM, Lutter R, Specht PA, et al. Acute respiratory distress syndrome leads to reduced ratio of ACE/ACE2 activities and is prevented by angiotensin-(1−7) or an angiotensin II receptor antagonist. *J Pathol.* 2011;225:618-627, with permission from Pathological Society of Great Britain and Ireland.)

angiotensin (Ang) II have been implicated in the pathogenesis of ARDS. A counter-regulatory enzyme of ACE, ie ACE2 that degrades Ang II to Ang-(1−7), offers a promising novel treatment modality for this syndrome. As the involvement of ACE and ACE2 in ARDS is still unclear, this study investigated the role of these two enzymes in an animal model of ARDS. ARDS

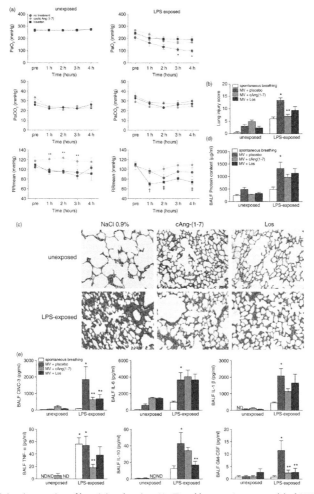

FIGURE 4.—Attenuation of lung injury by cAng-(1−7) and losartan in a rat model of ARDS. (a) Physiological parameters (PaO_2 levels, $PaCO_2$ levels, and blood pressure) of unexposed and LPS-exposed mechanically ventilated animals treated with saline, cAng-(1−7) or losartan. $n = 6$ per group. $*p < 0.05$ compared with animals treated with cAng-(1−7) or losartan, $**p < 0.05$ compared with placebo group and animals treated with losartan; $^{†}p < 0.05$ compared with placebo group and animals treated with cAng-(1−7); $^{‡}p < 0.05$ compared with animals treated with cAng-(1−7). (b) Lung injury scores. $*p < 0.05$ compared with unexposed animals; $**p < 0.05$ compared with ventilated LPS-exposed animals treated with saline (placebo). (c) Lung histopathology. Representative images are shown. Original magnification 20×. (d) BALF levels of total protein content. $*p < 0.05$ compared with unexposed and non-ventilated LPS-exposed animals. (e) BALF levels of CINC-3, interleukin (IL)-6, IL-1β, TNF-α, IL-10, and granulocyte macrophage-colony stimulating factor (GM-CSF) in BALF from unexposed and LPS-exposed non-ventilated (spontaneously breathing) and mechanically ventilated (MV) animals treated with saline (placebo), cAng-(1−7) or losartan. $n = 6$ per group. $*p < 0.01$ compared with unexposed and non-ventilated LPS-exposed animals; $**p < 0.05$ compared with ventilated LPS-exposed animals treated with saline. (Reprinted from Wösten-van Asperen RM, Lutter R, Specht PA, et al. Acute respiratory distress syndrome leads to reduced ratio of ACE/ACE2 activities and is prevented by angiotensin-(1−7) or an angiotensin II receptor antagonist. *J Pathol.* 2011;225:618-627, with permission from Pathological Society of Great Britain and Ireland.)

was induced in rats by intratracheal administration of LPS followed by mechanical ventilation. During ventilation, animals were treated with saline (placebo), losartan (Ang II receptor antagonist), or with a protease-resistant, cyclic form of Ang-(1−7) [cAng-(1−7)]. In bronchoalveolar lavage fluid (BALF) of ventilated LPS-exposed animals, ACE activity was enhanced, whereas ACE2 activity was reduced. This was matched by enhanced BALF levels of Ang II and reduced levels of Ang-(1−7). Therapeutic intervention with cAng-(1−7) attenuated the inflammatory mediator response, markedly decreased lung injury scores, and improved lung function, as evidenced by increased oxygenation. These data indicate that ARDS develops, in part, due to reduced pulmonary levels of Ang-(1−7) and that repletion of this peptide halts the development of ARDS (Figs 2 and 4).

▶ Acute respiratory distress syndrome (ARDS) is a devastating disorder that carries considerable morbidity and mortality. To this day, no pharmacologic treatment is available, and the treatment remains supportive. Previous studies have found that renin angiotensin system (RAS) plays an important role in the pathogenesis of ARDS. This is supported by the fact that BALF ACE activity was increased in animal models and human ARDS. Angiotensin-converting enzyme (ACE) and ACE2 are homologues with different key functions in the RAS. ACE cleaves Ang 1 to generate the activator Ang II, whereas ACE2 acts as negative regulator of the system by inactivating angiotensin II and generating Ang-(1−7). The current study extends the previous finding of others by showing that in a rat model of ARDS, the ACE2 activity is reduced paralleled by low amounts of Ang-(1−7). A characteristic feature of this study is that restoring the equilibrium of ACE/ACE2 activity after induction of ARDS mimics therapeutic options in the clinical situation.

M. Mathru, MD

Alternative Fluids for Prehospital Resuscitation: "Pharmacological" Resuscitation Fluids
Cotton BA (Univ of Texas Health Science Ctr at Houston)
J Trauma 70:S30-S31, 2011

Background.—Injured patients with severe hemorrhage often receive immediate resuscitation using intravenous fluids and blood products to boost blood pressure. Rapid replacement of large fluid volumes, however, increases hemorrhage volume and lowers survival compared to low-volume or delayed fluid replacement. Apparently, inadequate tissue perfusion produces gross metabolic disorders, mitochrondrial dysfunction and energy failure, severe acidosis, and free radical generation plus the consumption of endogenous antioxidants. To prevent or reduce shock-related damage, novel agents that maintain intracellular and extracellular status during active resuscitation but require no large fluid volumes have been proposed. These include pyruvate, sodium ion/hydrogen ion exchange (NHE) inhibitors, valproic acid, and dihydroepiandrosterone (DHEA). The qualities of these various "pharmacological" resuscitative fluids were evaluated.

Pyruvate.—Structurally similar to lactate but offering antioxidant and anti-inflammatory properties, pyruvate is associated with a survival benefit in hemorrhage but its use is limited by toxicity and instability. A stable lipophilic derivative, ethyl pyruvate, has been tested in animal models of hemorrhagic shock. In mice, adding ethyl pyruvate to conventional resuscitation fluids reduced tumor necrosis factor levels and improved survival, possibly because it is a reactive oxygen species scavenger. Hemorrhage-induced gut barrier dysfunction and hepatic lipid peroxidation were also reduced.

NHE Inhibitors.—NHE inhibition with methanesulfonate attenuated cardiovascular dysfunction and delayed the progression of circulatory collapse related to hypovolemia. In adult rat models of hemorrhagic shock the hemodynamic response to fluid resuscitation, blood oxygen content, and mortality at 6 and 24 hours were all improved by using an NHE-1 inhibitor.

DHEA.—The benefits of DHEA shown in male rats after hemorrhage appear to include restoring cardiac performance, improving organ perfusion, and preventing reperfusion injury. Androstenediol, a DHEA metabolite, limited cytokine production and neutrophil cell activation and attenuated liver injury in rats subjected to trauma and hemorrhagic shock, but more importantly it reduced mortality from 50% to 6%. Porcine models of DHEA supplementation, however, showed no benefit for DHEA over lactated Ringer's solution.

Valproic Acid.—Survival has also been improved with valproic acid in several animal models. Administering valproic acid rather than performing fluid resuscitation after shock improved early survival in rat models of hemorrhagic shock. In a large animal model, valproic acid treatment improved early survival, seemingly by preserving the Akt pathway, which promotes cell survival and opposes apoptosis.

Conclusions.—None of the agents described has been tested in human subjects. However, animal tests suggest a possible role for these pharmacological agents in patients suffering major hemorrhages. They eliminate the risks of blood transfusion, remove the harmful effects of cystalloids, and reduce the burden on prehospital providers and medics who carry the products, making them especially attractive for military medical uses.

▶ Aggressive fluid resuscitation is utilized to restore hemodynamics in traumatic hemorrhagic shock. However, rapid replacement of large amounts of fluid leads to increased bleeding and decreased survival compared with either low-volume or delayed fluid replacement. Organ failure following resuscitation is attributed to positive fluid balance and the global ischemia-reperfusion event. To reduce the organ failure related to fluid therapy, several novel pharmacological resuscitative fluids are designed to protect from global ischemia-reperfusion event. These fluids include ethyl pyruvate, Na^+/H^+ exchange (NHE) inhibitors, valproic acid, and dehydroepiandrosterone (DHEA).

The protective effects of ethyl pyruvate include anti-inflammation, antioxidation, and reduction in hemorrhage-induced gut barrier dysfunction.

Fluids containing NHE-3 inhibitors are protective against ischemia-reperfusion injury and are cardioprotective.

DHEA an intermediary in the synthesis of testosterone and estrogen prevents ischemia-reperfusion injury and has potent anti-inflammatory effects and has shown improved survival in experimental models. Valproic acid also improved survival in hemorrhagic shock models.

Although none of these pharmacological fluids have been tested in clinical trials, the potential for resuscitating injured patients with hemorrhagic shock without the need for blood or blood products remains quite attractive.

M. Mathru, MD

An association between decreased cardiopulmonary complications (transfusion-related acute lung injury and transfusion-associated circulatory overload) and implementation of universal leukoreduction of blood transfusions
Blumberg N, Heal JM, Gettings KF, et al (Univ of Rochester Med Ctr, NY)
Transfusion 50:2738-2744, 2010

Background.—Cardiopulmonary adverse events after transfusion include transfusion-related acute lung injury (TRALI) and transfusion-associated circulatory overload (TACO), which are potentially lethal and incompletely understood.

Study Design and Methods.—To determine whether the incidence of TRALI and TACO was affected by leukoreduction we conducted a retrospective, before-and-after study of acute transfusion reactions for the 7 years before and after introduction of universal leukoreduction in 2000, involving 778,559 blood components.

Results.—Substantial decreases occurred in the rates of TRALI (-83%; from 2.8 cases per 100,000 components before to 0.48 after universal leukoreduction; $p = 0.01$), TACO (-49%; 7.4 to 3.8 cases per 100,000; $p = 0.03$), and febrile reactions (-35%; 11.4 to 7.4 cases per 10,000; $p < 0.0001$). The incidence of allergic reactions remained unchanged (7.0 per 100,000 before and after universal leukoreduction). These outcomes were primarily attributable to decreased TRALI and/or TACO associated with red blood cell (RBC) and platelet (PLT) transfusions (-64%) with notably smaller decreases associated with fresh-frozen plasma or cryoprecipitate transfusions (-29%). The incidence of TRALI and/or TACO after 28,120 washed RBC and 69,325 washed transfusions was zero.

Conclusion.—These data suggest novel hypotheses for further testing in animal models, in prospective clinical trials, and via the new US hemovigilance system: 1) Is TACO or TRALI mitigated by leukoreduction? 2) Is the mechanism of TACO more complex than excessive blood volume? and

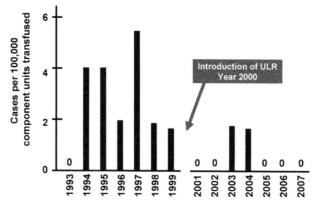

FIGURE 1.—The annual incidence of TRALI before (1993-1999) and after (2001-2007) the introduction of universal leukoreduction (ULR) in the year 2000 is shown. No cases of TRALI were reported in 5 of the 7 years after the introduction of ULR, compared with only 1 of 7 years before the introduction of ULR in which cases of TRALI were not reported. (Reprinted from Blumberg N, Heal JM, Gettings KF, et al. An association between decreased cardiopulmonary complications (transfusion-related acute lung injury and transfusion-associated circulatory overload) and implementation of universal leukoreduction of blood transfusions. *Transfusion*. 2010;50:2738-2744, with permission from John Wiley and Sons. [www.interscience. wiley.com])

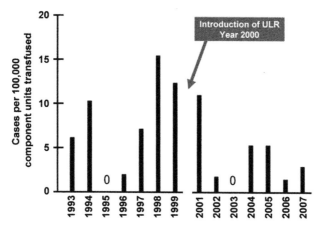

FIGURE 2.—The annual incidence of TACO before (1993-1999) and after (2001-2007) the introduction of universal leukoreduction (ULR) in the year 2000 is shown. The incidence rate was five or fewer cases per 100,000 components transfused in 6 of the 7 years after the introduction of ULR, compared with only 2 of the 7 years before the introduction of ULR. (Reprinted from Blumberg N, Heal JM, Gettings KF, et al. An association between decreased cardiopulmonary complications (transfusion-related acute lung injury and transfusion-associated circulatory overload) and implementation of universal leukoreduction of blood transfusions. *Transfusion*. 2010;50:2738-2744, with permission from John Wiley and Sons. [www.interscience.wiley.com])

3) Does washing mitigate TRALI and TACO due to PLT and RBC transfusions? (Figs 1 and 2).

▶ Transfusion-related acute lung injury (TRALI) carries high morbidity and mortality. The primary mechanism that results in TRALI includes white cell antibodies (the donors) reacting with antigen-positive cells, platelet-activating factor, and platelet-derived CD40L. Universal leukoreduction has been associated with decreased incidence of acute lung injury (ALI) in a cohort of critically ill patients. The odds ratio (OR) for mortality in ALI patients was 1.06 in recipients of leukoreduced red blood cells compared with 1.14 in recipients of nonleukoreduced RBCs in a recent cohort study. The authors examined whether leukoreduction might influence the occurrence of TRALI and transfusion-associated circulatory overload (TACO). The authors observed a significant overall decrease in the absolute number of cases and incidence per component transfused of TRALI and TACO associated with the introduction of universal leukoreduction. This raises the possibility that leukoreduction of whole blood donations influences TRALI mediated by white blood cells, platelets, and their mediators in fresh-frozen plasma as well as in red blood cells and platelets. White blood cell and platelet-derived mediators have been proposed and are increasingly accepted as potential contributors to TRALI. The authors' findings are interesting, but the study results are limited by the small sample size and retrospective nature of their data. Further investigations are necessary in a larger sample to determine whether these associations are causal and whether leukoreducton and/or washing has a significant beneficial effect in reducing the incidence of TRALI and TACO.

M. Mathru, MD

Angiotensin-Converting Enzyme N-Terminal Inactivation Alleviates Bleomycin-Induced Lung Injury
Li P, Xiao HD, Xu J, et al (Cedars-Sinai Med Ctr, Los Angeles, CA; Emory Univ, Atlanta, GA; et al)
Am J Pathol 177:1113-1121, 2010

Bleomycin has potent anti-oncogenic properties for several neoplasms, but drug administration is limited by bleomycin-induced lung fibrosis. Inhibition of the renin-angiotensin system has been suggested to decrease bleomycin toxicity, but the efficacy of such strategies remains uncertain and somewhat contradictory. Our hypothesis is that, besides angiotensin II, other substrates of angiotensin-converting enzyme (ACE), such as the tetrapeptide N-acetyl-seryl-aspartyl-lysyl-proline (AcSDKP), play a significant role in controlling fibrosis. We studied bleomycin-induced lung injury in normotensive mice, termed N-KO and C-KO, which have point mutations inactivating either the N- or C-terminal catalytic sites of ACE, respectively. N-KO, but not C-KO mice, have a marked resistance to bleomycin lung injury as assessed by lung histology and hydroxyproline content. To determine the importance of the ACE N-terminal peptide substrate AcSDKP in the resistance to bleomycin injury, N-KO mice were treated with S-17092, a prolyl-oligopeptidase inhibitor that inhibits the formation of AcSDKP. In response to bleomycin injection, S-17092-treated N-KO mice developed lung fibrosis similar to wild-type mice. In

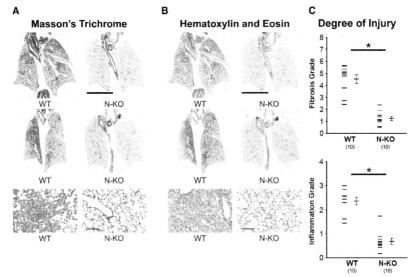

FIGURE 1.—Evaluation of bleomycin-induced lung fibrosis. **A** and **B**: Bleomycin-induced lung injury in wild-type (WT) and N-KO mice 14 days after drug administration. Whole lung sections were stained with Masson's trichrome (**A**) or H&E (**B**). These representative sections show focal inflammation and fibrosis in lungs from wild-type mice. In contrast, lungs from N-KO mice show a near-normal appearance. The line represents 5 mm. The **lower panels** are pictures of lesions taken at a higher magnification (the line is 20 μm). **C**: Lung histology was graded by a pathologist who was blinded to mouse genotype. Fibrosis was graded using a scale described by Ashcroft et al,[24] varying from 0 (normal lung) to 8 (total fibrosis). Inflammation was graded using the 0 (normal lung) to 4 (maximum inflammation) scale described by Sur et al.[25] The inactivation of the N-terminal catalytic site of ACE significantly reduced the lung injury scores for both fibrosis and inflammation ($n = 10$ per group; $*P < 0.001$). *Editor's Note*: Please refer to original journal article for full references. (Reprinted from Li P, Xiao HD, Xu J, et al. Angiotensin-converting enzyme N-terminal inactivation alleviates bleomycin-induced lung injury. *Am J Pathol.* 2010;177:1113-1121, with permission from American Society for Investigative Pathology.)

contrast, the administration of AcSDKP to wild-type mice reduced lung fibrosis due to bleomycin administration. This study shows that the inactivation of the N-terminal catalytic site of ACE significantly reduced bleomycin-induced lung fibrosis and implicates AcSDKP in the mechanism of protection. These data suggest a possible means to increase tolerance to bleomycin and to treat fibrosing lung diseases (Figs 1, 2, and 8).

▶ Despite its beneficial anti-oncogenic effects, bleomycin, a chemotherapeutic drug, can produce severe pulmonary fibrosis. Angiotensin-converting enzyme (ACE) II has been implicated in the genesis of pulmonary fibrosis. To further clarify the role of ACE in lung fibrosis, the authors investigated the role of ACE in genetically engineered mice with point mutations eliminating zinc binding in 1 of the 2 catalytic domains of ACE. Their results convincingly demonstrate that the inactivation of the N-terminal site of ACE protects N-KO mice against bleomycin-induced lung injury and fibrosis. These mice developed substantially less pulmonary inflammation and collagen deposition compared with either C-KO or wild-type

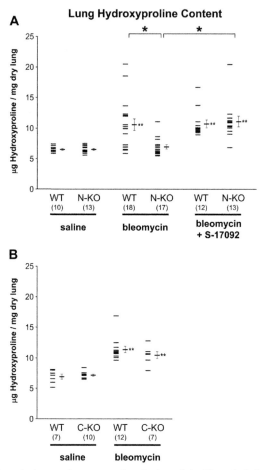

FIGURE 2.—Lung hydroxyproline content. Inactivation of the N-terminal site of ACE prevents collagen deposition in the lung after bleomycin injection. Lung hydroxyproline content was measured in wild-type (WT) and N-KO mice (**A**) or C-KO mice (**B**) two weeks after intratracheal injection of either saline or bleomycin. Because N-KO and C-KO mice are on a mixed 129-C57BL/6 genetic background, appropriate littermate wild-type mice were used for each strain. N-KO and wild-type littermates were also treated with a combination of bleomycin and S-17092, a prolyl-oligopeptidase inhibitor, to reduce the production of AcSDKP. Data points for individual mice are shown, as well as the group means ± SEM. The number of animals per group is indicated in parentheses. *$P < 0.01$; **$P < 0.01$ when a group is compared with the saline-treated group of the same genotype (ie, N-KO mice treated with bleomycin/S-17092 versus N-KO mice treated with saline alone). The inactivation of the N-terminal catalytic site of ACE in N-KO mice prevents bleomycin-induced lung collagen deposition. Inhibition of prolyl-oligopeptidase with S-17092 increases bleomycin-induced lung collagen in N-KO mice. (Reprinted from Li P, Xiao HD, Xu J, et al. Angiotensin-converting enzyme N-terminal inactivation alleviates bleomycin-induced lung injury. *Am J Pathol.* 2010;177:1113-1121, with permission from American Society for Investigative Pathology.)

mice. Furthermore, these mice showed enhanced survival when exposed to a dose of bleomycin lethal to wild-type mice. The clinical implication of this translational study is this: manipulation of N-acetyl-seryl-aspartyl-lysyl-proline and/or ACE

Survival to High Dose of Bleomycin

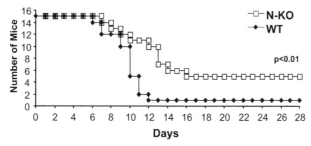

FIGURE 8.—Survival after a high dose of bleomycin. Kaplan-Mayer-type survival analysis of wild-type mice (WT) and N-KO mice treated with 5 mg/kg of bleomycin. N-KO mice have a significantly better survival than wild-type littermate mice ($n = 15$ for each group; $P < 0.01$). (Reprinted from Li P, Xiao HD, Xu J, et al. Angiotensin-converting enzyme N-terminal inactivation alleviates bleomycin-induced lung injury. *Am J Pathol.* 2010;177:1113-1121, with permission from American Society for Investigative Pathology.)

will be a novel therapeutic strategy to reduce the progression of pulmonary fibrosis associated with bleomycin therapy.

M. Mathru, MD

Arterial pressure-based cardiac output monitoring: a multicenter validation of the third-generation software in septic patients

De Backer D, Marx G, Tan A, et al (Erasme Univ Hosp, Brussels, Belgium; Aachen Univ Hosp, Germany; Queen's Med Ctr, Honolulu, HI; et al)
Intensive Care Med 37:233-240, 2011

Purpose.—Second-generation FloTrac software has been shown to reliably measure cardiac output (CO) in cardiac surgical patients. However, concerns have been raised regarding its accuracy in vasoplegic states. The aim of the present multicenter study was to investigate the accuracy of the third-generation software in patients with sepsis, particularly when total systemic vascular resistance (TSVR) is low.

Methods.—Fifty-eight septic patients were included in this prospective observational study in four university-affiliated ICUs. Reference CO was measured by bolus pulmonary thermodilution (iCO) using 3–5 cold saline boluses. Simultaneously, CO was computed from the arterial pressure curve recorded on a computer using the second-generation (CO_{G2}) and third-generation (CO_{G3}) FloTrac software. CO was also measured by semi-continuous pulmonary thermodilution (CCO).

Results.—A total of 401 simultaneous measurements of iCO, CO_{G2}, CO_{G3}, and CCO were recorded. The mean (95%CI) biases between CO_{G2} and iCO, CO_{G3} and iCO, and CCO and iCO were -10 (-15 to -5)%

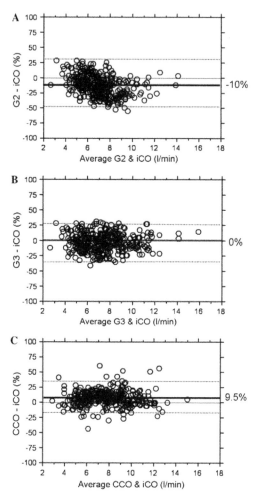

FIGURE 1.—Bland & Altman representations of CO_{G2}, CO_{G3}, and CCO versus iCO. Panel **A** shows relation between CO_{G2} and iCO, panel **B** CO_{G3} and iCO, and panel **C** CCO and iCO. The bias and limits of agreements, computed with correction for multiple measurements [23, 24], are provided in Table 2. *Editor's Note*: Please refer to original journal article for full references. (Reprinted from De Backer D, Marx G, Tan A, et al. Arterial pressure-based cardiac output monitoring: a multicenter validation of the third-generation software in septic patients. *Intensive Care Med*. 2011;37:233-240, with permission from Springer Science+Business Media: Intensive Care Medicine.)

[−0.8 (−1.1 to −0.4) L/min], 0 (−4 to 4)% [0 (−0.3 to 0.3) L/min], and 9 (6−13)% [0.7 (0.5−1.0) L/min], respectively. The percentage errors were 29 (20−37)% for CO_{G2}, 30 (24−37)% for CO_{G3}, and 28 (22−34)% for CCO. The difference between iCO and CO_{G2} was significantly correlated with TSVR ($r^2 = 0.37$, $p < 0.0001$). A very weak ($r^2 = 0.05$) relationship was also observed for the difference between iCO and CO_{G3}.

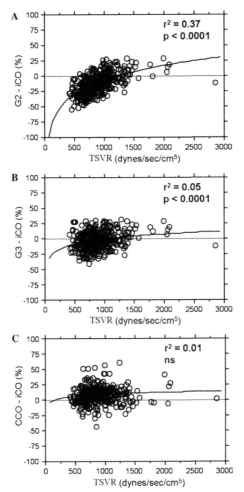

FIGURE 2.—Logarithmic relationships between total systemic vascular resistance (TSVR) and the differences between CO_{G2} and iCO, CO_{G3} and iCO, and CCO and iCO using all patient data. Panel **A** shows relation between CO_{G2} and iCO, panel **B** CO_{G3} and iCO, and panel **C** CCO and iCO. (Reprinted from De Backer D, Marx G, Tan A, et al. Arterial pressure-based cardiac output monitoring: a multicenter validation of the third-generation software in septic patients. *Intensive Care Med.* 2011;37:233-240, with permission from Springer Science+Business Media: Intensive Care Medicine.)

Conclusions.—In patients with sepsis, the third-generation FloTrac software is more accurate, as precise, and less influenced by TSVR than the second-generation software (Figs 1 and 2).

▶ Devices utilizing arterial pressure cardiac output CO are often used to monitor fluid responsiveness in critically ill patients. A commonly used device is FlowTrac, in which CO is derived from the following equation: CO = pulse rate × APsd × K, where APsd is the standard deviation of arterial pressure, and K is an autocalibration factor derived from a proprietary multivariate equation. This equation is influenced by compliance of the vasculature. Several recent studies have shown that FlowTrac may underestimate CO in hyperdynamic and vasoplegic states. To address this limitation, this study was undertaken to validate the third-generation software that was developed from a larger human database. The current study convincingly demonstrates that this third-generation FlowTrac software is more accurate and is less influenced by systemic vascular resistance (SVR).

It has been hypothesized that significant gradients between central and peripheral arterial pulse pressures may be responsible for the underestimation of CO with second-generation FlowTrac software in patients with low SVR. Decoupling of aortic and radial pulse pressure may be responsible for an underestimation when it is computed from a peripheral arterial pressure curve. Consistent with this hypothesis, the authors found that a bias and a percentage error tended to be higher in the radial than the femoral site for CO.

The current study has several limitations: (1) gold standard references for CO such as flow probe—derived CO were not used in this study; (2) the authors studied septic and vasoplegic patients, and whether their findings can be extrapolated to other populations such as patients with drug-induced hypotension and reperfusion states remains to be determined. Nevertheless, the third-generation FlowTrac software is more accurate and precise and is influenced much less by SVR.

M. Mathru, MD

Brain Death: Evaluation of Cerebral Blood Flow by Use of Arterial Spin Labeling

Yun TJ, Sohn C-H, Yoon B-W, et al (Seoul Natl Univ Med Res Ctr, Republic of Korea; Seoul Natl Univ Hosp, Republic of Korea)
Circulation 124:2572-2573, 2011

Background.—The cardinal requirements to diagnose brain death include coma, absence of brain stem reflexes, and apnea. Additional tests may be needed to declare a person brain dead when the results of any components of clinical testing cannot be evaluated reliably. Arterial spin labeling (ASL) offers a noninvasive means for measuring cerebral blood flow (CBF) and determining brain death.

> *Case Report.*—Woman, 48, was admitted to the emergency department having experienced nuchal rigidity, tonic seizure, and loss of consciousness. No pupil reaction to light was observed 5 hours after lumbar puncture for diagnostic purposes. In addition, the patient had apnea. Magnetic resonance imaging (MRI) showed tonsillar impaction in the foramen magnum, loss of signal void in the bilateral internal carotid arteries (suggesting a lack of flow), severe swelling in the gyri, and extensive intravenous thrombi filling the vessel lumens. On the twentieth day in the hospital clinical examinations to determine brain death produced results consistent with that

diagnosis. At 22 days an electroencephalogram demonstrated electro-cerebral silence consistent with brain death. Neurologists requested that conventional or radionuclide angiography be done to determine CBF, but the family refused further invasive tests. At 23 days unavoidable MRI using the ASL technique was performed, revealing severe perfusion defect in the entire brain. The mean value of CBF in the gray matter was 7.9 mL/100g/min. The accepted lower limit of CBF required by the human brain is 10 to 15 mL/100 g/min for regional CBF. The patient showed no improvement by day 25. Mechanical ventilation and other life support were removed in the operating

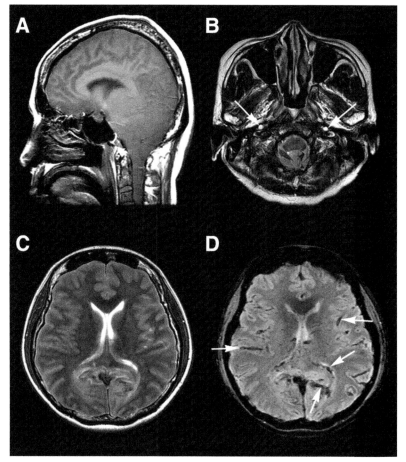

FIGURE 1.—Sagittal T1-weighted image (A) shows tonsillar impaction in the foramen magnum. Axial T2-weighted images (B and C) reveal loss of signal void in the bilateral distal internal carotid arteries (arrows) suggesting arrest in flow and severe gyral swelling with decreased ventricle size. Gradient echo image (D) reveals extensive intravenous thrombi filling vessel lumens (arrows). (Reprinted from Yun TJ, Sohn C-H, Yoon B-W, et al. Brain death: evaluation of cerebral blood flow by use of arterial spin labeling. *Circulation.* 2011;124:2572-2573. © American Heart Association, Inc.)

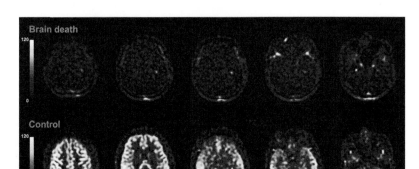

FIGURE 2.—CBF maps (scale unit of mL · 100 g^{-1} · min^{-1}) using ASL of the patient in brain death (upper row) reveal a severe perfusion defect in the whole brain. Mean value and standard deviation of CBF measured in the all pixels composing the gray matter were 7.9 and 3.4 mL · 100 g^{-1} · min^{-1}. Comparison with normal intracranial blood flow on ASL images acquired from a 27-year-old medical school student (bottom row) enhances severely impaired cerebral perfusion in the patient. CBF indicates cerebral blood flow; ASL, arterial spin labeling. (Reprinted from Yun TJ, Sohn C-H, Yoon B-W, et al. Brain death: evaluation of cerebral blood flow by use of arterial spin labeling. *Circulation.* 2011;124:2572-2573. © American Heart Association, Inc.)

room after 1 month of hospitalization, with organ donations made to five other patients.

Conclusions.—ASL is completely noninvasive and provides valuable information concerning absolute CBF. With ASL MRI, protons in arterial water are labeled magnetically in the vessels feeding the brain, then flow through the vascular tree and exchange water with unlabeled brain tissue. By subtracting an image in which incoming arterial spins are labeled from an image without spin labeling, a perfusion-weighted image is generated. ASL has proven validity in gray matter but tends to underestimate CBF in white matter. The ASL technique offers potential as a noninvasive imaging tool for determining CBF and thus brain death (Figs 1 and 2).

▶ Here the authors describe a magnetic resonance imaging (MRI) technique that can determine the absolute levels of cerebral blood flow at the tissue level to confirm brain death. Confirmation of brain death still remains a clinical diagnosis. Clinical tests include coma, absence of brain stem reflexes, and apnea. Cerebral blood flow to confirm brain death is usually performed using radionuclide angiography and conventional angiography. However, these tests are not acceptable to the next of kin because they are invasive. The arterial spin labeling (ASL) technique is a noninvasive emerging technique comparable to MRI and is capable of measuring the absolute amount of cerebral blood flow. The ASL technique is capable of measuring cerebral blood flow less than mL/100 g/min.

M. Mathru, MD

Brain Monitoring After Subarachnoid Hemorrhage: Lessons Learned
Spiotta AM, Provencio JJ, Rasmussen PA, et al (Cleveland Clinic, OH)
Neurosurgery 69:755-766, 2011

Aneurysmal subarachnoid hemorrhage is a serious condition with a high morbidity and mortality rate despite advances in neurocritical care. Intraparenchymal monitors providing continuous bedside physiological data have been introduced into the care of the neurocritically ill and are the focus of clinical research. We review the available technology for bedside brain monitoring and the knowledge that has been gathered and its clinical utility by organizing it into 3 main areas: detecting vasospasm early, establishing end points to resuscitation in the management of cerebral vasospasm, and developing insights into the pathophysiology of the disease. Finally, we discuss its implications for the field and future directions (Table 1).

▶ This is an excellent state-of-the-art review describing the potential usefulness of multimodality monitoring techniques (MMTs) in patients with subarachnoid hemorrhage (SAH). MMTs include cerebral perfusion pressure measurement, thermal diffusion cerebral blood flow, brain tissue oxygen tension (Pbto2), and microdialysis. The clinical benefits of MMTs in SAH include early detection of vasospasm, which could extend the therapeutic window during which multiple strategies could be used to augment cerebral oxygen delivery. MMTs also provide an unique opportunity to understand the pathophysiology of the disease by studying the response of the various brain parameters being measured to medical and interventional therapies. Thermal dilution cerebral blood flow measurement is valuable in early detection and predicts symptomatic vasospasm. Cerebral tissue oxygen tension could be used to measure the integrity of cerebral autoregulation by the bedside. Pbto2 can be considered as a surrogate for

TABLE 1.—Summary of Available Intraparenchymal Technologies That Have Been Studied in the Clinical Setting for Brain Monitoring[a,b]

Monitor	Parameter	Method	Sampling	Summary
External ventricular drain	Intracranial pressure	Fluid-coupled transducer	Intermittent or continuous	Gold standard for ICP monitoring, both diagnostic and therapeutic modality
Licox (2001)	Partial pressure oxygen	Clark-type electrode	Continuous	Most widely used brain tissue oxygen monitor; extensive use in TBI and SAH
Microdialysis (2003)	Glucose glutamate lactate pyruvate pH	Reagent analysis of the dialysate	Intermittent (hourly)	Extensive use in TBI and SAH
Hemedex (2002)	Cerebral blood flow	Thermal diffusion	Continuous	Limited clinical data, largely in the SAH population

[a]ICP, intracranial pressure; SAH, subarachnoid hemorrhage; TBI, traumatic brain injury.
[b]Dates in parentheses correspond to the year that the device received US Food and Drug Administration approval for human use.

regional blood flow; thus, variation in Pbto2 can be related to changes in cerebral perfusion pressure to estimate the degree of impairment of autoregulation. It can be inferred that patients with impaired autoregulation would therefore benefit from cerebral pressure-driven management to restore cerebral oxygenation. Pbto2 is also helpful in determining the efficacy of red blood cell transfusion on cerebral oxygenation. Lactate/pyruvate ratio and lactate/glutamate ratio have been shown to be helpful in predicting non-insulin-dependent diabetic patients in SAH. This article is a significant contribution to the neurocritical care literature.

M. Mathru, MD

Cardiac and central vascular functional alterations in the acute phase of aneurysmal subarachnoid hemorrhage

Papanikolaou J, Makris D, Karakitsos D, et al (Univ of Thessaly, Greece; General State Hosp of Athens, Greece; et al)
Crit Care Med 40:223-232, 2012

Objectives.—To investigate aortic functional alterations in the acute phase of aneurysmal subarachnoid hemorrhage and to evaluate the relationship between potential cardiovascular alterations and delayed cerebral infarctions or poor Glasgow Outcome Scale score at discharge from critical care unit.

Design.—Prospective observational study.

Setting.—Critical Care Departments of two tertiary centers.

Patients.—Thirty-seven patients with aneurysmal subarachnoid hemorrhage.

Interventions.—Patients were evaluated at two time points: on admission (acute aneurysmal subarachnoid hemorrhage phase) and at least 21 days later (stable aneurysmal subarachnoid hemorrhage state). At baseline, the severity of aneurysmal subarachnoid hemorrhage was assessed clinically (Hunt and Hess scale) and radiologically (brain computed tomography Fisher grading). Aortic elasticity was evaluated by Doppler-derived pulse-wave velocity and left ventricular function by echocardiography. Serum B-type natriuretic peptide and troponin I were also assessed at the same time points.

Measurements and Main Results.—At the acute phase, 23 patients (62%) were found to present supranormal pulse-wave velocity and 14 patients (38%) presented left ventricular systolic dysfunction; there were significant associations between pulse-wave velocity values and left ventricular ejection fraction ($p < .001$). Left ventricular ejection fraction and pulse-wave velocity were both associated with Hunt and Hess ($p \leq .004$) and Fisher grading ($p \leq .03$). Left ventricular ejection fraction and pulse-wave velocity were improved between acute aneurysmal subarachnoid hemorrhage and stable state ($p \leq .005$); changes ($\Delta\%$) were greater in patients who initially had regional wall motion abnormalities compared to patients who had not ($28.7\% \pm 10.2\%$ vs. $2.4\% \pm 1.8\%$ [$p = .002$]

and −17.9% ± 3.7% vs. −3.5% ± 4.7% [$p = .045$], respectively). Pulse-wave velocity/left ventricular ejection fraction ratio was the only independent predictor for delayed cerebral infarctions. Left ventricular ejection fraction, B-type natriuretic peptide, pulse-wave velocity, and pulse-wave velocity/left ventricular ejection fraction showed significant diagnostic performance for predicting delayed cerebral infarctions or poor Glasgow Outcome Scale score (1−3).

Conclusions.—Our findings suggest that significant cardiovascular alterations in left ventricular function and in aortic stiffness occur during the early phase of aneurysmal subarachnoid hemorrhage. These phenomena were associated with adverse outcomes in this study and their role in the pathogenesis of delayed neurologic complications warrants further investigation (Figs 2 and 3).

▶ Subarachnoid hemorrhage (SAH) in the acute phase is a very stressful state, characterized by sympathetic overstimulation and excessive catecholamine secretion. The sympathetic overstimulation may cause direct myocardial damage and may acutely affect the elastic properties of the aorta by increasing aortic stiffness. In this study, the authors examined the incidence of aortic stiffness and left

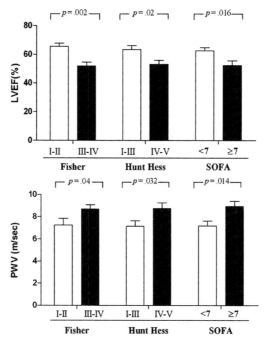

FIGURE 2.—Left ventricular ejection fraction (*LVEF*) and carotid femoral pulse wave velocity (*PWV*) according to clinical severity indices of aneurysmal subarachnoid hemorrhage patients on admission. *SOFA*, Sequential Organ Failure Assessment. (Reprinted from Papanikolaou J, Makris D, Karakitsos D, et al, Cardiac and central vascular functional alterations in the acute phase of aneurysmal subarachnoid hemorrhage. *Crit Care Med.* 2012;40:223-232, with permission from the Society of Critical Care Medicine and Lippincott Williams & Wilkins.)

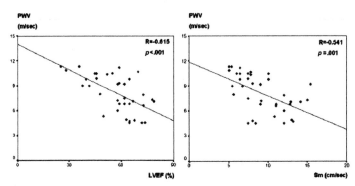

FIGURE 3.—Relationship between carotid femoral pulse wave velocity (*PWV*, m/sec) measurements (*x-axis*) and left ventricular ejection fraction (*LVEF* %) and tissue Doppler imaging-derived peak systolic velocity (*Sm*; cm/sec; *y-axis*) in aneurysmal subarachnoid hemorrhage patients (n = 37) at the acute phase of aneurysmal subarachnoid hemorrhage. (Reprinted from Papanikolaou J, Makris D, Karakitsos D, et al, Cardiac and central vascular functional alterations in the acute phase of aneurysmal subarachnoid hemorrhage. *Crit Care Med.* 2012;40:223-232, with permission from the Society of Critical Care Medicine and Lippincott Williams & Wilkins.)

ventricular (LV) systolic dysfunction in the acute phase of SAH. Aortic stiffness was evaluated by Doppler-derived pulse wave velocity and left ventricular function by echocardiography. In addition, serum B-type natriuretic peptide and troponin were also evaluated at the same time. In the present study, significant cardiovascular alterations, mainly systolic cardiac dysfunction and aortic stiffness, were observed during the acute phase of SAH. Global LV hypokinesis and aortic stiffness occurred in 32.4% and in 62% of patients, respectively. Both LV systolic function and aortic stiffness improved at follow-up. This might suggest a common underlying mechanism for their pathogenesis, potentially hypersecretion of catecholamines due to sympathetic stimulation during the acute phase of SAH.

M. Mathru, MD

Citrulline: A potential immunomodulator in sepsis

Asgeirsson T, Zhang S, Nunoo R, et al (Spectrum Health Res, Grand Rapids, MI; Guangxi Med Univ, Nanning Guangxi, China; et al)
Surgery 150:744-751, 2011

Background.—Sepsis leads to a complex systemic response of cytokines (both pro- and anti-inflammatory) and more recently recognized adipokine mediators. Endothelial nitric oxide (NO) may be a key component in regulating this response, but the pharmacologic manipulation of endothelial NO via L-arginine supplementation or inhibitors has provided inconsistent clinical data related to outcomes. These failures are related to the metabolism of L-arginine in the liver, toxicity of L-arginine, and asymmetric dimethylarginine inhibition, all of which may explain the "arginine paradox." L-citrulline (CIT) offers a potentially valuable means of supplementing arginine and therefore impacting favorably NO availability. The goal of

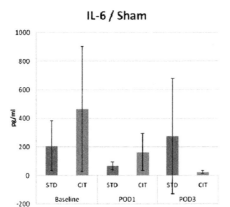

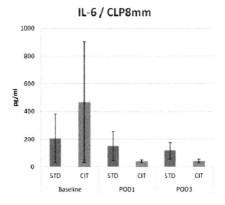

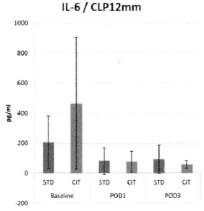

FIGURE 3.—Mean serum interleukin-6 (IL-6) values (pg/mL ± SD) comparing standard rodent diet (STD) to citrulline supplemented diet (CIT) in sham, 8-mm cecal ligation and puncture (CLP 8mm), and 12-mm cecal ligation and puncture (CLP 12mm) models of sepsis. *POD1*, Postoperative day 1; *POD3*, postoperative day 3. (Reprinted from Asgeirsson T, Zhang S, Nunoo R, et al. Citrulline: a potential immunomodulator in sepsis. *Surgery.* 2011;150:744-751, Copyright 2011, with permission from Mosby, Inc.)

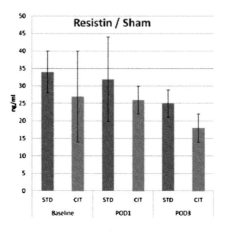

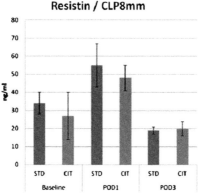

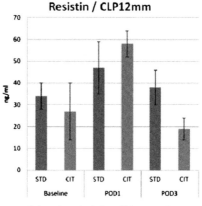

FIGURE 4.—Mean serum resistin values (ng/mL ± SD) comparing standard rodent diet (STD) to citrulline supplemented diet (CIT) in sham, 8-mm cecal ligation and puncture (CLP 8mm), and 12-mm cecal ligation and puncture (CLP 12mm) models of sepsis. *POD1*, Postoperative day 1; *POD3*, postoperative day 3. (Reprinted from Asgeirsson T, Zhang S, Nunoo R, et al. Citrulline: a potential immunomodulator in sepsis. *Surgery.* 2011;150:744-751, Copyright 2011, with permission from Mosby, Inc.)

this study was to determine whether CIT supplementation altered the systemic response of mediators and cytokines in a rat model of sepsis with varying degrees of severity.

Methods.—Sepsis was induced with 2 models of cecal ligation and puncture (CLP) of varying severity in Wistar rats. CIT supplementation was provided to half the animals as 8% CIT-supplemented feed for 3 weeks. Baseline mediator levels were assessed in the Wistar rats followed by comparison of the following groups at days 0, 1, and 3: sham-operated; CLP 8-mm (localized); and CLP 12-mm (extensive). The following analyses were performed in the groups: interleukin-6 (IL-6), IL-8, IL-10, resistin, and adiponectin levels (enzyme-linked immunosorbent assay performed in duplicate). L-arginine and CIT were measured with high-performance liquid chromatography combined with mass spectrometry.

Results.—Ninety-eight Wistar rats were evaluated, and survival was similar in both sepsis models with and without CIT. Serum IL-6 levels were lower in the CIT/CLP 8-mm group compared to the standard rat chow (STD)/CLP 8-mm group (41 vs 117 pg/mL; $P = .011$) on postoperative day 3. Serum IL-8 and IL-10 responses were similar across all groups. Serum resistin levels were lower in the CIT/CLP 12-mm group compared to the STD/CLP 12-mm group in the more severe sepsis model on day 3 (19 vs 38 ng/mL; $P < .0001$). The levels of serum L-arginine were greater in the CIT-supplemented animals compared to STD rodent diet animals before surgical insult (86.3 vs 294.0 μM; $P = .004$). Adiponectin was not affected by CIT supplementation.

Conclusion.—CIT may decrease the proinflammatory mediator response (IL-6 and resistin) without impairing the secretion of anti-inflammatory mediators (IL-10 and adiponectin) and thereby provide a safe means of immunomodulation that preserves the anti-inflammatory mediator response (Figs 3 and 4).

▶ The authors examined whether citrulline supplementation alters L-arginine levels and a panel of systemic proinflammatory mediators in a rat model of sepsis with varying degrees of severity. The investigators convincingly show citrulline supplementation enhanced arginine in control Wistar rats. However, the amino acid levels decline initially and recover only partially in septic rats. The authors also found significant reduction in interleukin (IL)-2, IL-6, and resistin levels in each of the experimental groups. They concluded that citrulline has the potential to reduce proinflammatory cytokines without any effect on anti-inflammatory cytokines. The authors did not measure the levels of IL-1, which has significant impact on the pathogenesis of sepsis. Furthermore, the authors have not produced any evidence that citrulline supplementation affected either arginine or nitric oxide levels. In the future, the authors should measure nitrite and arginine/AVM ratio, which can act as a surrogate for nitric oxide measurement.

M. Mathru, MD

Comparisons of predictive performance of breathing pattern variability measured during T-piece, automatic tube compensation, and pressure support ventilation for weaning intensive care unit patients from mechanical ventilation

Bien M-Y, Lin YS, Shih C-H, et al (Taipei Med Univ Hosp, Taiwan; et al)

Crit Care Med 39:2253-2262, 2011

Objective.—To investigate the influence of different ventilatory supports on the predictive performance of breathing pattern variability for extubation outcomes in intensive care unit patients.

Design and Setting.—A prospective measurement of retrospectively analyzed breathing pattern variability in a medical center.

Patients.—Sixty-eight consecutive and ready-for-weaning patients were divided into success (n = 45) and failure (n = 23) groups based on their extubation outcomes.

Measurements.—Breath-to-breath analyses of peak inspiratory flow, total breath duration, tidal volume, and rapid shallow breathing index were performed for three 30-min periods while patients randomly received T-piece, 100% inspiratory automatic tube compensation with 5 cm H_2O positive end-expiratory pressure, and 5 cm H_2O pressure support ventilation with 5 cm H_2O positive end-expiratory pressure trials. Coefficient of variations and data dispersion (standard descriptor values SD_1 and SD_2 of the Poincaré plot) were analyzed to serve as breathing pattern variability indices.

Main Results.—Under all three trials, breathing pattern variability in extubation failure patients was smaller than in extubation success patients. Compared to the T-piece trial, 100% inspiratory automatic tube compensation with 5 cm H_2O positive end-expiratory pressure and 5 cm H_2O pressure support ventilation with 5 cm H_2O positive end-expiratory pressure decreased the ability of certain breathing pattern variability indices to discriminate extubation success from extubation failure. The areas under the receiver operating characteristic curve of these breathing pattern variability indices were: T-piece (0.73−0.87) > 100% inspiratory automatic tube compensation with 5 cm H_2O positive end-expiratory pressure (0.60−0.79) >5 cm H_2O pressure support ventilation with 5 cm H_2O positive end-expiratory pressure (0.53−0.76). Analysis of the classification and regression tree indicated that during the T-piece trial, a SD_1 of peak inspiratory flow >3.36 L/min defined a group including all extubation success patients. Conversely, the combination of a SD_1 of peak inspiratory flow ≤3.36 L/min and a coefficient of variations of rapid shallow breathing index ≤0.23 defined a group of all extubation failure patients. The decision strategies using SD_1 of peak inspiratory flow and coefficient of variations of rapid shallow breathing index measured during 100% inspiratory automatic tube compensation with 5 cm H_2O positive end-expiratory pressure and 5 cm H_2O pressure support ventilation with 5 cm H_2O positive end-expiratory pressure trials achieved a less clear separation of extubation failure from extubation success.

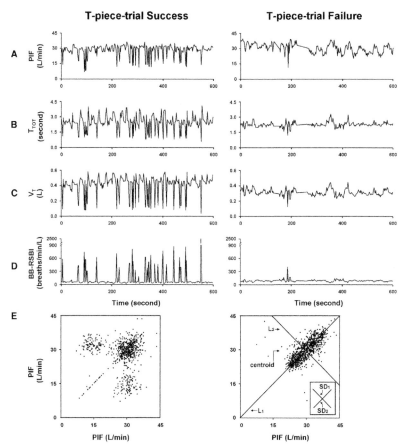

FIGURE 1.—Breath-to-breath analysis of peak inspiratory flow (*PIF*), total breath duration (T_{TOT}), tidal volume (V_T), and rapid shallow breathing index (*BB-RSBI*) measured in one patient from the extubation success group and one patient from the failure group during T-piece spontaneous breathing trial. Panels *A-D* are tracings from continuous measurements of data over 10 mins. Note that the tracings are less irregular in the patient from the failure group as compared to the patient from the success group. Panel *E* is a Poincaré plot using >300 successive breaths of PIF from data in *A*. Quantitative analyses of the plots yield two standard descriptor values, SD_1 and SD_2. SD_2 is defined as the dispersion of points along the line-of-identity (L_1), whereas SD_1 is defined as the dispersion of points perpendicular to the line-of-identity (L_2) through the centroid of the plot. The centroid is located at the coordinates in the plot expressed mathematically as (PIF_{aver}, PIF_{aver}), where PIF_{aver} is the average value for PIF of the predetermined segment (30 min). Note that the distribution of the data points in the success group are more scattered than those in the failure group. (Reprinted from Bien M-Y, Shui Lin Y, Shih C-H, et al. Comparisons of predictive performance of breathing pattern variability measured during T-piece, automatic tube compensation, and pressure support ventilation for weaning intensive care unit patients from mechanical ventilation. *Crit Care Med.* 2011;39:2253-2262, with permission from the Society of Critical Care Medicine and Lippincott Williams & Wilkins.)

Conclusions.—Since 100% inspiratory automatic tube compensation with 5 cm H_2O positive end-expiratory pressure and 5 cm H_2O pressure support ventilation with 5 cm H_2O positive end-expiratory pressure reduce the predictive performance of breathing pattern variability, breathing pattern variability measurement during the T-piece trial is the best choice

TABLE 4.—Area Under the Receiver Operating Characteristic Curve for Variability Indices of Peak Inspiratory Flow, Total Breath Duration, Tidal Volume, and Breath-by-Breath Rapid Shallow Breathing Index Measured During Three Different Spontaneous Breathing Trials

Variability Indices	T-piece	100% Inspiratory Automatic Tube Compensation with 5 cm H_2O Positive End-Expiratory Pressure Trial	5 cm H_2O Pressure Support Ventilation with 5 cm H_2O Positive End-Expiratory Pressure Trial
Peak inspiratory flow			
Coefficient of variation	0.85 ± 0.05	0.76 ± 0.06	0.67 ± 0.07
Poincaré plot			
SD_1	0.87 ± 0.04	0.79 ± 0.06	0.70 ± 0.07^a
SD_2	0.82 ± 0.05	0.71 ± 0.07	0.67 ± 0.07
Total breath duration			
Coefficient of variation	0.73 ± 0.07	0.64 ± 0.07	0.62 ± 0.08
Poincaré plot			
SD_1	0.75 ± 0.06	0.70 ± 0.07	0.67 ± 0.07
SD_2	0.73 ± 0.07	0.67 ± 0.07	0.64 ± 0.07
Tidal volume			
Coefficient of variation	0.85 ± 0.05	0.77 ± 0.06	0.71 ± 0.07^a
Poincaré plot			
SD_1	0.80 ± 0.05	0.75 ± 0.06	0.76 ± 0.06
SD_2	0.84 ± 0.05	0.75 ± 0.06	0.72 ± 0.06
Breath-by-breath rapid shallow breathing index			
Coefficient of variation	0.83 ± 0.05	0.66 ± 0.08^a	0.57 ± 0.08^a
Poincaré plot			
SD_1	0.78 ± 0.06	0.62 ± 0.07^a	0.54 ± 0.08^a
SD_2	0.79 ± 0.05	0.60 ± 0.07^a	0.53 ± 0.08^a

SD, standard descriptors in Poincaré plot; SD_1, instantaneous variability; SD_2, long-term continuous variability.
Breath-by-breath rapid shallow breathing index was calculated as 60 (secs)/total breath duration (secs)/expired tidal volume (L). Breathing pattern variability indices were measured by analyses of coefficient of variation and Poincaré plot of the 30-min weaning trial. Coefficient of variation is a normalized measure of dispersion of a probability distribution.
Values were derived from the data set comparing 45 patients who had successful extubation and 23 patients who failed to extubate.
[a]$p < .05$ vs. T-piece trial in the same variability index. Data are presented as mean $\pm$ SE.

for predicting extubation outcome in intensive care unit patients (Fig 1, Table 4).

▶ Traditional static weaning indices have been replaced by dynamic indices because of the lack of sensitivity and specificity. The frequency to tidal volume ratio (f/Vt), or rapid shallow breathing index, is considered superior to other weaning parameters. However, a single value of any of these measurements is of little value in determining weaning predictability. Successful spontaneous breathing trials are the standard of care and give valuable information regarding weaning predictability. During spontaneous breathing trials, the application of pressure support ventilation (PSV) and PSV with Positive end-expiratory pressure (PEEP) can modify the breathing pattern, inspiratory work, and cardiovascular responses compared with a spontaneous breathing trial (SBT) during T-piece. The use of 2 levels of support, PSV and PSV plus PEEP may mislead clinicians about the clinical tolerance of a spontaneous breathing trial. In this study, Bien and colleagues examined the evolution of f/Vt over a 30-minute SBT using a T-piece, automatic tube compensation (ATC) with 5 cm H_2O PEEP and PSV 5 cm H_2O with 5 cm of PEEP. They monitored the breath-to-breath variability of breathing pattern (inspiratory flow, f/Vt, and breath duration). The study showed that greater breathing pattern variability is associated with successful liberation from the ventilator. During ATC, breathing pattern variability is preserved, but the predictive value is reduced compared with measurements made during spontaneous breathing. The mechanistic basis for this observation is not clear from this study. This is a well-done study. With future availability of microprocessor-controlled ventilators, breathing pattern variability could be monitored on line during SBT.

M. Mathru, MD

Conditional Deletion of *Nrf2* in Airway Epithelium Exacerbates Acute Lung Injury and Impairs the Resolution of Inflammation

Reddy NM, Potteti HR, Mariani TJ, et al (Johns Hopkins Bloomberg School of Public Health, Baltimore, MD; Univ of Rochester Med Ctr, NY)
Am J Respir Cell Mol Biol 45:1161-1168, 2011

Oxidant stress, resulting from an excess of reactive electrophiles produced in the lung by both resident (epithelial and endothelial) and infiltrated leukocytes, is thought to play an obligatory role in tissue injury and abnormal repair. Previously, using a conventional (whole-body) knockout model, we showed that antioxidative gene induction regulated by the transcription factor Nrf2 is critical for mitigating oxidant-induced (hyperoxic) stress, as well as for preventing and resolving tissue injury and inflammation *in vivo*. However, the contribution to pathogenic acute lung injury (ALI) of the cellular stress produced by resident versus infiltrated leukocytes remains largely undefined *in vivo*. To address this critical gap in our knowledge, we generated mice with a conditional deletion of Nrf2 specifically in Clara cells, subjected these mice to hyperoxic insult, and allowed them to recover. We report that a deficiency of Nrf2 in airway epithelia alone is sufficient to contribute to the development and progression of ALI. When exposed to hyperoxia, mice lacking Nrf2 in Clara cells showed exacerbated lung injury, accompanied by greater levels of cell death and epithelial sloughing than in their wildtype littermates. In addition, we found that an Nrf2 deficiency in Clara cells is associated with a persistent inflammatory response and epithelial sloughing in the lungs during recovery from sublethal hyperoxic insult. Our results demonstrate (for the first time, to the best of our knowledge) that Nrf2 signaling in Clara cells is critical for conferring protection from hyperoxic lung injury and for resolving inflammation during the repair process (Figs 2 and 3).

▶ The transcription factor Nrf2 regulates the expression of several antioxidant enzymes and proteins that are required by cells to protect against oxidant injury. Nrf2 is normally located in the cytoplasm. However, during cellular stress it is translocated to the nucleus and binds to an antioxidant-responsive element in the regulatory regions of various antioxidant genes and activates their transcription. The conventional disruption of Nrf2 leads to greater vulnerability to

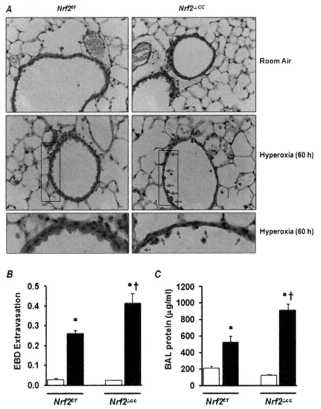

FIGURE 2.—Hyperoxia-induced lung injury in $Nrf2^{f/f}$ and $Nrf2^{\Delta cc}$ mice. $Nrf2^{f/f}$ and $Nrf2^{\Delta cc}$ mice were exposed to room air (RA) or hyperoxia for 60 hours and killed, and their left lungs were inflated and fixed in 1.5% paraformaldehyde. Lung tissue sections were prepared and stained with hematoxylin and eosin (H&E). (A) Representative images of H&E-stained lungs sections of three mice are shown. *Bottom:* Enlarged images of lung tissue sections of $Nrf2^{f/f}$ and $Nrf2^{\Delta cc}$ mice exposed to 60 hours of hyperoxia. *Arrows* indicate epithelial sloughing in $Nrf2^{\Delta cc}$ mice. (B) Evans blue dye (EBD) was injected intraperitoneally into the mice 2 hours before they were killed. Lungs were perfused, and lung EBD and serum EBD were extracted into formamide. Lungs were dried, and the ratios of lung EBD/serum EBD/dry ratios were calculated. The data shown represent means ± SEM ($n = 5$). (C) Bronchoalveolar lavage (BAL) fluid was collected from the right lung, and total protein was estimated in BAL fluids with a Bio-Rad protein assay. Data represent means ± SEM ($n = 6$). Significance was calculated using the Student t test. *$P \leq 0.05$, room air versus hyperoxia or recovery. †$P \leq 0.05$, $Nrf2^{f/f}$ mice versus $Nrf2^{\Delta cc}$ mice. *Open bars*, room-air controls; *solid bars*, hyperoxia. (Reprinted from Reddy NM, Potteti HR, Mariani TJ, et al. Conditional deletion of Nrf2 in airway epithelium exacerbates acute lung injury and impairs the resolution of inflammation. *Am J Respir Cell Mol Biol.* 2011;45:1161-1168, with permission from the Official Journal of the American Thoracic Society.)

injurious insults including hyperoxia. The oxidant-induced cellular injury to the lung endothelium and alveolar epithelium is known to contribute to lung injury. This study examined the contribution of Nrf2 toward lung injury in the presence of hyperoxic states. To determine this contribution, the investigators generated mice bearing a floxed allele of Nrf2 and deleted Nrf2 specifically in Clara cells and then exposed the mice to hyperoxic insult. In this elegant experimental study, the authors provide convincing evidence to support the critical role for

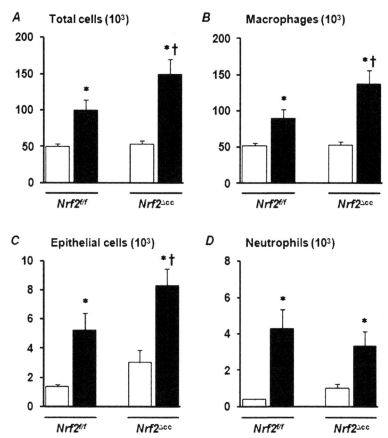

FIGURE 3.—Deletion of *Nrf2* in Clara cells exacerbates hyperoxia-induced lung inflammation. *Nrf2*^{f/f} mice and *Nrf2*^{Δcc} mice were exposed to room air or hyperoxia for 60 hours. BAL fluid was collected from the right lung, centrifuged, and stained with a Diff-Quik stain kit. Differential cell counts were performed to analyze total cells (*A*), macrophages (*B*), epithelial cells (*C*), and neutrophils (*D*), and are expressed as means ± SEM. One-way ANOVA, followed by Newman-Keuls *post hoc* analysis, was performed for multiple group comparisons, whereas two-way ANOVA with a Bonferroni correction was used to compare interactions between genotype and hyperoxia. In both cases, $P \leq 0.05$ was considered statistically significant. *Room air versus hyperoxia. †*Nrf2*^{f/f} versus *Nrf2*^{Δcc} counterparts. *Open bars*, room-air controls; *solid bars*, hyperoxia. (Reprinted from Reddy NM, Potteti HR, Mariani TJ, et al. Conditional deletion of *Nrf2* in airway epithelium exacerbates acute lung injury and impairs the resolution of inflammation. *Am J Respir Cell Mol Biol.* 2011;45:1161-1168, with permission from the Official Journal of the American Thoracic Society.)

airway epithelial—specific (Clara cell) Nrf2 signaling in conferring protection from oxidant-induced acute lung injury. Perturbation in the Nrf2-regulated antioxidant defense system in Clara-cell secretory protein—expressing cells exacerbated lung injury. Activation of the Nrf2 signaling pathway may offer a novel therapeutic strategy to attenuate lung injury and inflammatory responses in acute respiratory distress syndrome.

M. Mathru, MD

Contrast Stress-Echocardiography Predicts Cardiac Events in Patients with Suspected Acute Coronary Syndrome but Nondiagnostic Electrocardiogram and Normal 12-Hour Troponin

Gaibazzi N, Squeri A, Reverberi C, et al (Parma Univ Hosp, Italy; et al)

J Am Soc Echocardiogr 24:1333-1341, 2011

Background.—No large study has demonstrated that any stress test can risk-stratify future hard cardiac events (cardiac death or myocardial infarction) in patients with suspected acute coronary syndromes (ACS), nondiagnostic electrocardiographic (ECG) findings, and normal troponin levels. The aim of this study was to test the hypothesis that combined contrast wall motion and myocardial perfusion echocardiographic assessment (cMCE) during stress echocardiography can predict long-term hard cardiac events in patients with suspected ACS, nondiagnostic ECG findings, and normal troponin.

Methods.—A total of 545 patients referred for contrast stress echocardiography from the emergency department for suspected ACS but nondiagnostic ECG findings and normal troponin levels at 12 hours were followed up for cardiac events. Patients underwent dipyridamole-atropine echocardiography with adjunctive myocardial perfusion imaging using a commercially available ultrasound contrast medium (SonoVue).

Results.—During a median follow-up period of 12 months, 25 cardiac events (4.6%) occurred (no deaths, 12 nonfatal myocardial infarctions, 13 episodes of unstable angina). Abnormal findings on cMCE were the most significant predictor of both hard cardiac events (hazard ratio, 22.8; 95% confidence interval, 2.9−176.7) and the combined (cardiac death, myocardial infarction, or unstable angina requiring revascularization) end point (hazard ratio, 10.7; 95% confidence interval, 3.7−31.3). The inclusion of the cMCE variable significantly improved multivariate models, determining lower Akaike information criterion values and higher discrimination ability.

Conclusions.—cMCE during contrast stress echocardiography provided independent information for predicting hard and combined cardiac events beyond that predicted by stress wall motion abnormalities in patients with suspected ACS, nondiagnostic ECG findings, and normal troponin levels (Fig 5, Table 3).

▶ Predicting cardiac events in patients who present with acute coronary syndrome (ACS), with normal or nondiagnostic electrocardiogram (EKG) and normal serial biomarkers, pose a considerable challenge to clinicians. Current guidelines recommend stress testing for this cohort of patients. Contrast stress echocardiography, which simultaneously evaluates both myocardial wall motion and myocardial perfusion, has been shown to be accurate for the assessment of coronary artery disease (CAD) and to provide information for the prediction of cardiac events over clinical data in suspected CAD. The current study examined the efficacy of contrast stress echocardiography in predicting cardiac events in patients presenting with ACS with normal EKG and normal

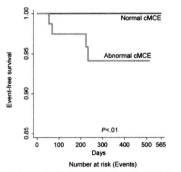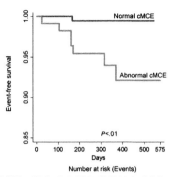

Number at risk (Events)

| Normal cMCE | 161 (0) 161 (0) 151 (0) 105 (0) 66 (0) 19(0) 1 |
| Abnormal cMCE | 79 (2) 77 (0) 63 (2) 32 (0) 11 (0) 4 (0) 0 |

| Normal cMCE | 190 (0) 190 (1) 180 (0) 139 (0) 91 (0) 26(0) 0 |
| Abnormal cMCE | 115 (1) 111 (4) 91 (0) 65 (2) 41 (0) 17(0) 1 |

FIGURE 5.—Kaplan-Meier survival curves for hard cardiac events in patients with normal versus abnormal cMCE findings and low (*left*) or intermediate (*right*) Thrombolysis In Myocardial Infarction risk scores. (Reprinted from Gaibazzi N, Squeri A, Reverberi C, et al. Contrast stress-echocardiography predicts cardiac events in patients with suspected acute coronary syndrome but nondiagnostic electrocardiogram and normal 12-hour troponin. *J Am Soc Echocardiogr.* 2011;24:1333-1341, Copyright 2011, with permission from the American Society of Echocardiography.)

TABLE 3.—Univariate Cox Regression Risk for Hard Cardiac Events

Variable	HR	95% CI	P
Age	1.037	(0.977−1.1)	.230
Three or more risk factors	0.990	(0.314−3.12)	.986
Cigarette smoking	0.981	(0.266−3.625)	.977
Hypercholesterolemia	0.701	(0.226−2.175)	.539
Diabetes	2.353	(0.747−7.416)	.144
Hypertension	1.571	(0.344−7.172)	.560
Previous AMI	0.520	(0.114−2.374)	.399
Statins	2.673	(0.723−9.882)	.140
Aspirin	7.383	(0.953−57.203)	.056
β-blockers	4.097	(0.897−18.708)	.069
Previous AMI, CAD, or revascularization	1.115	(0.354−3.512)	.853
TIMI risk score low/intermediate	1.530	(0.46−5.085)	.488
Abnormal rest ECG findings	1.325	(0.399−4.399)	.646
Rest WM abnormalities	1.374	(0.414−4.563)	.604
Abnormal vs normal WM	4.916	(1−583−15.268)	.006
Abnormal vs normal cMCE findings	22.778	(2.936−176.730)	.003

HR, Hazard ratio; *TIMI*, Thrombolysis In Myocardial Infarction.

troponin levels. The results show that in this cohort of patients there was a hard cardiac event rate of 2.2% per year and a combined event rate of 4.6% per year The study also shows that clinical risk factors, EKG findings, and rest wall motion abnormalities did not significantly affect the risk for hard cardiac events, while a contrast stress echocardiogram was the most significant predictor, at least in terms of model fitting and discrimination. Contrast echocardiography is readily available in most institutions and should be used routinely in patients who present with ACS with a normal EKG and normal biomarkers.

M. Mathru, MD

CPAP for acute cardiogenic pulmonary oedema from out-of-hospital to cardiac intensive care unit: a randomised multicentre study

Ducros L, on behalf of the CPAP collaborative study group (Hôpital Universitaire Lariboisiére, Paris, France; et al)
Intensive Care Med 37:1501-1509, 2011

Purpose.—Continuous positive airway pressure (CPAP) is a useful treatment for patients with acute cardiogenic pulmonary oedema (CPE). However, its usefulness in the out-of-hospital setting has been poorly investigated and only by small and single-centre studies. We designed a multicentre randomised study to assess the benefit of CPAP initiated out of hospital.

Methods.—A total of 207 patients with CPE were randomly allocated by emergency mobile medical units to receive either standard treatment alone or standard treatment plus CPAP. CPAP was maintained after admission to the intensive care unit (ICU). Inclusion criteria were orthopnoea, respiratory rate greater than 25 breaths/min, pulse oximetry less than 90% in room air and diffuse crackles. The primary end point was assessed during the first 48 h and combined: death, presence of intubation criteria, persistence of either all inclusion criteria or circulatory failure at the second hour or their reappearance before 48 h. Absence of all criteria defined successful treatment.

Results.—CPAP was used for 60 min [40, 65] (median [Q1, Q3]) in the pre-hospital setting and 120 min [60, 242] in ICU and was well tolerated in all patients. Treatment was successful in 79% of patients in the CPAP group and 63% in the control group ($p = 0.01$), especially for persistence of inclusion criteria after 2 h (12 vs. 26%) and for intubation criteria (4 vs. 14%). CPAP was beneficial irrespective of the initial $PaCO_2$ or left ventricular ejection fraction.

Conclusion.—Immediate use of CPAP in out-of-hospital treatment of CPE and until CPE resolves after admission significantly improves early outcome compared with medical treatment alone (Tables 2-4).

▶ Application of continuous positive airway pressure (CPAP) and the concomitant increases in intrathoracic pressure (ITP) have a salutary effect on the heart. This is attributed to the ITP-induced decreases in preload, afterload, and reduced sympathetic traffic. In addition, CPAP improves gas exchange and minimizes work of breathing. Several randomized clinical trials have shown therapeutic benefits in cardiogenic pulmonary edema (CPE). However, only one prospective, randomized study showed benefit of early and short application of CPAP in severe CPE. In this prospective, multicenter, randomized study the authors examined the impact of early application of CPAP when started in an out-of-hospital setting and continued in hospital in a cardiac intensive care unit. The authors hypothesized that the respiratory and circulatory perturbations should disappear more quickly and permanently in the CPAP group. The study

TABLE 2.—Physiological Parameters at Study Entry and Echocardiographic Findings

Parameters	Control Group (N = 100)	CPAP Group (N = 107)
SpO$_2$ in air (%)	84 [78, 88]	84 [80, 88]
pH	7.30 [7.22, 7.36]	7.30 [7.25, 7.37]
PO$_2$ (mmHg)	127 [86, 177]	114 [79, 183]
PCO$_2$ (mmHg)	49 [41, 57]	46 [39, 55]
Bicarbonates (mmol/L)	23 [20, 26]	24 [20, 26]
Respiratory rate (per min)	35 [30, 40]	36 [30, 40]
Systolic arterial blood pressure (mmHg)	170 [143, 193]	170 [150, 195]
Diastolic arterial blood pressure (mmHg)	97 [80, 103]	95 [82, 110]
Heart rate (bpm)	101 [90, 116]	102 [83, 116]
Encephalopathy	7 (7)	13 (12)
Circulatory failure	18 (18)	17 (16)
Echocardiographic findings LVEF	35 [30, 60]	45 [35, 60]
Syst. PAP (mmHg)	40 [32, 45]	38 [31, 43]
E/A ratio	0.9 [1, 1]	0.9 [1, 2]

Data are expressed as median with 25th and 75th interquartile range [Q1, Q3] or number and percentage n (%); *SpO$_2$* pulse oximetry; arterial blood gases were sampled under O$_2$ mask with a reservoir at 15 L/min. *LVEF* left ventricular ejection fraction, *Syst PAP* systolic pulmonary arterial pressure (mmHg); *E/A ratio* flow velocity ratio across the mitral valve between early diastole and atrial contraction.

TABLE 3.—Overall Outcome of the Study Groups: Primary End Point

	Control Group (n = 100)	CPAP Group (n = 107)	OR [95% CI] Control/CPAP
Primary end point (combined criteria)	37 (37)	23 (21)	2.1 [1.2, 4.0]
Death	5 (5)	4 (4)	1.4 [0.4, 5.2]
Persistence of inclusion criteria[a] at H2	23 (26)	12 (12)	2.5 [1.2, 5.5]
Reappearance of inclusion criteria[a] after H2	1 (1)	3 (3)	0.4 [0, 3.5]
Persistence of circulatory failure at H2	6 (6)	1 (1)	7.0 [0.8, 58.9]
Reappearance of circulatory failure after H2	6 (6)	1 (1)	6.8 [0.8, 57.7]
Presence of intubation criteria	13 (14)	4 (4)	3.9 [1.2, 12.5]

Data are expressed as number and percentage n (%), and odds ratio with their 95% CI. Primary end point is evaluated between inclusion and H48.

p value = 0.01 for primary end point comparison between groups.

[a]Inclusion criteria are orthopnoea, diffuse crackles (Killip score at least III), respiratory rate greater than 25/min, and SpO$_2$ less than 90% with room air.

found complete and more frequent resolution of CPE when CPAP was applied early. However, this trial did not show benefit on early mortality. This trial also shows benefits in correcting hypercapnia in patients with severe circulatory failure. This study is the first to show that CPAP is beneficial in hypercapnic patients compared with standard treatment alone. A limitation of this study is that it was not blinded. A second limitation was that the investigators could not prevent physicians from crossing over from standard therapy to CPAP once patients met the intubation criteria. Nevertheless, the results of this study strengthen the previous data and support the widespread use of CPAP early as

TABLE 4.—Overall Outcome of the Study Groups: Secondary Criteria

	Control Group (n = 100)	CPAP Group (n = 107)	OR [95% CI] Control/CPAP	p Value
Primary end point without intubation criteria	36 (36)	23 (21)	2.1 [1.1, 3.8]	0.02
ICU length of stay (days)	2 [1, 3]	2 [1, 3]		0.67
Death at day 7	7 (7)	4 (3.7)	1.9 [0.5, 6.8]	0.30
In-hospital mortality	9 (9)	8 (8.5)	0.9 [0.4, 2.5]	0.90
SBP (mmHg)				
H0.5	153 [129, 177]	147 [131, 169]		0.52[†]
H1	142 [125, 167]	142 [133, 160]		
H2	133 [110, 154]	135 [118, 150]		
H6	118 [102, 137]	128 [112, 143]		
DBP (mmHg)				
H0.5	87 [73, 100]	82 [74, 96]		0.035[†]
H1	80 [69, 90]	83 [69, 95]		
H2	68 [59, 78]	73 [60, 85]		
H6	62 [55, 70]	66 [58, 76]		
HR (bpm)				
H0.5	100 [82, 114]	94 [79, 108]		0.023[†]
H1	94 [80, 110]	88 [72, 106]		
H2	86 [71, 101]	80 [70, 98]		
H6	80 [69, 98]	78 [70, 87]		
RR (cpm)				
H0.5	30 [26, 36]	30 [25, 36]		0.001[†]
H1	29 [24, 34]	27 [22, 32]		
H2	26 [20, 33]	24 [20, 29]		
H6	24 [21, 30]	22 [18, 27]		
pH at ICU admission	7.35 [7.27, 7.40]	7.37 [7.33, 7.41]		0.048
PCO_2 at ICU admission	45 [39, 53]	41 [36, 45]		0.011
BNP (pg/mL)				
T0	842 [413, 1620]	641 [371, 996]		
H6	772 [391, 2000]	675 [401, 1230]		
H24	409 [262, 901]	497 [239, 887]		
BNP variation T0−H24 (%)	−28 [−46, 11]	−14 [−58, 31]		0.93
Peak troponin I (ng/mL)	0.20 [0.08, 0.92]	0.29 [0.09, 1.45]		0.35
Total dose of diuretics (mg)				
Furosemide	200 [120, 280]	180 [120, 270]		0.65
Bumetanide	2 [2, 3]	2 [2, 2]		0.09
Total dose of nitrates (mg)				
Bolus	3 [2, 6]	3 [2, 6]		0.68
Continuous infusion	21 [6, 42]	27 [12, 51]		0.08
Inotropic support	9 (9)	5 (5)		0.22

Data are expressed as median with 25th and 75th interquartile range [Q1, Q3], number and percentage n (%) and odds ratio with their 95% CI
SBP systolic blood pressure, DBP diastolic blood pressure, HR heart rate, RR respiratory rate
[†]Interaction between treatment effect and time from T0 to H6.

soon as CPE is diagnosed, irrespective of the presence or absence of hypercapnia and left ventricular ejection fraction.

M. Mathru, MD

Cyclooxygenase-2 Deficiency Leads to Intestinal Barrier Dysfunction and Increased Mortality during Polymicrobial Sepsis

Fredenburgh LE, Velandia MMS, Ma J, et al (Brigham and Women's Hosp, Boston, MA; et al)

J Immunol 187:5255-5267, 2011

Sepsis remains the leading cause of death in critically ill patients, despite modern advances in critical care. Intestinal barrier dysfunction may lead to secondary bacterial translocation and the development of the multiple organ dysfunction syndrome during sepsis. Cyclooxygenase (COX)-2 is highly upregulated in the intestine during sepsis, and we hypothesized that it may be critical in the maintenance of intestinal epithelial barrier function during peritonitis-induced polymicrobial sepsis. $COX-2^{-/-}$ and $COX-2^{+/+}$ BALB/c mice underwent cecal ligation and puncture (CLP) or sham surgery. Mice chimeric for COX-2 were derived by bone marrow transplantation and underwent CLP. C2BBe1 cells, an intestinal epithelial cell line, were treated with the COX-2 inhibitor NS-398, PGD_2, or vehicle and stimulated with cytokines. $COX-2^{-/-}$ mice developed exaggerated bacteremia and increased mortality compared with $COX-2^{+/+}$ mice following CLP. Mice chimeric for COX-2 exhibited the recipient phenotype, suggesting that epithelial COX-2 expression in the ileum attenuates bacteremia following CLP. Absence of COX-2 significantly increased epithelial permeability of the ileum and reduced expression of the tight junction proteins zonula occludens-1, occludin, and claudin-1 in the ileum following CLP. Furthermore, PGD_2 attenuated cytokine-induced hyperpermeability and zonula occludens-1 downregulation in NS-398—treated C2BBe1 cells. Our findings reveal that absence of COX-2 is associated with enhanced intestinal epithelial permeability and leads to exaggerated bacterial translocation and increased mortality during peritonitis-induced sepsis. Taken together, our results suggest that epithelial expression of COX-2 in the ileum is a critical modulator of tight junction protein expression and intestinal barrier function during sepsis (Fig 3).

▶ Sepsis is the leading cause of death in critically ill patients. Furthermore, intra-abdominal sepsis accounts for 20% of the cases of sepsis, which has a substantial mortality of up to 60%. Several lines of experimental evidence suggest that loss of integrity of the epithelial barrier function plays a significant role in the development of multiple organ dysfunction syndrome in patients with sepsis. This is supported by the finding that increased intestinal permeability has been demonstrated in a wide variety of critically ill patients. A growing body of evidence also suggests that COX-2—derived prostaglandins (PG) play a pivotal role in both PG production and mucosal defense of the gastrointestinal tract in the setting of mucosal injury. This current study examined the role of COX-2, the inducible isoform of COX in a murine model of sepsis. The authors' findings suggest that COX-2 deficiency produces profound shock with very high systemic overload of bacteria. Pharmacological inhibition of COX-2 leads to disruption of epithelial tight junctions and loss of intestinal

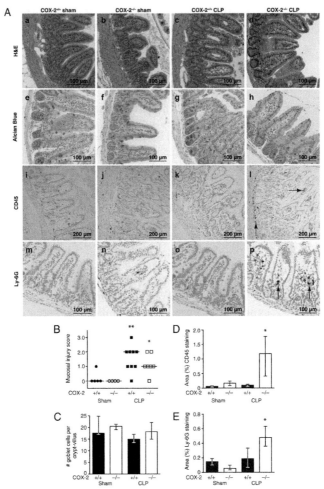

FIGURE 3.—COX-2−deficient mice have increased ileal inflammation following peritonitis-induced polymicrobial sepsis. COX-2$^{+/+}$ and COX-2$^{-/-}$ mice underwent CLP with a 19-g needle (one hole). Ileums were harvested 48 h following CLP. *A*, Representative H&E staining (*a−d*), Alcian blue staining (*e−h*), CD45 immunostaining (*i−l*), and Ly-6G immunostaining (*m−p*) in COX-2$^{+/+}$ and COX-2$^{-/-}$ mice following sham surgery (*left two panels*) and CLP (*right two panels*). Arrows indicate cells staining positive for CD45 (*l*) and Ly-6G (*p*) in COX-2$^{-/-}$ mice following CLP. *B*, Histologic scoring of mucosal injury in H&E-stained ileums following sham (COX-2$^{-/-}$, $n = 4$; COX-2$^{+/+}$, $n = 5$) and CLP (COX-2$^{-/-}$, $n = 7$; COX-2$^{+/+}$, $n = 9$) from two independent experiments. *$p < 0.05$, versus COX-2$^{-/-}$ sham, **$p < 0.05$, versus COX-2$^{+/+}$ sham, χ^2 test for trend). *C*, Quantitation of goblet cell number (three mice/condition) per crypt-villus in COX-2$^{-/-}$ and COX-2$^{+/+}$ mice following sham and CLP. Quantitation of CD45 (*D*) and Ly-6G (*E*) immunostaining in ileums of COX-2$^{-/-}$ and COX-2$^{+/+}$ mice (two to five mice/condition) demonstrates that COX-2$^{-/-}$ mice have significantly increased neutrophilic inflammation in the ileum compared with COX-2$^{+/+}$ mice following CLP. *$p < 0.05$, COX-2$^{-/-}$ mice after CLP versus COX-2$^{-/-}$ mice after sham and versus COX-2$^{+/+}$ mice after CLP, Mann−Whitney U test. For interpretation of the references to color in this figure legend, the reader is referred to web version of this article. (Reprinted from Fredenburgh LE, Velandia MMS, Ma J, et al. Cyclooxygenase-2 deficiency leads to intestinal barrier dysfunction and increased mortality during polymicrobial sepsis. *J Immunol.* 2011;187:5255-5267, with permission from The American Association of Immunologists, Inc.)

barrier function during bacterial sepsis. This suggests that in addition to atten-uating inflammation, PGD_2 plays a critical role in preserving intestinal barrier function by regulating epithelial expression of tight junction proteins in the small intestine during peritonitis-induced polymicrobial sepsis. Accordingly, therapeutic strategies that modulate the epithelial expression of COX-2 and PGD_2 may lead to novel therapeutic approaches to combat fatal sepsis. Future clinical studies should address this issue.

M. Mathru, MD

Death during Intensive Glycemic Therapy of Diabetes: Mechanisms and Implications
Cryer PE (Washington Univ in St Louis, MO)
Am J Med 124:993-996, 2011

Background.—Intensive glycemic therapy has documented microvascular and potential macrovascular benefits for patients with type 1 and type 2 dia-betes, but the three most recent randomized clinical trials have not found any macrovascular or survival benefits. Intensive glycemic therapy can increase mortality in type 2 diabetes patients and critically ill persons. Giving insulin or an insulin secretagogue can cause fatal hypoglycemia in diabetic patients. As a result, it is reasonable to suspect that iatrogenic hypoglycemia may cause excess mortality during intensive glycemic therapy. It was proposed that when the target A1C of less than 6% was not attained, more aggressive glycemic therapy was instituted and excess mortality resulted.

Analysis of Evidence.—Severe hypoglycemia may directly cause death or indicate vulnerability to another cause of death. Finding excess mortality or cardiovascular events in patients with type 2 diabetes whose A1C levels are lower or higher suggests that hypoglycemia exerts a direct effect. Prolonged, profound hypoglycemia can cause brain death, possibly through sustained increased glutamate release and receptor activation when plasma glucose concentrations fall below 18 mg/dL, the electroencephalogram is isoelectric, and brain glucose and glycogen levels are too low to measure. Because these conditions are rare in patients with diabetes, most fatal hypoglycemic episodes result from other mechanisms, usually cardiac arrhythmias. Impaired ventricular repolarization, reflected in a prolonged corrected QT (QTc) interval, is associated with lethal ventricular arrhythmias and seen in experimental and clinical hypoglycemia in type 1 diabetes.

Relationships to Diabetes.—When therapeutic hyperinsulinemia and compromised defenses against the fall in plasma glucose concentrations interact, iatrogenic hypoglycemia can occur in diabetics. The presence of hypoglycemia also reduces baroreflex sensitivity. Iatrogenic hypoglycemia with sympathoadrenal activation can trigger a ventricular arrhythmia and sudden death. Thus iatrogenic hypoglycemia is a limiting factor in the gly-cemic management of diabetes, causing recurrent morbidity and possibly death. Diabetics cannot maintain euglycemia over a lifetime of diabetes, defenses against declines in plasma glucose concentrations are impaired, and recurrent hypoglycemia ensues. There are therefore compelling reasons to minimize the risk of hypoglycemia in diabetic patients.

Recommendations.—It may be appropriate to reconsider glycemic goals for diabetic patients. The glycemic goal for a given person at a given point should be based on the drug regimen and the risk of hypoglycemia. A generic glycemic goal is the lowest A1C that does not cause severe hypoglycemia, preserves hypoglycemia awareness, and allows an acceptable number of episodes of symptomatic hypoglycemia as the worst outcome. The patient's regimen would be altered to eliminate problems or the glycemic goal could be adjusted. Initial therapy is seldom effective for a lifetime of type 2 diabetes and ineffective for patients with type 1 diabetes.

Conclusions.—If the treatment performed to maintain a patient's A1C level cannot be achieved safely, there is some evidence that the A1C can be reevaluated and raised or lowered. Glycemic control is just one component to consider; interventions against multiple risk factors are needed to achieve microvascular and macrovascular benefits (Fig).

▶ Landmark studies from Leuven, Belgium, suggested that targeting normoglycemia (a blood glucose concentration of 80—110 mg/dL) reduced mortality and morbidity, but other investigators have not been able to replicate those findings. This is attributed to the association between therapeutic insuline-induced hypoglycemia and the subsequent sympathetic nervous system activation. Iatrogenic hypoglycemia in critically ill patients leads to hypoglycemia-associated autonomic failure (HAFF), including reduced baroreflex activity, and the resulting increased vulnerability to a ventricular arrhythmia. Furthermore, recent antecedent hypoglycemia causes metabolic HAFF with an increased risk for an episode of

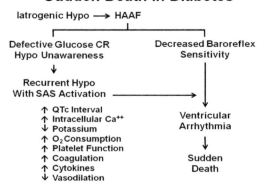

Sudden Death in Diabetes

FIGURE.—Potential mechanism of iatrogenic hypoglycemia-induced hypoglycemia-associated autonomic failure (HAAF) mediated sudden death in diabetes: cardiovascular HAAF causing reduced baroreceptor sensitivity and metabolic HAAF, leading to an episode of hypoglycemia that increases sympathoadrenal system activity, which triggers a fatal ventricular arrhythmia in the setting of reduced baroreflex sensitivity. (Reprinted from The American Journal of Medicine. Cryer PE. Death during intensive glycemic therapy of diabetes: mechanisms and implications. *Am J Med.* 2011;124:993-996, Copyright 2011, with permission from Elsevier.)

iatrogenic hypoglycemia with sympathoadrenal activation, which through an array of mechanisms including abnormal cardiac repolarization could trigger a ventricular arrhythmia and sudden death. Based on the current evidence, tight glycemic control in critically ill patients is not recommended. This article nicely summarizes the possible mechanisms behind death associated with intensive glycemic control.

M. Mathru, MD

Effects of Hypertonic Saline on CD4+CD25+Foxp3+ Regulatory T Cells After Hemorrhagic Shock in Relation to iNOS and Cytokines
Isayama K, Murao Y, Saito F, et al (Kansai Med Univ, Osaka, Japan; Kinki Univ Faculty of Medicine, Osaka, Japan)
J Surg Res 172:137-145, 2012

Background.—Hemorrhagic shock and resuscitation induce immunosuppression. CD4+CD25+Foxp3+ regulatory T Cells (Foxp3+ Tregs), iNOS and cytokines may affect these severe conditions such as acute respiratory distress syndrome and multiple organ failure after hemorrhagic shock and resuscitation. Foxp3+ Tregs have been described to be specific and play a key role in the control of the immune system. Immune condition may be restored by hypertonic saline resuscitation that inhibits pro-inflammatory effects of cytokine. Our aim was to investigate how hypertonic saline resuscitation affected Foxp3+ Tregs after hemorrhagic shock and resuscitation in relation to iNOS and cytokines.

Methods.—Male C57BL6/J and B6.129P2-NOS2^{tm1Lau}/J (iNOS gene knockout) mice were used in creating hemorrhagic shock model. Mice were divided into two groups, each according to the type of resuscitation. (1) Wild HS: resuscitation with hypertonic saline (4 mL/Kg of 7.5% NaCl) and the shed blood (SB); (2) wild 2LR: resuscitation with lactated Ringer's solution and the SB; (3) iNOS knockout HS: similarly resuscitated as wild HS; (4) iNOS knockout 2LR: similarly resuscitated as wild 2LR. Samples of thymus and spleen were harvested at 2, 6, 24, 48, and 72 h after resuscitation. CD4+ T cells and Foxp3+ Tregs were analyzed at 24, 48, and 72 h. At 2, 6, 24, and 48 h, plasma cytokines were assayed and expression of iNOS (NOS2) was also measured by immunofluorescence.

Results.—NOS2 of HS and 2LR wild groups at 2 and 6 h in spleen increased compared with the control group. At 6 h, NOS2 in HS wild group was significantly lower than in 2LR wild group. Plasma levels of interleukin (IL)-6, TNF-α, MCP-1, and IL-10 increased at 2 h. Both in wild type and iNOS knockout mice, hypertonic saline resuscitation decreased plasma IL-6, TNF-α, and MCP-1 levels at 2 h; CD4+ T cells in spleen and thymus decreased at 24, 48, and 72 h, and Foxp3+ Tregs in spleen at 48 h increased, however, hypertonic saline resuscitation did not affect the Foxp3+.

Conclusions.—These results show that in early phase, the inflammatory cytokines in plasma might affect iNOS expression and cytokines. Further,

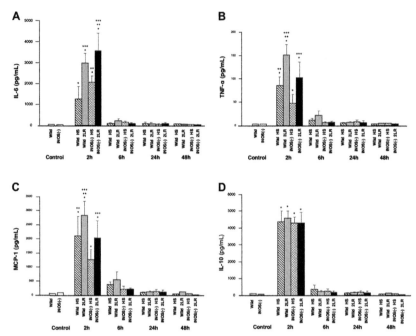

FIGURE 3.—(A) IL-6 levels in plasma. Wild: wild type, iNOS (−): iNOS knockout mice. Data are mean ± SEM; $n = 6$ per group; *$P < 0.01$ *versus* controls. **$P < 0.05$ *versus* Wild. ***$P < 0.01$ *versus* HS. (B) TNF-α levels in plasma. Wild: wild type, iNOS (−): iNOS knockout mice. Data are mean ± SEM; $n = 6$ per group; *$P < 0.01$ *versus* controls. **$P < 0.05$ *versus* iNOS (−). ***$P < 0.01$ *versus* HS. (C) MCP-1 levels in plasma. Wild: wild type, iNOS (−): iNOS knockout mice. Data are mean ± SEM; $n = 6$ per group; *$P < 0.01$ *versus* controls. **$P < 0.05$ *versus* iNOS (−). $P < 0.01$ *versus* HS. (D) IL-10 levels in plasma. Wild: wild type, iNOS (−): iNOS knockout mice. Data are mean ± SEM; $n = 6$ per group; *$P < 0.01$ *versus* controls. (Reprinted from Isayama K, Murao Y, Saito F, et al. Effects of hypertonic saline on CD4⁺CD25⁺Foxp3⁺ regulatory T cells after hemorrhagic shock in relation to iNOS and cytokines. *J Surg Res.* 2012;172:137-145, with permission from Elsevier.)

this study showed that hypertonic saline resuscitation and suppression of iNOS might improve immunosuppressive reaction after hemorrhagic shock (Figs 3 and 6).

▶ Previous studies have shown that hypertonic saline resuscitation reduces organ damage and apoptosis. iNOS worked as an accelerating factor for immunosuppressive conditions, affected apoptosis, and reaction of hypertonic saline. In the current study, the authors investigated how Fox3 Tregs in relation to iNOS and cytokines affect hemorrhagic shock resuscitation. In this study, the proinflammatory cytokines such as TNF-α and MCP-1 increased, but interleukin (IL)-6 decreased significantly in the presence of iNOS. However, the level of IL-10 did not show any difference. Hypertonic saline suppressed IL-6, TNF-α, and MCP-1 without any effect on Fox-3 Tregs. This indicates that the effects of hypertonic saline were reduced by cross talk between iNOS and cytokines toward Fox3 Tregs. This study shows hypertonic saline in combination with

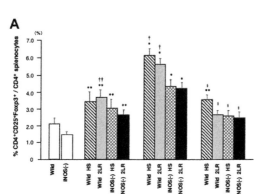

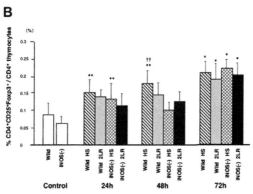

FIGURE 6.—(A) % CD4$^+$CD25$^+$Foxp3$^+$ Treg cells of total CD4$^+$ splenocytes. Wild: wild type, iNOS (−): iNOS knockout mice. Data are mean 6 SEM; $n = 6$ per group; $*P < 0.01$ *versus* controls. $**P < 0.05$ *versus* controls. $^†P < 0.01$ *versus* iNOS (−). $^{††}P < 0.05$ *versus* iNOS (−). $^§P < 0.01$ *versus* 48 h. (B) % CD4$^+$CD25$^+$Foxp3$^+$ Treg cells of total CD4$^+$ thymocytes. Wild: wild type, iNOS (−): iNOS knockout mice. Data are mean ± SEM; $n = 6$ per group; $*P < 0.01$ *versus* controls. $**P < 0.05$ *versus* controls. $^†P < 0.01$ *versus* iNOS (−). $^{††}P < 0.05$ *versus* iNOS (−). (Reprinted from Isayama K, Murao Y, Saito F, et al. Effects of hypertonic saline on CD4$^+$CD25$^+$Foxp3$^+$ regulatory T cells after hemorrhagic shock in relation to iNOS and cytokines. *J Surg Res.* 2012;172:137-145, with permission from Elsevier.)

iNOS suppression may have salutatory effects in hemorrhagic shock. This novel therapeutic strategy needs to be explored in future studies.

M. Mathru, MD

Efficacy of ventilator waveforms observation in detecting patient—ventilator asynchrony
Colombo D, Cammarota G, Alemani M, et al (Università del Piemonte Orientale "Amedeo Avogadro," Novara, Vercelli, Italy; et al)
Crit Care Med 39:2452-2457, 2011

Objectives.—The value of visual inspection of ventilator waveforms in detecting patient—ventilator asynchronies in the intensive care unit has never been systematically evaluated. This study aims to assess intensive care unit physicians' ability to identify patient–ventilator asynchronies through ventilator waveforms.

Design.—Prospective observational study.

Setting.—Intensive care unit of a University Hospital.

Patients.—Twenty-four patients receiving mechanical ventilation for acute respiratory failure.

Intervention.—Forty-three 5-min reports displaying flow-time and airway pressure-time tracings were evaluated by 10 expert and 10 nonexpert, i.e., residents, intensive care unit physicians. The asynchronies identified by experts and nonexperts were compared with those ascertained by three independent examiners who evaluated the same reports displaying, additionally, tracings of diaphragm electrical activity.

Measurements and Main Results.—Data were examined according to both breath-by-breath analysis and overall report analysis. Sensitivity, specificity, and positive and negative predictive values were determined. Sensitivity and positive predictive value were very low with breath-by-breath analysis (22% and 32%, respectively) and fairly increased with report analysis (55% and 44%, respectively). Conversely, specificity and negative predictive value were high with breath-by-breath analysis (91% and 86%, respectively) and slightly lower with report analysis (76% and 82%, respectively). Sensitivity was significantly higher for experts than for nonexperts for breath-by-breath analysis (28% vs. 16%, $p < .05$), but not for report analysis (63% vs. 46%, $p = .15$). The prevalence of asynchronies increased at higher ventilator assistance and tidal volumes ($p < .001$ for both), whereas it decreased at higher respiratory rates and diaphragm electrical activity ($p < .001$ for both). At higher prevalence, sensitivity decreased significantly ($p < .001$).

Conclusions.—The ability of intensive care unit physicians to recognize patient–ventilator asynchronies was overall quite low and decreased at higher prevalence; expertise significantly increased sensitivity for breath-by-breath analysis, whereas it only produced a trend toward improvement for report analysis (Fig 1).

▶ Asynchronies during mechanical ventilation are known to occur in 80% of mechanically ventilated patients. Several clinical studies have demonstrated that bedside interpretation of airflow and airway pressure waveforms are helpful for recognizing patient-ventilator asynchrony and optimizing ventilator settings. In this study, the authors examined the capability of clinicians to detect patient–ventilator asynchrony (PVA) by simple inspection of ventilator waveforms from 24 patients at 2 levels of pressure support ventilation (> 3000 breaths recorded) operated independently by 20 physicians (10 attendings and 10 residents). The authors mainly assessed 2 aspects: the effect of experience among observers and the capability of the ventilator waveforms to reveal the presence of asynchronies. Their results demonstrate that 20 physicians were unable to detect the majority of true asynchronies by using ventilator waveforms analysis alone. A major limitation of this study is that the 20 physicians who participated in this

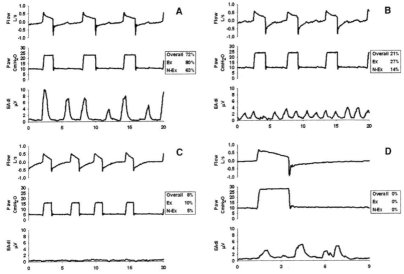

FIGURE 1.—Portions of four representative reports are presented in the four panels. In each panel tracings of flow, airways pressure (*Paw*) and diaphragm electrical activity (*EAdi*) are shown from top to bottom. In addition, sensitivity for expert (*Ex*), nonexpert (*N-Ex*), and the overall group of intensive care unit (*ICU*) physicians is reported in each lateral box. *A,* A typical example of ineffective efforts that can be recognized by the decrease in expiratory flow and the corresponding drop in airway pressure. Sensitivity is, in fact, quite high. *B,* An example of ineffective efforts; their detection, however, is more problematic and sensitivity is much lower than in the previous case. *C,* A series of autotriggered breaths that are recognized by a small fraction of physicians. *D,* An extreme form of asynchrony (one autotriggered breath associated with four ineffective efforts) that remains undetected at all. (Reprinted from Colombo D, Cammarota G, Alemani M, et al. Efficacy of ventilator waveforms observation in detecting patient—ventilator asynchrony. *Crit Care Med.* 2011;39:2452-2457, with permission from the Society of Critical Care Medicine and Lippincott Williams & Wilkins.)

study had access only to pressure and flow tracings. Clinical signs of asynchronies such as respiratory efforts, comfort, and other indicators of asynchronies (heart rate, blood pressure) were not available. Hopefully in the near future, ventilator manufacturers will be able to come up with predictive algorithms to detect asynchronies derived by using ventilator wave patterns and clinical signs.

M. Mathru, MD

Emulsified Isoflurane Preconditioning Protects Against Liver and Lung Injury in Rat Model of Hemorrhagic Shock

Zhang L, Luo N, Liu J, et al (Sichuan Univ, Chengdu, China)
J Surg Res 171:783-790, 2011

Background.—Isoflurane has demonstrated protective effects against ischemia/reperfusion injury in some organs. In this study, using the hemorrhagic shock model, we investigated whether emulsified isoflurane preconditioning protected against liver and lung injury caused by massive surgical blood loss.

Methods.—Male Sprague-Dawley (SD) rats were randomly divided into five groups: a control group, a hemorrhagic shock (HS) group, an intralipid (IL) group, an isoflurane (Iso) group, and an emulsified isoflurane (E-Iso) group. Saline, intralipid, isoflurane, or emulsified isoflurane were administered over 15 min. Forty-five min after injection, hemorrhage was initiated in the experimental group. Four h after resuscitation alanine aminotransferase (ALT), protein and white blood cell (WBC) in bronchoalveolar lavage fluid (BAL), and the liver and lung histopathology were measured. The malondialdehyde (MDA) and superoxide dismutase (SOD) in the liver and lung mitochondria were tested. The survival was also observed in hemorrhagic shocked rats.

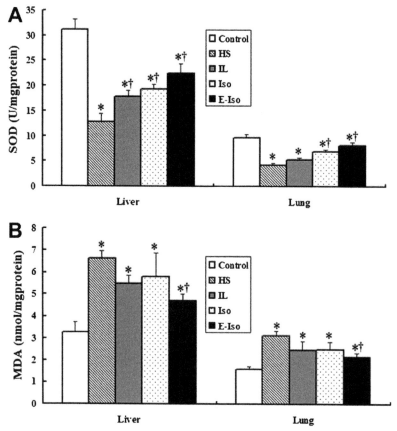

FIGURE 2.—(A) SOD activity in mitochondria. (B) MDA levels in mitochondria. Control = without hemorrhage; HS = saline; IL = intralipid; Iso = isoflurane; E-Iso = emulsified isoflurane. Values were presented as mean 6 SEM, $n = 8$ for each group. *$P < 0.05$ *versus* Control group and †$P < 0.05$ *versus* HS group. (Reprinted from Zhang L, Luo N, Liu J, et al. Emulsified isoflurane preconditioning protects against liver and lung injury in rat model of hemorrhagic shock. *J Surg Res.* 2011;171:783-790, with permission from Elsevier.)

Results.—Emulsified isoflurane enhanced survival and decreased ALT, protein and WBC in BAL, liver and lung apoptosis, and the histologic score. It also decreased MDA and increased SOD activity in mitochondria. In the IL group, liver mitochondrial SOD activity increased, while ALT, liver apoptosis and histological score decreased. In the Iso group liver and lung mitochondrial SOD activity increased, while liver and lung apoptosis decreased.

Conclusion.—Emulsified isoflurane preconditioning has a protective effect against liver and lung injury as well as improving the survival in hemorrhagic shock. The potential mechanisms involved are the inhibition of cell death and improvement of antioxidation in mitochondria (Figs 2-4).

▶ Isoflurane, an anesthetic agent, is known to have tissue-protective effects in several models of ischemia-reperfusion injury. This tissue-protective effect has been demonstrated in heart and liver. This protective effect is attributed to anesthetic-induced ischemic preconditioning, one of the most potent strategies available for organ protection. Recently refined emulsified isoflurane has been shown to have protective effects against ischemia-reperfusion injury in several organs. This protective effect involves inhibition of cell death and improvement in mitochondrial function. This study examined the impact of emulsified isoflurane in a global ischemia-reperfusion (hemorrhage/resuscitation) model. In this model,

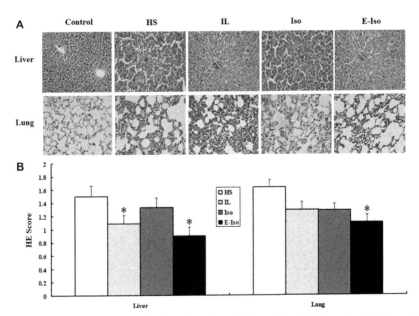

FIGURE 3.—(A) Representative histological sections of a liver and lung. (B) The grade of the liver and lung injury. Control = without hemorrhage; HS = saline; IL = intralipid; Iso = isoflurane; E-Iso = emulsified isoflurane. Values were presented as mean ± SEM, *n* = 8 for each group. *P < 0.05 *versus* HS group. Original magnification ×400. (Reprinted from Zhang L, Luo N, Liu J, et al. Emulsified isoflurane preconditioning protects against liver and lung injury in rat model of hemorrhagic shock. *J Surg Res.* 2011;171:783-790, with permission from Elsevier.)

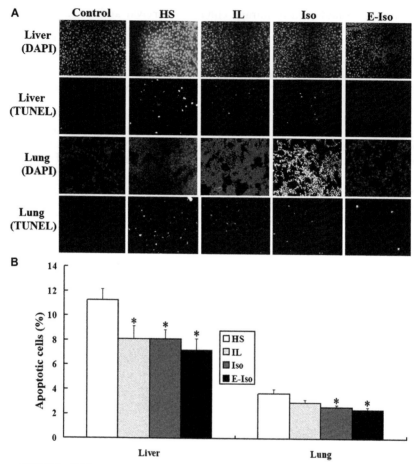

FIGURE 4.—(A) Representative TUNEL-sections of a liver and lung. (B) The cell apoptosis of liver and lung. Control = without hemorrhage; HS = saline; IL = intralipid; Iso = isoflurane; E-Iso = emulsified isoflurane. Values were presented as mean ± SEM, n = 8 for each group. *P < 0.05 *versus* HS group. Original magnification ×400. (Reprinted from Zhang L, Luo N, Liu J, et al. Emulsified isoflurane preconditioning protects against liver and lung injury in rat model of hemorrhagic shock. *J Surg Res.* 2011;171: 783-790, with permission from Elsevier.)

emulsified isoflurane improved survival and reduced malondialdehyde (MDA) and increased superoxide dismutase (SOD) activity. In addition, emulsified iso-flurane reduce cell death in lung and liver. Furthermore, there was a substantial decrease in plasma levels of alanine aminotransferase, amelioration of liver injury caused by hemorrhage, and resuscitation. The increases in MDA imply a protective effect of the membrane structure of the mitochondria, and increases in SOD imply an increased antioxidant effect. These findings suggest that emulsified isoflurane preconditioning could protect the normal structure of the mitochondrial mem-brane and enhance the activity of SOD in mitochondria, thereby attenuating mito-chondrial injury and dysfunction. Emulsified isoflurane is an attractive therapeutic strategy for preconditioning because it can be administered intravenously rather than by inhalation, which makes it easier to control the depth of anesthesia.

M. Mathru, MD

Enteral Omega-3 Fatty Acid, γ-Linolenic Acid, and Antioxidant Supplementation in Acute Lung Injury

Rice TW, for the NHLBI ARDS Clinical Trials Network (Vanderbilt Univ School of Medicine, Nashville, TN; et al)
JAMA 306:1574-1581, 2011

Context.—The omega-3 (n-3) fatty acids docosahexaenoic acid and eicosapentaenoic acid, along with γ-linolenic acid and antioxidants, may modulate systemic inflammatory response and improve oxygenation and outcomes in patients with acute lung injury.

Objective.—To determine if dietary supplementation of these substances to patients with acute lung injury would increase ventilator-free days to study day 28.

Design, Setting, and Participants.—The OMEGA study, a randomized, double-blind, placebo-controlled, multicenter trial conducted from January 2, 2008, through February 21, 2009. Participants were 272 adults within 48 hours of developing acute lung injury requiring mechanical ventilation whose physicians intended to start enteral nutrition at 44 hospitals in the National Heart, Lung, and Blood Institute ARDS Clinical Trials Network. All participants had complete follow-up.

Interventions.—Twice-daily enteral supplementation of n-3 fatty acids, γ-linolenic acid, and antioxidants compared with an isocaloric control. Enteral nutrition, directed by a protocol, was delivered separately from the study supplement.

Main Outcome Measure.—Ventilator-free days to study day 28.

Results.—The study was stopped early for futility after 143 and 129 patients were enrolled in the n-3 and control groups. Despite an 8-fold increase in plasma eicosapentaenoic acid levels, patients receiving the n-3 supplement had fewer ventilator-free days (14.0 vs 17.2; $P=.02$) (difference, -3.2 [95% CI, -5.8 to -0.7]) and intensive care unit—free days (14.0 vs 16.7; $P=.04$). Patients in the n-3 group also had fewer non-pulmonary organ failure—free days (12.3 vs 15.5; $P=.02$). Sixty-day hospital mortality was 26.6% in the n-3 group vs 16.3% in the control group ($P=.054$), and adjusted 60-day mortality was 25.1% and 17.6% in the n-3 and control groups, respectively ($P=.11$). Use of the n-3 supplement resulted in more days with diarrhea (29% vs 21%; $P=.001$).

Conclusions.—Twice-daily enteral supplementation of n-3 fatty acids, γ-linolenic acid, and antioxidants did not improve the primary end point of ventilator-free days or other clinical outcomes in patients with acute lung injury and may be harmful.

Trial Registration.—clinicaltrials.gov Identifier: NCT00609180.

▶ Rice and colleagues report the results from the Omega clinical trials involving patients with acute lung injury (ALI) who were randomly assigned to receive either placebo or a supplement, comparing the omega-3 fatty acids and antioxidants. The authors postulated that the pharmaconutrient supplementation would decrease ventilator-free days (primary outcome), favorably influence inflammation, and have other salutary effects on clinical endpoints.

In contrast to the previous trials in this study, pharmaconutrient administration did not improve lung physiology or clinical outcome in patients with ALI compared with supplementation of an isocaloric control. Furthermore, n-3 supplementation did not protect from nosocomial infections or improve nonpulmonary organ function.

There are several possible explanations for their results: the bolus administration in this trial could have blunted the modulation of inflammatory response, and the amount of protein received in the control group could have modified the results. A recent study found that 30 g/d of protein administered in mechanically ventilated patients increased the ventilator-free days and lowered mortality. Furthermore, in catabolic patients who were relatively "underfed," the administered fish oil could have been oxidized to meet the caloric requirements rather than stored in membranes where it could influence the subsequent inflammatory response.

M. Mathru, MD

Evaluation of new acute kidney injury biomarkers in a mixed intensive care unit
Doi K, Negishi K, Ishizu T, et al (The Univ of Tokyo, Japan; et al)
Crit Care Med 39:2464-2469, 2011

Objective.—Biomarkers for detection of acute kidney injury and prediction of mortality will be useful to improve the outcomes of critically ill patients. Although several promising acute kidney injury biomarkers have been reported, evaluation in heterogeneous disease-oriented populations is necessary to confirm their reliability before their translation to clinical use. This study was undertaken to evaluate the reliability of new acute kidney injury biomarkers including urinary L-type fatty acid-binding protein with heterogeneous intensive care unit populations.

Design.—Prospective observational cohort study.

Setting.—Single-center study, 15-bed medical–surgical mixed intensive care unit at a university hospital.

Patients.—Three hundred thirty-nine adult critically ill patients who had been admitted to the intensive care unit were studied prospectively.

Interventions.—None.

Measurements and Main Results.—Five urinary biomarkers (L-type fatty acid-binding protein, neutrophil gelatinase-associated lipocalin, interleukin-18, N-acetyl-β-D-glucosaminidase, and albumin) were measured at intensive care unit admission. By the RIFLE (Risk, Injury, Failure, Loss, End-stage kidney disease) criteria, 131 patients (39%) were diagnosed as acute kidney injury. Urinary L-type fatty acid-binding protein detected acute kidney injury better than the other biomarkers did (the area under the receiver operating characteristic curves for L-type fatty acid-binding protein 0.75, neutrophil gelatinase-associated lipocalin 0.70, interleukin-18 0.69, N-acetyl-β-D-glucosaminidase 0.62, albumin 0.69). Urinary L-type fatty acid-binding protein predicted later-onset acute kidney injury after intensive care unit admission with the highest area under the receiver operating characteristic

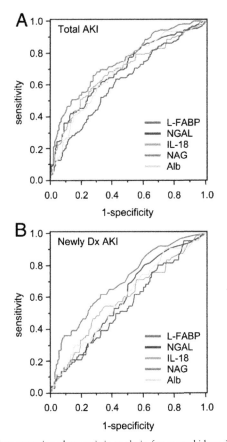

FIGURE 1.—Receiver operating characteristic analysis for acute kidney injury (*AKI*) diagnosis. Receiver operating characteristic curves for total AKI and newly diagnosed AKI are shown. Among 339 adult critically ill patients, 131 patients (38.6%) were diagnosed as AKI (*A*, total AKI). Of 131 patients with AKI, 66 patients were not diagnosed as AKI at intensive care unit admission, but reached the modified Risk, Injury, Failure, Loss, End-stage kidney disease criteria within 1 week (*B*, newly diagnosed AKI). The area under the curve-receiver operating characteristic values are presented in Table 2. *L-FABP*, L-type fatty acid-binding protein; *NGAL*, neutrophil gelatinase-associated lipocalin; *IL*, interleukin; *NAG*, N-acetyl-β-D-glucosaminidase; *Alb*, albumin. (Reprinted from Doi K, Negishi K, Ishizu T, et al. Evaluation of new acute kidney injury biomarkers in a mixed intensive care unit. *Crit Care Med.* 2011;39:2464-2469, with permission from the Society of Critical Care Medicine and Lippincott Williams & Wilkins.)

curve value of 0.70. Furthermore, L-type fatty acid-binding protein, neutrophil gelatinase-associated lipocalin, and interleukin-18 were able to predict 14-day mortality with higher area under the receiver operating characteristic curves than acute kidney injury detection (area under the receiver operating characteristic curve for L-type fatty acid-binding protein 0.90, neutrophil gelatinase-associated lipocalin 0.83, interleukin-18 0.83). The combination of L-type fatty acid-binding protein and neutrophil gelatinase-associated lipocalin improved mortality prediction (area under the receiver operating characteristic curve 0.93).

Conclusion.—This prospective observational study with a cohort of heterogeneous patients treated in a mixed intensive care unit revealed that new acute kidney injury biomarkers have a significantly and moderately predictive use for acute kidney injury diagnosis and that urinary L-type fatty acid-binding protein and neutrophil gelatinase-associated lipocalin can serve as new biomarkers of mortality prediction in critical care (Figs 1-3).

▶ Acute kidney injury (AKI) is traditionally diagnosed using serum creatinine concentration. However, serum creatinine has been recognized as a late and

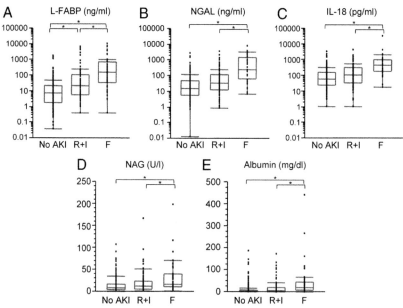

FIGURE 2.—Five urinary biomarker values grouped by acute kidney injury (*AKI*) severity. Values of five urinary biomarkers (L-type fatty acid-binding protein [*L-FABP*] [*A*], neutrophil gelatinase-associated lipocalin [*NGAL*] [*B*], interleukin [*IL*]-18 [*C*], N-acetyl-β-D-glucosaminidase [*NAG*] [*D*], and albumin [*E*]) measured at intensive care unit admission are shown in each AKI severity category (no AKI [n = 208], risk and injury [*R+I*] [n = 87], failure [*F*] [n = 44]). Dots show individual values. Boxes enclose the range of lower to upper quartile values; lines inside the boxes represent the median values. Error bars represent the lowest datum still within 1.5 interquartile range of the lower quartile, and the highest datum still within 1.5 interquartile range of the upper quartile *$p < .05$ using Tukey–Kramer *post hoc* analysis. (Reprinted from Doi K, Negishi K, Ishizu T, et al. Evaluation of new acute kidney injury biomarkers in a mixed intensive care unit. *Crit Care Med.* 2011;39:2464-2469, with permission from the Society of Critical Care Medicine and Lippincott Williams & Wilkins.)

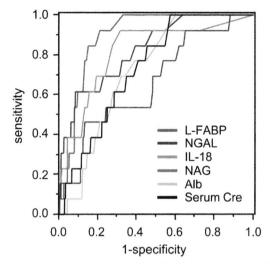

FIGURE 3.—Receiver operating characteristic analysis for 14-day mortality. Receiver operating characteristic curves for 14-day mortality are shown. Among 339 adult critically ill patients, 14 patients (4.1%) died within 2 weeks after intensive care unit admission. The area under the curve-receiver operating characteristic values are presented in Table 3. *L-FABP*, L-type fatty acid binding protein; *NGAL*, neutrophil gelatinase associated lipocalin; *IL*, interleukin; *NAG*, N-acetyl-β-D-glucosaminidase; *Alb*, albumin. (Reprinted from Doi K, Negishi K, Ishizu T, et al. Evaluation of new acute kidney injury biomarkers in a mixed intensive care unit. *Crit Care Med*. 2011;39:2464-2469, with permission from the Society of Critical Care Medicine and Lippincott Williams & Wilkins.)

inaccurate renal injury marker for detecting decreased glomerular filtration rate and tubular injury. Furthermore, serum creatinine concentration is influenced by nonrenal factors including sepsis, hypervolemia, and liver disease. In this study, the authors evaluated the use of new AKI biomarkers, including urinary L-type fatty acid-binding protein (L-FABP), neutrophil gelatinase-associated lipocalin (NGAL), and interleukin-18, in a mixed medical-surgical intensive care unit population by comparing them with the urinary biomarkers of N-acetyl-B-D glucosaminidase (NAG) and albumin, which are currently in clinical use. In their heterogeneous population, urinary L-FABP and NGAL were able to detect AKI, showing good discrimination capability and showing even better performance for mortality prediction. The study limitations include that it was performed in single center, and urinary biomarkers were measured only at single time point. Further investigation for the optimal combination of candidate urinary biomarkers including kidney injury molecule-1, and cystatin C, and gamma glutamyl transferase will be needed to establish the best biomarker panel for AKI diagnosis and mortality prediction.

M. Mathru, MD

Gender and Acute Respiratory Distress Syndrome in Critically Injured Adults: A Prospective Study

Heffernan DS, Dossett LA, Lightfoot MA, et al (Rhode Island Hosp, Providence; et al)
J Trauma 71:878-885, 2011

Background.—The acute respiratory distress syndrome (ARDS) is a pro-inflammatory condition that often complicates trauma and critical illness. Animal studies have shown that both gender and sex hormones play an important role in inflammatory regulation. Human data are scant regarding the role of gender and sex hormones in developing ARDS. Our objective was to describe gender and hormonal differences in patients who develop ARDS in a large cohort of critically injured adults.

Methods.—A prospective cohort study of adult trauma patients requiring intensive care unit admission for at least 48 hours was performed. Demographic and clinical data were collected prospectively, and sex hormones were assayed at study entry (48 hours). The primary outcome was the development of ARDS. Multivariate logistic regression was used to determine the adjusted odds of death associated with differences in gender.

Results.—Six hundred forty-eight patients met entry criteria, and 180 patients developed ARDS (31%). Women were more likely to develop ARDS (35% vs. 25%, $p = 0.02$). This association remained after adjusting for age, mechanism of injury, injury severity, and blood product transfusion (odds ratio, 1.6; 95% confidence interval: 1.1–2.4; $p = 0.02$). Of patients with ARDS, there was no difference in mortality related to gender (22% mortality in women with ARDS vs. 20% in men; $p = $ not significant). A proinflammatory sex hormone profile (low testosterone and high estradiol) was associated with ARDS in both men and women.

Conclusion.—Women are more likely than men to develop ARDS after critical injury. Despite the increased incidence in ARDS, the mortality in patients with ARDS does not differ according to gender. The inflammatory properties of sex hormones may contribute to ARDS, but they do not fully explain observed gender differences (Fig 1).

▶ Adult respiratory distress syndrome (ARDS) carries a high morbidity and mortality. The lung injury following trauma is attributed to the proinflammatory response associated with trauma. Evidence suggests that gender can modify the inflammatory and immune response following trauma, particularly in the laboratory setting. Several lines of experimental evidence suggest that the proestrous state is proinflammatory and is associated with improved survival. However, 2 recent clinical studies demonstrated increased mortality in critically ill patients with elevated endogenous estrogens, regardless of sex. The current study examined the possible role of gender and sex hormones after severe traumatic injury on the development of ARDS. It reported a 10% higher incidence of ARDS in females. This was associated with increased estradiol and reduced testosterone concentrations. The study does not provide any details regarding ventilator management (ie, number of patients requiring mechanical ventilation

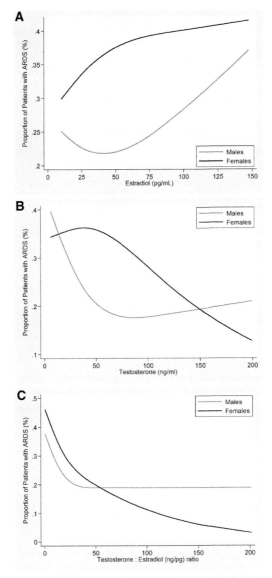

FIGURE 1.—The relationship between sex hormones and ARDS stratified by gender. (A) For both genders, rates of ARDS increase with increasing estradiol. The higher rates of ARDS observed in women are not fully explained by estrogens; however, for all estradiol levels, the rate of ARDS is higher in females. (B) For both genders, rates of ARDS decrease with increasing testosterone. (C) Relationship between testosterone and estradiol (testosterone to estradiol ratio) and rates of ARDS. For both genders, a higher ratio appears protective, with the lowest rates of ARDS being expected in patients with ratios greater than 50. (Reprinted from Heffernan DS, Dossett LA, Lightfoot MA, et al. Gender and acute respiratory distress syndrome in critically injured adults: a prospective study. *J Trauma*. 2011;71:878-885, with permission from Lippincott Williams & Wilkins.)

or number of ventilator-free days). The number of blood transfusions has been confirmed to be an independent risk factor for ARDS. However, no data are provided on blood transfusion. Nevertheless, the authors are to be congratulated for this interesting prospective study. Physicians should look forward to future studies by this group in the area of gender and hormonal impact on trauma outcomes.

M. Mathru, MD

Hemorrhagic Shock in Polytrauma Patients: Early Detection with Renal Doppler Resistive Index Measurements
Corradi F, Brusasco C, Vezzani A, et al (Universitá degli Studi di Genova, Italy; Azienda Ospedaliera Universitaria di Parma, Italy; et al)
Radiology 260:112-118, 2011

Purpose.—To investigate whether renal Doppler resistive index (RI) changes occur early during posttraumatic bleeding and may be predictive of occult hypoperfusion—and thus hemorrhagic shock—in patients with polytrauma.

Materials and Methods.—This study was approved by the institutional ethics committee, and informed consent was obtained from all patients. The renal Doppler RI was measured in 52 hemodynamically stable adult patients admitted to the emergency department (ED) because of polytrauma. Renal Doppler RI, hemoglobin, standard base excess, lactate, systolic blood pressure, pH, heart rate, and inferior vena cava diameter values were recorded at admittance and correlated with outcome (progression or nonprogression to hemorrhagic shock). Logistic regression analysis was performed to assess the risk factors for progression to hemorrhagic shock.

Results.—Twenty-nine patients developed hemorrhagic shock, and 23 did not. At univariable analysis, the hemorrhagic shock group, as compared with the nonhemorrhagic shock group, had higher renal Doppler RI (mean, 0.80 ± 0.10 [standard deviation] vs 0.63 ± 0.03; $P < .01$), injury severity score (mean, 36 ± 11 vs 26 ± 5; $P < .01$), and standard base excess (mean, -4.0 mEq/L ± 4 vs 1 mEq/L ± 3; $P = .04$) values. At logistic regression analysis, a renal Doppler RI greater than 0.7 (vs less than or equal to 0.7) was the only independent risk factor for progression to hemorrhagic shock (odds ratio, 57.8; 95% confidence interval: 10.5, 317.0) ($P < .001$).

Conclusion.—In polytrauma patients who are hemodynamically stable at admittance to the ED, renal cortical blood flow redistribution occurs very early in response to occult bleeding and might be noninvasively detected by using the renal Doppler RI. A renal Doppler RI greater than 0.7 is predictive of progression to hemorrhagic shock in polytrauma patients (Fig 1, Table 2).

▶ Uncontrolled occult bleeding in trauma patients contributes to high mortality. Commonly used indices to determine the endpoint of resuscitation include injury

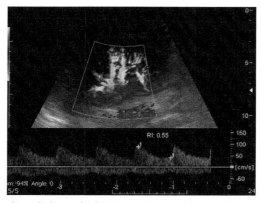

FIGURE 1.—Renal Doppler longitudinal US image in 38-year-old man with normal renal cortical blood flow and renal Doppler RI values who did not develop hemorrhagic shock. (Reprinted from Corradi F, Brusasco C, Vezzani A, et al. Hemorrhagic shock in polytrauma patients: Early detection with renal Doppler resistive index measurements. *Radiology.* 2011;260:112-118. Copyright by the Radiological Society of North America.)

TABLE 2.—Independent Variables Predictive of Hemorrhagic Shock and Bleeding

Independent Variable	Odds Ratio*	*P* Value
Renal Doppler RI	57.8 (10.5, 317.0)	<.001
ISS	5.89 (0.61, 56.9)	.67
Standard base excess	3.5 (0.97, 12.9)	.60

*Numbers in parentheses are 95% confidence intervals.

severity score, mean arterial pressure, base-deficit, lactate, hematocrit, and urine output. However, all these indices have poor sensitivity in recognizing occult hypoperfusion. Recently, functional hemodynamic monitoring indices have been used to determine the endpoint of resuscitation. In experimental models, increases in renal vascular resistance have been consistently demonstrated during hemorrhage. In this study, the investigators examined whether the renal Doppler resistance index (RI) occurs early in post traumatic bleeding and whether renal Doppler RI may enable accurate prediction of occult hypoperfusion. Their results show that, in normotensive polytrauma patients, renal Doppler RI > 0.7 at admittance into the emergency department was predictive of hemorrhagic shock within the first 24 hours (odds ratio, 57.8; 95% confidence interval, 10.5, 317.0; *P* < .001). A high renal Doppler RI is an early sign of hypoperfusion in apparently stable polytrauma patients and may facilitate accurate prediction of the occurrence of hemorrhagic shock and thus help to activate aggressive resuscitation strategies or surgical/radiologic interventions.

M. Mathru, MD

Identification of Cardiac Dysfunction in Sepsis with B-Type Natriuretic Peptide

Turner KL, Moore LJ, Todd SR, et al (The Methodist Hosp Res Inst, Houston, TX)

J Am Coll Surg 213:139-147, 2011

Background.—B-type natriuretic peptide (BNP) is secreted in response to myocardial stretch and has been used clinically to assess volume overload and predict death in congestive heart failure. More recently, BNP elevation has been demonstrated with septic shock and is predictive of death. How BNP levels relate to cardiac function in sepsis remains to be established.

Study Design.—Retrospective review of prospectively gathered sepsis database from a surgical ICU in a tertiary academic hospital. Initial BNP levels, patient demographics, baseline central venous pressure levels, and in-hospital mortality were obtained. Transthoracic echocardiography was performed during initial resuscitation per protocol.

Results.—During 24 months ending in September 2009, two hundred and thirty-one patients (59 ± 3 years of age, 43% male) were treated for sepsis. Baseline BNP increased with initial sepsis severity (ie, sepsis vs severe sepsis vs septic shock, by ANOVA; $p < 0.05$) and was higher in those who died vs those who lived (by Fisher's exact test; $p < 0.05$). Of these patients, 153 (66%) had early echocardiography. Low ejection fraction (<50%) was associated with higher BNP (by Fisher's exact test; $p < 0.05$) and patients with low ejection fraction had a higher mortality (39% vs 20%; odds ratio = 3.03). We found no correlation between baseline central venous pressure (12.7 ± 6.10 mmHg) and BNP (526.5 ± 82.10 pg/mL) (by Spearman's ρ, $R_s = .001$) for the entire sepsis population.

Conclusions.—In surgical sepsis patients, BNP increases with sepsis severity and is associated with early systolic dysfunction, which in turn is associated with death. Monitoring BNP in early sepsis to identify occult systolic dysfunction might prompt earlier use of inotropic agents (Figs 1-4).

▶ Systolic and diastolic dysfunction have been described in sepsis models and in septic patients. Right ventricular dysfunction has also been described in 30% of septic patients independent of the afterload. Proinflammatory cytokines, mitochondrial dysfunction, and alterations in calcium currents have been implicated in the pathogenesis of myocardial dysfunction associated with sepsis.

B-type natriuretic peptide (BNP) has been used extensively as a marker of cardiac dysfunction and volume overload in chronic heart failure. In this study, the predictive value of BNP was evaluated in myocardial dysfunction associated with sepsis.

The results of this study demonstrate a strong correlation of BNP levels with sepsis severity, which has not been demonstrated previously. This study also demonstrated a binary difference between normal and abnormal systolic function, but also as a continuum with worsening ejection fraction. The investigators

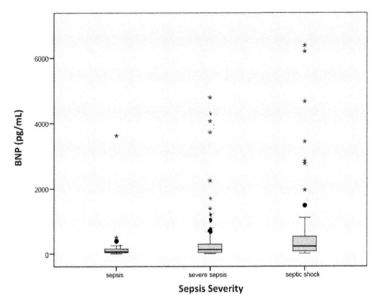

FIGURE 1.—B-type natriuretic peptide (BNP) by sepsis category. BNP expressed as median and inter-quartile ranges per sepsis severity category. (Reprinted from Turner KL, Moore LJ, Todd SR, et al. Identifi-cation of cardiac dysfunction in sepsis with B-type natriuretic peptide. *J Am Coll Surg.* 2011;213:139-147, with permission from the American College of Surgeons.)

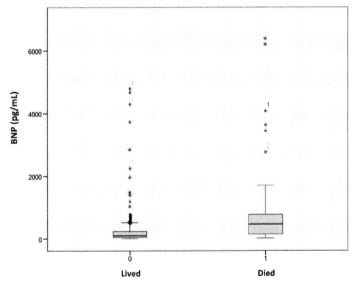

FIGURE 2.—B-type natriuretic peptide (BNP) by mortality. BNP expressed as median and interquar-tile ranges per mortality category. (Reprinted from Turner KL, Moore LJ, Todd SR, et al. Identification of cardiac dysfunction in sepsis with B-type natriuretic peptide. *J Am Coll Surg.* 2011;213:139-147, with permission from the American College of Surgeons.)

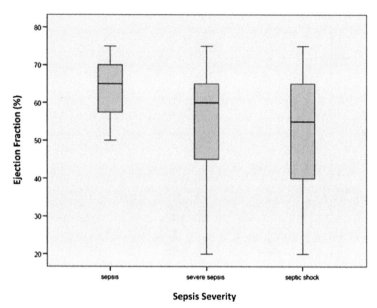

FIGURE 3.—Ejection fraction by sepsis category. Left ventricular ejection fraction percent expressed as median and interquartile ranges per sepsis severity category. (Reprinted from Turner KL, Moore LJ, Todd SR, et al. Identification of cardiac dysfunction in sepsis with B-type natriuretic peptide. *J Am Coll Surg.* 2011;213:139-147, with permission from the American College of Surgeons.)

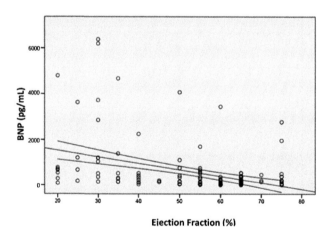

FIGURE 4.—B-type natriuretic peptide (BNP) and ejection fraction. Test for correlation between left ventricular ejection fraction and BNP with best fit line and confidence intervals. Correlation coefficient −0.381. Significant at 0.0001 level. (Reprinted from Turner KL, Moore LJ, Todd SR, et al. Identification of cardiac dysfunction in sepsis with B-type natriuretic peptide. *J Am Coll Surg.* 2011;213:139-147, with permission from the American College of Surgeons.)

concluded that in surgical sepsis patients, BNP increases with sepsis severity and is associated with early cardiac dysfunction and subsequent death. This study suggests that monitoring BNP in early sepsis may be a marker for occult systolic dysfunction, which could be useful in prompting early use of inotropes in septic patients.

M. Mathru, MD

Identification of lipids that accumulate during the routine storage of prestorage leukoreduced red blood cells and cause acute lung injury

Silliman CC, Moore EE, Kelher MR, et al (Denver Health Med, CO; Univ of Colorado Denver, Aurora)
Transfusion 51:2549-2554, 2011

Background.—Lipids accumulate during the storage of red blood cells (RBCs), prime neutrophils (PMNs), and have been implicated in transfusion-related acute lung injury (TRALI). These lipids are composed of two classes: nonpolar lipids and lysophosphatidylcholines based on their retention time on separation by high-pressure liquid chromatography. Prestorage leukoreduction significantly decreases white blood cell and platelet contamination of RBCs; therefore, it is hypothesized that prestorage leukoreduction changes the classes of lipids that accumulate during storage, and these lipids prime PMNs and induce acute lung injury (ALI) as the second event in a two-event in vivo model.

Study Design and Methods.—RBC units were divided: 50% was leukoreduced (LR-RBCs), stored, and sampled on Day 1 and at the end of storage, Day 42. Priming activity was evaluated on isolated PMNs, and the purified lipids from Day 1 or Day 42 were used as the second event in the in vivo model.

Results.—The plasma and lipids from RBCs and LR-RBCs primed PMNs, and the LR-RBC activity decreased with longer storage. Unlike RBCs, nonpolar lipids comprised the PMN-priming activity from stored LR-RBCs. Mass spectroscopy identified these lipids as arachidonic acid and 5-, 12-, and 15-hydroxyeicosatetraenoic acid. At concentrations from Day 42, but not Day 1, three of four of these lipids individually, and the mixture, primed PMNs. The mixture also caused ALI as the second event in a two-event model of TRALI.

Conclusion.—We conclude that the nonpolar lipids that accumulate during LR-RBC storage may represent the agents responsible for antibody-negative TRALI (Figs 2 and 3).

▶ In this article, Silliman and his colleagues report that nonpolar lipids accumulate in stored leukoreduced red blood cell (RBC) components. These nonpolar lipids include arachidonic acid and hydroxyeicosatetraenoic acids. These nonpolar lipids prime neutrophils and induce lung injury in rats previously primed with lipopolysaccharides. This study convincingly demonstrates that nonpolar lipid levels are elevated in RBC components after 14 days of storage and reach higher levels by 28 days and remain stable until day 42. The findings need to be confirmed by future clinical studies. Case control studies are needed, and

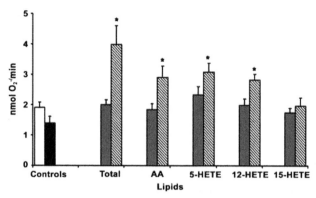

FIGURE 2.—PMN-priming activity and ALI induced by purified lipids from fresh (Day 1) versus stored (Day 42) LR-RBCs. The priming activity, the maximal rate of O_2^- production (nmol O_2^-/min), is depicted as a function of treatment group. The controls consist of albumin- (■) or buffer-primed (□) PMNs, and the priming activity from both the lipid mixtures and the individual lipid moieties from Day 1 (■) or Day 42 (▨) of LR-RBC storage are shown. *p < 0.05 versus the controls, both buffer and albumin treated, and the concentrations of the individual lipid moieties or mixture on Day 1 of storage. Each bar represents a sample size of seven. AA = arachidonic acid. (Reprinted from Silliman CC, Moore EE, Kelher MR, et al. Identification of lipids that accumulate during the routine storage of prestorage leukoreduced red blood cells and cause acute lung injury. *Transfusion*. 2011;51:2549-2554, with permission from John Wiley and Sons. [www.interscience.wiley.com])

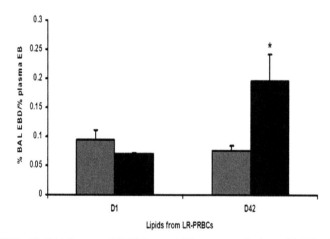

FIGURE 3.—The lipids from stored LR-RBCs cause ALI in a two-event in vivo model. ALI is shown as the percentage of EBD leak from the plasma into the bronchoalveolar lavage (BAL) as a function of treatment group. *p < 0.05 versus the NS/lipids from Day 1 LR-RBCs, LPS/lipids from Day 1 LR-RBCs, and NS/lipids from Day 42 LR-RBCs. Each bar represents five different rats that underwent identical treatment protocols with differing first and second insults. (■) NS; (■) LPS. (Reprinted from Silliman CC, Moore EE, Kelher MR, et al. Identification of lipids that accumulate during the routine storage of prestorage leukoreduced red blood cells and cause acute lung injury. *Transfusion*. 2011;51:2549-2554, with permission from John Wiley and Sons. [www.interscience.wiley.com])

issues that should be addressed should include what proportion of transfusion-related acute lung injury (TRALI) cases are caused by the transfusion of RBC components with high levels of nonpolar lipids. Future studies should also address what concentration of nonpolar lipids in stored RBC components places the transfusion recipients at risk for TRALI. This is an interesting study with potential clinical implications.

M. Mathru, MD

Inhaled Nitric Oxide for Acute Respiratory Distress Syndrome and Acute Lung Injury in Adults and Children: A Systematic Review with Meta-Analysis and Trial Sequential Analysis

Afshari A, Brok J, Møller AM, et al (Juliane Marie Centre, Copenhagen, Denmark; Hvidovre Hosp, Denmark; Copenhagen Univ Hosp, Denmark)
Anesth Analg 112:1411-1421, 2011

Background.—Acute hypoxemic respiratory failure, defined as acute lung injury and acute respiratory distress syndrome, are critical conditions associated with frequent mortality and morbidity in all ages. Inhaled nitric oxide (iNO) has been used to improve oxygenation, but its role remains controversial. We performed a systematic review with meta-analysis and trial sequential analysis of randomized clinical trials (RCTs). We searched CENTRAL, Medline, Embase, International Web of Science, LILACS, the Chinese Biomedical Literature Database, and CINHAL (up to January 31, 2010). Additionally, we hand-searched reference lists, contacted authors and experts, and searched registers of ongoing trials. Two reviewers independently selected all parallel group RCTs comparing iNO with placebo or no intervention and extracted data related to study methods, interventions,

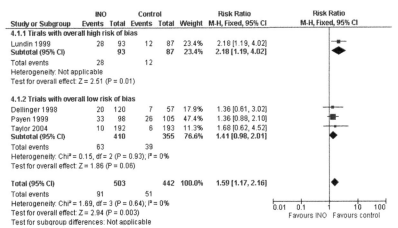

FIGURE 4.—Forest plot of the effect of inhaled nitric oxide on renal function suggested by the randomized controlled trials; subgroup analysis based on the overall quality of the included trials. Risk ratio with 95% confidence interval (CI), fixed effects model. df = degrees of freedom; I^2 = heterogeneity; iNO = inhaled nitric oxide; M-H = Mantel-Haenszel. (Reprinted from Afshari A, Brok J, Møller AM, et al. Inhaled nitric oxide for acute respiratory distress syndrome and acute lung injury in adults and children: a systematic review with meta-analysis and trial sequential analysis. *Anesth Analg.* 2011;112:1411-1421, with permission from International Anesthesia Research Society.)

TABLE 2.—Effects of Inhaled Nitric Oxide Versus Control on Clinical and Physiological Outcomes in Patients with Acute Hypoxemic Respiratory Failure

Outcome or Subgroup	No. of Trials (Patients)	Statistical Method	Effect Estimate & I^2
Mortality (longest follow-up)	14 (1250)	Risk ratio (M-H, fixed, 95% CI)	1.06 [0.93–1.22], $I^2 = 0$
Mortality (28–30 days)	9 (1082)	Risk ratio (M-H, fixed, 95% CI)	1.12 [0.95–1.31], $I^2 = 0$
Mortality (paediatric subgroup)	3 (162)	Risk ratio (M-H, fixed, 95% CI)	0.97 [0.67–1.38], $I^2 = 0$
Mortality (adult subgroup)	11 (1088)	Risk ratio (M-H, fixed, 95% CI)	1.08 [0.93–1.25], $I^2 = 0$
Mortality (only AECC criteria trials)	11 (864)	Risk ratio (M-H, fixed, 95% CI)	1.08 [0.93–1.25], $I^2 = 0$
Mortality (abstracts excluded)	12 (1028)	Risk ratio (M-H, fixed, 95% CI)	1.06 [0.91–1.24], $I^2 = 0$
Mortality (shorter than median duration of iNO)[a]	6 (424)	Risk ratio (M-H, fixed, 95% CI)	1.05 [0.86–1.28], $I^2 = 0$
Mortality (longer than median duration of iNO)[a]	8 (826)	Risk ratio (M-H, fixed, 95% CI)	1.07 [0.90–1.29], $I^2 = 0$
Bleeding events	5 (614)	Risk ratio (M-H, fixed, 95% CI)	0.88 [0.43–1.79], $I^2 = 0$
Renal impairment	4 (945)	Risk ratio (M-H, fixed, 95% CI)	1.59 [1.17–2.16], $I^2 = 0$
Pao2/Fio2 up to 24 hours	11 (614)	Mean difference (IV, random, 95% CI)	15.91 [8.25–23.56], $I^2 = 25\%$
Pao2/Fio2 up to 48 hours	5 (416)	Mean difference (IV, random, 95% CI)	8.65 [−2.80–20.11], $I^2 = 37\%$
Pao2/Fio2 up to 72 hours	5 (450)	Mean difference (IV, fixed, 95% CI)	6.88 [−3.91–17.68], $I^2 = 0$
Pao2/Fio2 up to 96 hours	4 (334)	Mean difference (IV, fixed, 95% CI)	14.51 [3.64–25.38], $I^2 = 0$
Ventilator free days (28–30 days)	5 (804)	Mean difference (IV, fixed, 95% CI)	−0.57 [−1.82–0.69], $I^2 = 0$
Duration of mechanical ventilation (days)	6 (390)	Mean difference (IV, Random, 95% CI)	1.02 [−2.08–4.12], $I^2 = 76\%$
Oxygenation index 24 hours	4 (317)	Mean difference (IV, fixed, 95% CI)	−2.31 [−2.74−−1.89], $I^2 = 0$
Oxygenation index 48 hours	2 (183)	Mean difference (IV, Random, 95% CI)	1.99 [−10.40–14.38], $I^2 = 74\%$
Oxygenation index 72 hours	2 (245)	Mean difference (IV, fixed, 95% CI)	−3.48 [−6.80−−0.15], $I^2 = 0$
MPAP up to 24 hours	5 (205)	Mean difference (IV, fixed, 95% CI)	−1.76 [−3.41−−0.12], $I^2 = 1\%$
MPAP up to 48 hours	3 (167)	Mean difference (IV, fixed, 95% CI)	−1.39 [−3.43−0.65], $I^2 = 0$
MPAP up to 72 hours	2 (111)	Mean difference (IV, fixed, 95% CI)	−1.92 [−4.36−−0.52], $I^2 = 0$
MPAP up to 96 hours	3 (130)	Mean difference (IV, fixed, 95% CI)	−1.74 [−3.77−−0.30], $I^2 = 0$

M-H = Mantel-Haenszel; CI = confidence interval; IV = inverse variance; MPAP = mean pulmonary arterial pressure; No. = number; Pao2/Fio2 = partial pressure of arterial oxygen/fraction of inspired oxygen; I2 = Cochrane's test of heterogeneity.
[a]Median duration of iNO was 1 week.

outcomes, bias risk, and adverse events. All trials, irrespective of blinding or language status were included. Retrieved trials were evaluated with Cochrane methodology. Disagreements were resolved by discussion. Our primary outcome measure was all-cause mortality. We performed subgroup and sensitivity analyses to assess the effect of iNO in adults and children and on various clinical and physiological outcomes. We assessed the risk of bias through assessment of trial methodological components. We assessed the risk of random error by applying trial sequential analysis.

Results.—We included 14 RCTs with a total of 1303 participants; 10 of these trials had a high risk of bias. iNO showed no statistically significant effect on overall mortality (40.2% versus 38.6%) (relative risks [RR] 1.06, 95% confidence interval [CI] 0.93 to 1.22; $I^2 = 0$) and in several subgroup and sensitivity analyses, indicating robust results. Limited data demonstrated a statistically insignificant effect of iNO on duration of ventilation, ventilator-free days, and length of stay in the intensive care unit and hospital. We found a statistically significant but transient improvement in oxygenation in the first 24 hours, expressed as the ratio of Po_2 to fraction of inspired oxygen (mean difference [MD] 15.91, 95% CI 8.25 to 23.56; $I^2 = 25\%$). However, iNO appears to increase the risk of renal impairment among adults (RR 1.59, 95% CI 1.17 to 2.16; $I^2 = 0$) but not the risk of bleeding or methemoglobin or nitrogen dioxide formation.

Conclusion.—iNO cannot be recommended for patients with acute hypoxemic respiratory failure. iNO results in a transient improvement in oxygenation but does not reduce mortality and may be harmful (Fig 4, Table 2).

▶ Inhaled nitric oxide (iNO) can cause selective pulmonary vasodilation and improve ventilation perfusion mismatch, and it has been shown that iNO could have potent anti-inflammatory effects locally and in remote tissues. This is attributed to the production of endogenous metabolites with biological activity similar to NO. Previous studies have shown that iNO has no effect on improving clinical outcome in acute respiratory distress syndrome (ARDS) but increased the incidence of renal dysfunction. In this systematic meta-analysis, benefits and harms of iNO were evaluated in children and adults with ARDS. In this systematic review of 14 trials and 1303 patients, the authors found no benefits of iNO on survival. However, iNO increased the risk of renal failure. There was some temporary improvement in oxygenation. Furthermore, the 3 pediatric trials with 162 patients were insufficient to demonstrate any benefits or harms of iNO therapy in pediatric acute lung injury (ALI) and ARDS. The lack of benefit could be attributed to the trials being conducted in an era in which protective ventilatory strategies were not used. In addition, the application of high positive end-expiratory pressure and administration of high oxygen toxicity could have biased the results of these trials. Currently there is insufficient evidence to use iNO in any categories of ARDS and ALI patients.

M. Mathru, MD

Patients' prediction of extubation success

Perren A, Previsdomini M, Llamas M, et al (Ospedale Regionale Bellinzona e Valli, Switzerland; Univ of Geneva, Switzerland; et al)
Intensive Care Med 36:2045-2052, 2010

Purpose.—The spontaneous breathing trial (SBT)—relying on objective criteria assessed by the clinician—is the major diagnostic tool to determine if patients can be successfully extubated. However, little is known regarding the patient's subjective perception of autonomous breathing.

Methods.—We performed a prospective observational study in 211 mechanically ventilated adult patients successfully completing a SBT. Patients were randomly assigned to be interviewed during this trial regarding their prediction of extubation success. We compared post-extubation outcomes in three patient groups: patients confident (*confidents*; $n = 115$) or not (*non-confidents*; $n = 38$) of their extubation success and patients not subjected to interview (*control group*; $n = 58$).

Results.—Extubation success was more frequent in *confidents* than in *non-confidents* (90 vs. 45%; $p < 0.001$/positive likelihood ratio $= 2.00$) or in the control group (90 vs. 78%; $p = 0.04$). On the contrary, extubation failure was more common in *non-confidents* than in *confidents* (55 vs. 10%; $p < 0.001$/negative likelihood ratio $= 0.19$). Logistic regression analysis showed that extubation success was associated with patient's prediction [OR (95% CI): 9.2 (3.74–22.42) for *confidents vs. non-confidents*] as well as to age [0.72 (0.66–0.78) for age 75 vs. 65 and 1.31 (1.28–1.51) for age 55 vs. 65].

Conclusions.—Our data suggest that at the end of a sustained SBT, extubation success might be correlated to the patients' subjective perception of autonomous breathing. The results of this study should be confirmed by a large multicenter trial.

▶ In light of the results of this study, it is important to remember that patient perception of readiness for extubation is an additional tool to be used in conjunction with other more conventional tests of whether it is appropriate to extubate a patient's trachea. This is a simple, easy-to-implement additional step in the process of extubation. Many clinicians are likely do this in a less structured way as they assess a patient's level of sedation and explain the gradual withdrawal of ventilator support.

Of note, patients questioned about their perceived readiness for extubation after they had met the requisite criteria more reliably predicted their success with extubation than they had prior to meeting extubation criteria. The interview did not replace the spontaneous breathing trial; it was done in addition.

Even after meeting extubation criteria and agreeing that they felt ready to have the endotracheal tube removed, some patients required postextubation ventilator support. The percentage of patients requiring support after extubation was, as noted in the article, in those patients who both met criteria and felt ready to have the endotracheal tube removed: 13 of 58 control patients, 21 of 38 who met extubation criteria but were not confident about their ability to breathe without support, and 12 of 115 who felt they were ready for extubation. Although not a guarantee, asking patients how they feel about having their endotracheal tube removed seems an easy way to increase the likelihood of success with extubation.

C. Lien, MD

Peripheral vascular decoupling in porcine endotoxic shock

Hatib F, Jansen JRC, Pinsky MR (Edwards Lifesciences, Irvine, CA; Leiden Univ Med Ctr, The Netherlands; Univ of Pittsburgh School of Medicine, PA)
J Appl Physiol 111:853-860, 2011

Cardiac output measurement from arterial pressure waveforms presumes a defined relationship between the arterial pulse pressure (PP), vascular compliance (C), and resistance (R). Cardiac output estimates degrade if these assumptions are incorrect. We hypothesized that sepsis would differentially alter central and peripheral vasomotor tone, decoupling the usual pressure wave propagation from central to peripheral sites. We assessed arterial input impedance (Z), C, and R from central and peripheral arterial pressures, and aortic blood flow in an anesthetized porcine model ($n = 19$) of fluid resuscitated endotoxic shock induced by endotoxin infusion ($7\ \mu g \cdot kg^{-1} \cdot h^{-1}$ increased to 14 and $20\ \mu g \cdot kg^{-1} \cdot h^{-1}$ every 10 min and stopped when mean arterial pressure <40 mmHg or Sv_{O_2} <45%). Aortic, femoral, and radial artery pressures and aortic and radial artery flows were measured. Z was calculated by FFT of flow and pressure data. R and C were derived using a two-element Windkessel model. Arterial PP increased from aortic to femoral and radial sites. During stable endotoxemia with fluid resuscitation, aortic and radial blood flows returned to or exceeded baseline while mean arterial pressure remained similarly decreased at all three sites. However, aortic PP exceeded both femoral and radial arterial PP. Although Z, R, and C derived from aortic and radial pressure and aortic flow were similar during baseline, Z increases and C decreases when derived from aortic pressure whereas Z decreases and C increases when derived from radial pressure, while R decreased similarly with both pressure signals. This central-to-peripheral vascular tone decoupling, as quantified by the difference in calculated Z and C from aortic and radial artery pressure, may explain the decreasing precision of peripheral arterial pressure profile algorithms in assessing cardiac output in septic shock patients and suggests that different algorithms taking this vascular decoupling into account may be necessary to improve their precision in this patient population.

▶ In this elegant experimental study in pigs, the authors convincingly demonstrate that endotoxemia induces a dissociation in calculated compliance (C) from central to peripheral vasculature, such that the central compartment behaves as if it is getting stiffer (less compliant), whereas the peripheral compartment becomes more compliant. The differences in input impedance and C with central and peripheral pressures become even more apparent following fluid resuscitation. The data derived from this study have important clinical implications in the management of critically ill patients. Many devices are used by the bedside to estimate cardiac output using pulse pressure—derived data with the premise that aortic compliance or pulse power transmission remain constant. These devices use a proprietary algorithm based on healthy vasculature. Thus algorithm calibration based on healthy vasculature without recalibration following significant nonhomogeneous vascular tone changes (ie, endotoxemia) may display a reporting bias, either underestimating or overestimating true cardiac output.

M. Mathru, MD

Pre-Ejection Period to Estimate Cardiac Preload Dependency in Mechanically Ventilated Pigs Submitted to Severe Hemorrhagic Shock

Giraud R, Siegenthaler N, Morel DR, et al (Intensive Care Unit, Geneva University Hospitals, CH-1211 Geneva 14; Division d'Investigations Anesthésiologiques, Geneva Medical School, Geneva)
J Trauma 71:702-707, 2011

Background.—Respiratory change in pre-ejection period (ΔPEP) has been described as a potential parameter for monitoring cardiac preload dependency in critically ill patients. This study was designed to describe the relationship between ΔPEP and pulse pressure variation (PPV) in pigs submitted to severe hemorrhagic shock.

Methods.—In 17 paralyzed, anesthetized mechanically ventilated pigs, electrocardiography, arterial pressure, and cardiac output derived from pulmonary artery catheter were recorded. Hemorrhagic shock was induced by removal of blood volume followed by restoration. PEP was defined as the time interval between the beginning of the Q wave on the electrocardiogram and the upstroke of the invasive radial arterial pressure curve.

Results.—At baseline, ΔPEP and PPVs were both <12% with PPV significantly correlated with ΔPEP ($r = 0.96$, $p < 0.001$). Volume loss induced by hemorrhage significantly increased PPV and ΔPEP values ($p < 0.05$). During severe hemorrhage, PPV correlated well with ΔPEP ($r = 0.88$, $p < 0.001$) with PPV values significantly higher than ΔPEP ($p < 0.05$). However, the reproducibility of ΔPEP measurements was significantly better than PPV during this step ($p < 0.05$). Retransfusion significantly decreased PPV and ΔPEP ($p < 0.05$) with PPV significantly correlated to ΔPEP ($r = 0.94$, $p < 0.001$).

Conclusion.—Available correlations between PPV and ΔPEP at each time of the study were observed, meaning that ΔPEP is a reliable parameter to estimate and track the changes in cardiac preload dependency. Moreover, during the severe hemorrhagic shock period, ΔPEP measurements were more reproducible than PPV values (Figs 1, 2, and 6).

▶ Functional hemodynamic monitoring indices such as pulse pressure variation (PPV) and stroke volume variation are often used in critically ill patients to determine fluid responsiveness. Recently, ventilator-induced variation in the

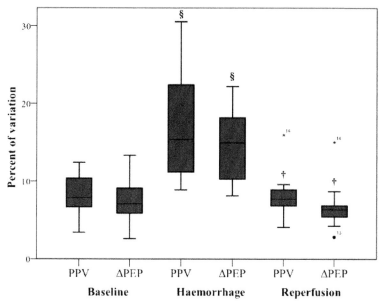

FIGURE 1.—*Box plot* representing PPV (%) and ΔPEP (%) at the three times of the protocol; § vs. corresponding "baseline" $p < 0.05$, † vs. corresponding "hemorrhage" $p < 0.05$ (*stars* and *point* describe the extreme values and the animal number). (Reprinted from Giraud R, Siegenthaler N, Morel DR, et al. Pre-ejection period to estimate cardiac preload dependency in mechanically ventilated pigs submitted to severe hemorrhagic shock. *J Trauma.* 2011;71:702-707, with permission from Lippincott Williams & Wilkins.)

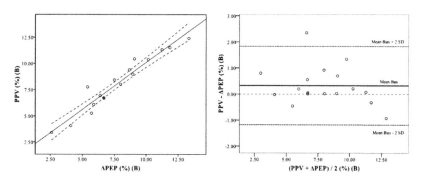

FIGURE 2.—Linear regression analysis and Bland-Altman analysis of the relationship between PPV (%) and ΔPEP (%) at baseline (B). (Reprinted from Giraud R, Siegenthaler N, Morel DR, et al. Pre-ejection period to estimate cardiac preload dependency in mechanically ventilated pigs submitted to severe hemorrhagic shock. *J Trauma.* 2011;71:702-707, with permission from Lippincott Williams & Wilkins.)

left ventricular pre-ejection period (ΔPEP) was found to be a reliable parameter for predicting fluid responsiveness in critically ill patients. Unlike the other indices, PEP is based on mechanical ventilation—induced nonstroke volume, whereas PPV is an index based on stroke volume variation. The current study compared the (ΔPEP) and (ΔPEV) in pigs submitted to hemorrhagic shock.

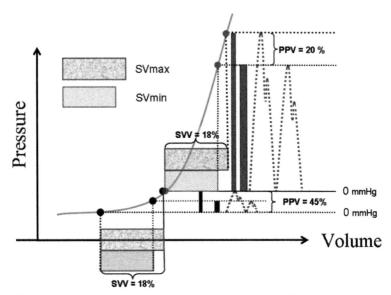

FIGURE 6.—A mathematical conception explaining how two different PPV values could be related to a same stroke volume variation (SVV) value as the aortic elastance (pressure volume relationship) is curvilinear. In case of low intra-aortic volume as in our severe hemorrhagic shock, PPV value increases, whereas SVV value has not changed; SVmax, maximal stroke volume; SVmin, minimal stroke volume. (Reprinted from Giraud R, Siegenthaler N, Morel DR, et al. Pre-ejection period to estimate cardiac preload dependency in mechanically ventilated pigs submitted to severe hemorrhagic shock. *J Trauma*. 2011;71:702-707, with permission from Lippincott Williams & Wilkins.)

The study demonstrated good correlation between (ΔPEP) and (ΔPPV) during various stages of hemorrhagic shock. However, (ΔPEP) measurement was more reproducible than (ΔPPV) assessment during severe hemorrhagic shock. Similar correlation has been demonstrated in cardiac surgical patients. In this setting, the authors found that PPV was larger than stroke volume variations at severe hypovolemia because of the changing relation of the stroke volume to the pulse pressure when the filling of the aorta greatly decreased.

M. Mathru, MD

Pulmonary artery catheters: Evolving rates and reasons for use
Koo KKY, Sun JCJ, Zhou Q, et al (Univ of Western Ontario, London, Canada; Harvard Univ, Boston, MA; McMaster Univ, Hamilton, Canada)
Crit Care Med 39:1613-1618, 2011

Objective.—Randomized trials have demonstrated risks and failed to establish a clear benefit for the use of the pulmonary artery catheter. We assessed rates of pulmonary artery catheter use in multiple centers over 5 yrs, variables associated with their use, and how these variables changed over time (2002—2006).

Design.—A multicenter longitudinal study using the Hamilton Regional Critical Care Database. A two-level multiple logistic regression analysis was used to determine significant variables associated with pulmonary artery catheter use and whether these varied over time.

Setting.—Academic intensive care units in Hamilton, Canada.

Patients.—We identified patients from five intensive care units who received a pulmonary artery catheter within the first 2 days of intensive care unit admission.

Interventions.—Pulmonary artery catheter use over a 5-yr period.

Measurements and Main Results.—Among 15,006 patients, 1,921 (12.8%) had a pulmonary artery catheter. Adjusted rates of pulmonary artery catheter use decreased from 16.4% to 6.5% over 5 yrs. Determinants of pulmonary artery catheter use included Acute Physiology and Chronic Health Evaluation II score (odds ratio [OR], 1.05; confidence interval [CI], 1.04–1.06; $p < .0001$), elective surgical status (OR, 2.82; CI, 2.29–3.48; $p < .0001$), postabdominal aortic aneurysm repair (OR, 10.91; CI, 8.24–14.45; $p < .0001$), cardiogenic shock (OR, 5.31; CI, 3.35–8.42; $p < .0001$), sepsis (OR, 2.83; CI, 1.94–4.13; $p < .0001$), vasoactive infusion use (OR, 4.04; CI, 3.47–4.71; $p < .0001$), and mechanical ventilation (OR,

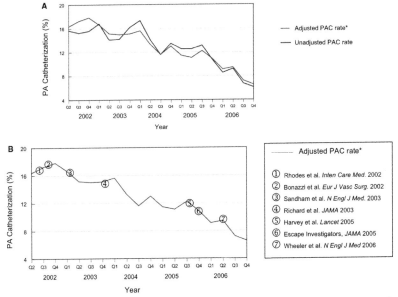

FIGURE 1.—*A,* Unadjusted and adjusted rates of pulmonary artery catheter (*PAC*), Hamilton Regional Critical Care Units (*HRCC*), 2002–2006. *B,* Publication of randomized trials evaluating PAC efficacy in relation to rates of pulmonary artery (*PA*) catheterization, HRCC, 2002–2006. *Adjusted PAC rates were adjusted for age, Acute Physiology and Chronic Health Evaluation II score, diagnosis at intensive care unit admission, and medical or surgical status. *Q1,* first quarter from January to March; *Q2,* second quarter from April to June; *Q3,* third quarter from July to September; *Q4,* fourth quarter from October to December. (Reprinted from Koo KKY, Sun JCJ, Zhou Q, et al. Pulmonary artery catheters: evolving rates and reasons for use. *Crit Care Med.* 2011;39:1613-1618, with permission from the Society of Critical Care Medicine and Lippincott Williams & Wilkins.)

2.21; CI, 1.86–2.63; $p < .0001$). Physician's base specialty and local intensive care unit were also associated with pulmonary artery catheter use ($p < .0001$). The determinants of pulmonary artery catheter use did not change over time.

Conclusions.—We observed a >50% reduction in the rate of pulmonary artery catheter use over 5 yrs. Patient factors predicting pulmonary artery catheter use were illness severity, specific diagnoses, and the need for advanced life support. Nonpatient factors predicting pulmonary artery

TABLE 3.—Logistic Regression Results: Determinants of Pulmonary Catheter Catheterization (n = 12,428)[a]

Variable	Regression Coefficient	p^c	Adjusted Odds Ratio (95% Confidence Interval)
Year	—	<.0001	[d]
Patient variables			
Age, yrs	−0.004	.08	—
Sex, female vs. male	0.05	.49	—
Acute Physiology and Chronic Health Evaluation II per point score	0.05	<.0001	1.05 (1.04–1.06)
Type, elective surgical vs. medical	1.04	<.0001	2.82 (2.29–3.48)
Emergent surgical vs. medical	0.41	<.0001	1.51 (1.25–1.81)
Diagnosis	0.66		
Myocardial infarction	1.67	<.0001	1.93 (1.48–2.52)
Cardiogenic shock	2.38	<.0001	5.31 (3.35–8.42)
Abdominal aortic aneurysm	0.21	<.0001	10.91 (8.24–14.45)
Other cardiovascular	−0.06	.28	—
Respiratory	−1.12	.54	—
Neurologic	0.14	<.0001	0.33 (0.21–0.52)
Gastrointestinal	1.04	.16	—
Sepsis	−0.02	<.0001	2.83 (1.94–4.13)
Trauma	−0.36	.95	—
Renal	−0.45	<.01	0.70 (0.51–0.97)
Metabolic/toxic	0.26	.02	—
Hematologic	−0.55	.26	—
Other primary diagnoses		<.01	0.57 (0.38–0.86)
Serum creatinine, low vs. high	−0.41	<.01	0.66 (0.50–0.88)
Urine output, high vs. low	0.57	<.0001	1.77 (1.38–2.26)
Use of mechanical ventilation, yes vs. no	0.79	<.0001	2.21 (1.86–2.63)
Use of vasoactive infusions, yes vs. no	1.40	<.0001	4.04 (3.47–4.71)
Physician variables			
Individual physician[b]	0.04	.08	—
Physician years of practice in ICU	0.36	.33	—
Physician base specialty			
Surgery vs. anesthesiology	−0.58	<.01	0.56 (0.39–0.81)
Medicine vs. anesthesiology	−0.36	<.01	0.70 (0.52–0.94)
ICU variables			
ICU site	1.19		
ICU-G vs. ICU-J	0.09	<.0001	3.29 (2.49–4.34)
ICU-H vs. ICU-J	−0.67	.58	—
ICU-M vs. ICU-J		<.01	0.51 (0.35–0.75)

ICU, intensive care unit.

[a]Multiple logistic regression results are based on the determined sample. The dependent variable is early pulmonary artery catheter use within the first 2 calendar days of ICU admission.

[b]Level one of regression included individual physicians using random effects. Level two included all patient, physician group, and ICU variables using fixed effects.

[c]Nonsignificant interaction terms removed ($p < .05$).

[d]There is not an adjusted odds ratio for year because the odds ratio was not constant.

catheter use were intensive care unit and the attending physician's base specialty (Fig 1, Table 3).

▶ Pulmonary artery catheters (PAC) were extensively used in the past in the management of critically ill patients. However, in recent years, several multinational trials have found little evidence to support routine use of PACs in the management of patients with acute coronary syndrome, high-risk cardiac surgery, refractory congestive heart failure, acute respiratory distress syndrome, and various forms of shock states. In this longitudinal study, the authors examined trends and determinants of early PAC use over a 5-year period during which landmark trials were published. In addition the authors addressed the influence of an attending intensivist on PAC insertion.

The authors found that the rates of PAC use declined among all patient, physician, and intensive care unit (ICU) groups. One standout feature of their results was that anesthesiology intensivists were more likely to use PACs in the ICU than were surgical or medical intensivists. This was attributed to disciplinary practice patterns rather than the level of comfort with PAC use. The authors also found that patient variables independently associated with PAC use were similar to the previous studies. The study was not able to discriminate between intraoperative and postoperative use, which could have potentially overestimated the use of PACs in surgical patients. The authors also did not investigate whether third-party payment schedule had influenced PAC use.

M. Mathru, MD

Randomized, Placebo-controlled Clinical Trial of an Aerosolized β2-Agonist for Treatment of Acute Lung Injury

The National Heart, Lung, and Blood Institute Acute Respiratory Distress Syndrome (ARDS) Clinical Trials Network (Univ of California, San Francisco; Johns Hopkins Univ, Baltimore, MD; Univ of North Carolina, Chapel Hill; et al)
Am J Respir Crit Care Med 184:561-568, 2011

Rationale.—β2-Adrenergic receptor agonists accelerate resolution of pulmonary edema in experimental and clinical studies.

Objectives.—This clinical trial was designed to test the hypothesis that an aerosolized β2-agonist, albuterol, would improve clinical outcomes in patients with acute lung injury (ALI).

Methods.—We conducted a multicenter, randomized, placebo controlled clinical trial in which 282 patients with ALI receiving mechanical ventilation were randomized to receive aerosolized albuterol (5 mg) or saline placebo every 4 hours for up to 10 days. The primary outcome variable for the trial was ventilator-free days.

Measurements and Main Results.—Ventilator-free days were not significantly different between the albuterol and placebo groups (means of 14.4 and 16.6 d, respectively; 95% confidence interval for the difference, −4.7 to 0.3 d; $P = 0.087$). Rates of death before hospital discharge were not significantly different between the albuterol and placebo groups (23.0 and 17.7%, respectively; 95% confidence interval for the difference, −4.0 to 14.7%; $P = 0.30$). In the subset of patients with shock before randomization, the number of ventilator-free days was lower with albuterol, although mortality was not different. Overall, heart rates were significantly higher in the albuterol group by approximately 4 beats/minute in the first 2 days after randomization, but rates of new atrial fibrillation (10% in both groups) and other cardiac dysrhythmias were not significantly different.

Conclusions.—These results suggest that aerosolized albuterol does not improve clinical outcomes in patients with ALI. Routine use of β_2- agonist therapy in mechanically ventilated patients with ALI cannot be recommended.

Clinical trial registered with www.clinicaltrials.gov (NCT 00434993) (Fig 2).

▶ Recovery from acute lung injury requires that the pulmonary edema resolves. The resolution of pulmonary edema is accomplished by active transport of sodium and chloride ions from the luminal space across both type I and type II alveolar cells, creating an osmotic gradient for the reabsorption of edema fluid. Experimental evidence suggests that the rate of alveolar fluid transport is augmented

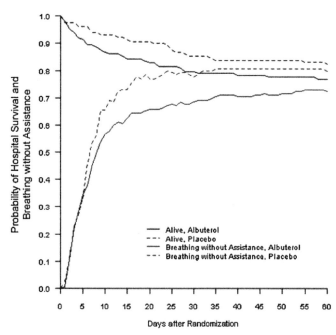

FIGURE 2.—Probabilities of survival and of discharge home and breathing without assistance, from the day of randomization (Day 0) to Day 60, according to whether patients received albuterol or placebo. (Reprinted from The National Heart, Lung, and Blood Institute Acute Respiratory Distress Syndrome (ARDS) Clinical Trials Network. Randomized, placebo-controlled clinical trial of an aerosolized β_2-agonist for treatment of acute lung injury. *Am J Respir Crit Care Med.* 2011;184:561-568, Official Journal of the American Thoracic Society © American Thoracic Society.)

by endogenous or exogenous cyclic adenosine monophosphate (AMP) stimulation. An ex vivo study in human lungs demonstrated that the rate of alveolar fluid clearance can be accelerated by an acyclic AMP β_2-adrenergic receptor agonist. This current study examined whether a β_2-adrenergic receptor agonist can accelerate the resolution of pulmonary edema and improve the outcome in patients with lung injury. The results of this randomized double-blind clinical trial demonstrate that aerosolized β_2-agonist therapy with albuterol did not improve clinical outcomes in patients with acute lung injury. The lack of improvement in outcome with the β_2-agonist could be attributed to the following: (1) inadequate delivery of aerosol in the presence of edema fluid, (2) failure of the injured epithelium to respond to the β_2-agonist, (3) possible downregulation of the β-adrenergic receptors occurring during the course of albuterol therapy, and, (4) the combination of fluid conservative and protective ventilatory strategies applied in this patient population provided very little opportunity to further enhance alveolar fluid clearance with albuterol. Another failed pharmacological therapy in acute lung injury!

M. Mathru, MD

Reducing ventilator-associated pneumonia in intensive care: Impact of implementing a care bundle

Morris AC, Hay AW, Swann DG, et al (Univ of Edinburgh, Scotland; Royal Infirmary Edinburgh, Scotland)
Crit Care Med 39:2218-2224, 2011

Objectives.—Ventilator-associated pneumonia is the most common intensive care unit-acquired infection. Although there is widespread consensus that evidenced-based interventions reduce the risk of ventilator-associated pneumonia, controversy has surrounded the importance of implementing them as a "bundle" of care. This study aimed to determine the effects of implementing such a bundle while controlling for potential confounding variables seen in similar studies.

Design.—A before-and-after study conducted within the context of an existing, independent, infection surveillance program.

Setting.—An 18-bed, mixed medical—surgical teaching hospital intensive care unit.

Patients.—All patients admitted to intensive care for 48 hrs or more during the periods before and after intervention.

Interventions.—A four-element ventilator-associated pneumonia prevention bundle, consisting of head-of-bed elevation, oral chlorhexidine gel, sedation holds, and a weaning protocol implemented as part of the Scottish Patient Safety Program using Institute of Health Care Improvement methods.

Measurements and Main Results.—Compliance with head-of-bed elevation and chlorhexidine gel were 95%—100%; documented compliance with "wake and wean" elements was 70%, giving overall bundle compliance rates of 70%. Compared to the preintervention period, there was a significant reduction in ventilator-associated pneumonia in the postintervention period (32 cases per 1,000 ventilator days to 12 cases per 1,000 ventilator days; $p < .001$). Statistical process control charts showed the decrease was most marked after bundle implementation. Patient cohorts staying ≥6 and ≥14 days had greater reduction in ventilator-associated pneumonia acquisition and also had reduced antibiotic use (reduced by 1 and 3 days; $p = .008/.007$, respectively). Rates of methicillin-resistant *Staphylococcus aureus* acquisition also decreased (10% to 3.6%; $p < .001$).

Conclusions.—Implementation of a ventilator-associated pneumonia prevention bundle was associated with a statistically significant reduction in ventilator-associated pneumonia, which had not been achieved with earlier ad hoc ventilator-associated pneumonia prevention guidelines in our unit. This occurred despite an inability to meet bundle compliance targets of 95% for all elements. Our data support the systematic approach to achieving high rates of process compliance and suggest systematic intro-duction can decrease both infection incidence and antibiotic use, especially for patients requiring longer duration of ventilation (Fig 2).

▶ Implementing a care bundle has been strongly advocated in ventilated inten-sive care patients, who are at the risk of developing ventilator-associated pneu-monia (VAP). "Bundling" multiple modalities into a single preventive strategy has become a standard of practice in critical care units. The authors introduced a 4-component bundle in their 18-bed medical-surgical intensive care unit that includes elevation of the head, oral care with chlorhexidine, a daily sedation hold, and a weaning protocol. The authors should be commended on their efforts in implementing the bundle, achieving relatively high compliance, and reducing a common hospital-acquired infection that is associated with high

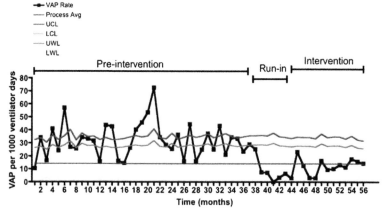

FIGURE 2.—A run chart showing the incidence of clinical ventilator-associated pneumonia (*VAP*), expressed per 1000 ventilator days, on a month-by-month basis. VAP indicates rate of VAP per 1000 venti-lator days. *LCL*, lower control line; *LWL*, lower warning line; *process avg*, process average; *UCL*, upper control line; *UWL*, upper warning line. (Reprinted from Morris AC, Hay AW, Swann DG, et al. Reducing ventilator-associated pneumonia in intensive care: impact of implementing a care bundle. *Crit Care Med.* 2011;39:2218-2224, with permission from the Society of Critical Care Medicine and Lippincott Williams & Wilkins.)

morbidity and mortality. This is one of those before-and-after studies that is inherently flawed because they do not control for other factors that change over time, and these are difficult to interpret when the condition being studied is a hospital-acquired infection. The microbiological VAP rate may have been lowered by the increased use of bronchoscopically obtained cultures rather than tracheal aspirate cultures. We need future randomized, controlled clinical trials to assess whether bundles or their specific elements have any role in decreasing infection rates.

M. Mathru, MD

Relation between brain interstitial and systemic glucose concentrations after subarachnoid hemorrhage

Zetterling M, Hillered L, Enblad P, et al (Uppsala Univ, Sweden)
J Neurosurg 115:66-74, 2011

Object.—The aim in the present investigation was to study the relation between brain interstitial and systemic blood glucose concentrations during the acute phase after subarachnoid hemorrhage (SAH). The authors also evaluated the effects of insulin administration on local brain energy metabolism.

Methods.—Nineteen patients with spontaneous SAH were prospectively monitored with intracerebral microdialysis (MD). The relation between plasma glucose and MD-measured interstitial brain glucose concentrations as well as the temporal pattern of MD glucose, lactate, pyruvate, glutamate, and glycerol was studied for 7 days after SAH. Using a target plasma glucose concentration of 5−10 mmol/L, the effect of insulin injection was also evaluated.

Results.—The mean (± SD) correlation coefficient between plasma glucose and MD glucose was 0.27 ± 0.27 (p = 0.0005), with a high degree of individual variation. Microdialysis glucose, the MD/plasma glucose ratio, and MD glutamate concentrations decreased in parallel with a gradual increase in MD pyruvate and MD lactate concentrations. There were no significant changes in the MD L/P ratio or MD glycerol levels. Insulin administration induced a decrease in MD glucose and MD pyruvate.

Conclusions.—After SAH, there was a positive correlation between plasma and MD glucose concentrations with a high degree of individual variation. A gradual decline in MD glucose and the MD/plasma glucose ratio and an increase in MD pyruvate and MD lactate concentrations during the 1st week after SAH suggest a transition to a hyperglycolytic state with increased cerebral glucose consumption. The administration of insulin was related to a lowering of MD glucose and MD pyruvate, often to low levels even though plasma glucose values remained above 6 mmol/L. After SAH, the administration of insulin could impede the glucose supply of the brain (Figs 2 and 3).

▶ Microdialysis (MD) of the brain and analysis of brain interstitial metabolites provide a unique window of opportunity to study the energy status of the

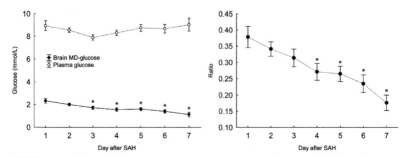

FIGURE 2.—**Left:** Graph demonstrating mean concentrations and 95% CIs for plasma glucose (728 measurements from 19 patients) and brain MD glucose (728 measurements from 19 patients). There was a significant decrease *(asterisk)* in MD glucose concentrations on Days 3–7 compared with Day 1. **Right:** Graph showing the mean concentrations and 95% CIs for the MPR (728 measurements from 19 patients). There was a significant decrease *(asterisk)* in the MPRs on Days 4–7 compared with Day 1. (Reprinted from Zetterling M, Hillered L, Enblad P, et al. Relation between brain interstitial and systemic glucose concentrations after subarachnoid hemorrhage. *J Neurosurg.* 2011;115:66-74, with permission from American Association for Neurological Surgeons, with Rockwater, Inc.)

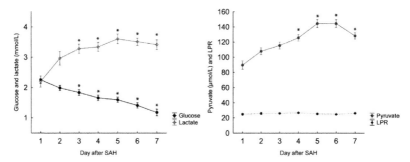

FIGURE 3.—**Left:** Graph demonstrating the mean concentrations and 95% CIs for MD glucose (2909 measurements from 19 patients) and MD lactate (2909 measurements from 19 patients). Compared with levels on Day 1, there was a significant decrease *(asterisk)* in MD glucose concentrations on Days 3–7 and a significant increase in MD lactate concentrations from Days 3 to 7. **Right:** Graph demonstrating the mean concentrations and 95% CIs for MD pyruvate (2909 measurements from 19 patients) and MD LPR (2992 measurements from 19 patients). There was a significant increase *(asterisk)* in MD pyruvate concentrations on Days 4–7 compared with Day 1. No significant change in MD LPR was found. (Reprinted from Zetterling M, Hillered L, Enblad P, et al. Relation between brain interstitial and systemic glucose concentrations after subarachnoid hemorrhage. *J Neurosurg.* 2011;115:66-74, with permission from American Association for Neurological Surgeons, with Rockwater, Inc.)

brain. Evidence suggests a better outcome in critically ill patients with tight glycemic control. In a subpopulation of critically ill patients with brain injury, Van den Berghe et al demonstrated that intensive insulin therapy decreased intracranial pressure seizure, seizure, frequency, and the incidence of diabetes insipidus. The relationship between hyperglycemia and poor neurological outcome is well established. However, the effect of tight glycemic control on the brain is not conclusive. Furthermore, the relationship between plasma glucose and brain glucose is shown to be poor. Previous studies have shown significant reduction in brain glucose levels after intensive insulin therapy in traumatic brain injury. In the current study, the investigators examined the temporal relationship between plasma glucose and interstitial brain glucose in patients with subarachnoid hemorrhage (SAH). The authors closely followed the biochemical changes that occur in the brain during the first 7 days of SAH. In this study, there was a progressive decrease in cerebral glucose levels despite relatively normal plasma glucose concentrations. Moreover, there was a decrease in glutamate as well as elevations in both pyruvate and lactate. In the absence of cellular stress, this reflects an increase in energy consumption following SAH. The correlation between plasma glucose and brain glucose improved with time. Finally, the authors also showed that insulin therapy caused cerebral hypoglycemia without any concomitant changes in lactate/pyruvate ratio, indicating alteration in glucose utilization rather than energy crisis. This study convincingly demonstrates that insulin administration in SAH patients may expose the brain to a risk of insufficient glucose supply, potentially aggravating preexisting brain injury. Therefore, insulin administration in neurosurgical patients should be done with caution.

M. Mathru, MD

8 Other Perioperative Patient Care Issues

Atelectasis as a Cause of Postoperative Fever: Where Is the Clinical Evidence?

Mavros MN, Velmahos GC, Falagas ME (Alfa Inst of Biomedical Sciences, Athens, Greece; Massachusetts General Hosp and Harvard Med School, Boston)
Chest 140:418-424, 2011

Background.—Atelectasis is considered to be the most common cause of early postoperative fever (EPF) but the existing evidence is contradictory. We sought to determine if atelectasis is associated with EPF by analyzing the relevant published evidence.

Methods.—We performed a systematic search in PubMed and Scopus databases to identify studies examining the association between atelectasis and EPF.

Results.—A total of eight studies, including 998 cardiac, abdominal, and maxillofacial surgery patients, were eligible for analysis. Only two studies specifically examined our question, and six additional articles reported sufficient data to be included. Only one study reported a significant association between postoperative atelectasis and fever, whereas the remaining studies indicated no such association. The performance of EPF as a diagnostic test for atelectasis was also assessed, and EPF performed poorly (pooled diagnostic OR, 1.40; 95% CI, 0.92-2.12). The significant heterogeneity among the studies precluded a formal meta analysis.

Conclusion.—The available evidence regarding the association of atelectasis and fever is scarce. We found no clinical evidence supporting the concept that atelectasis is associated with EPF. More so, there is no clear evidence that atelectasis causes fever at all. Large studies are needed to precisely evaluate the contribution of atelectasis in EPF.

▶ For decades, early postoperative fever (EPF) has been attributed to atelectasis, which has served as a convenient diagnostic scapegoat. These authors critically evaluated existing literature and found just 8 studies that used sensitive and specific diagnostic criteria for atelectasis while simultaneously documenting postoperative patient temperatures. Five of these studies and nearly 60% of the patients were cardiac surgical. The authors performed a variant of meta-analysis but admit that the heterogeneity of the data preclude reliable lumping of studies. Considered individually or collectively, the presumed association between atelectasis and EPF just doesn't hold up statistically, although there is a suggestion of an association. An association makes sense, because both atelectasis and low-grade fever are common early postoperative occurrences. A better theory is that patients release inflammatory cytokines in response to surgery and that these may cause fever. Because early postoperative cardiac surgical patients may tolerate fever poorly, both avoidance and rapid treatment are desirable. Presumptive prophylaxis against, diagnosis of, or treatment of atelectasis does not appear to be a productive approach to the problem.

G. P. Gravlee, MD

Prevalence of Heavy Smoking in California and the United States, 1965-2007

Pierce JP, Messer K, White MM, et al (Univ of California San Diego, La Jolla; et al)
JAMA 305:1106-1112, 2011

Context.—The intensity of smoking, not just prevalence, is associated with future health consequences.

Objective.—To estimate smoking intensity patterns over time and by age within birth cohorts for California and the remaining United States.

Design, Setting, and Participants.—Two large population-based surveys with state estimates: National Health Interview Surveys, 1965-1994; and Current Population Survey Tobacco Supplements, 1992-2007. There were 139 176 total respondents for California and 1 662 353 for the remaining United States.

Main Outcome Measure.—Number of cigarettes smoked per day (CPD), high-intensity smokers (≥20 CPD); moderate-intensity smokers (10-19 CPD); low-intensity smokers (0-9 CPD).

Results.—In 1965, 23.2% of adults in California (95% confidence interval [CI], 19.6%-26.8%) and 22.9% of adults in the remaining United States (95% CI, 22.1%-23.6%) were high-intensity smokers, representing 56% of all smokers. By 2007, this prevalence was 2.6% (95% CI, 0.0%-5.6%) or 23% of smokers in California and 7.2% (95% CI, 6.4%-8.0%) or 40% of smokers in the remaining United States. Among individuals (US residents excluding California) born between 1920-1929, the prevalence of moderate/high-intensity smoking (≥10 CPD) was 40.5% (95% CI, 38.3%-42.7%) in 1965. Moderate/high-intensity smoking declined across successive birth cohorts, and for the 1970-1979 birth cohort, the highest rate of moderate/high-intensity smoking was 9.7% (95% CI, 7.7%-11.7%) in California and 18.3% (95% CI, 16.4%-20.2%) in the remaining United States. There was a marked decline in moderate/high-intensity smoking at older ages in all cohorts, but this was greater in California. By age 35 years, the prevalence of moderate/high-intensity smoking in the 1970-1979 birth cohort was 4.6% (95% CI, 3.0%-6.1%) in California and 13.5% (95% CI, 11.8%-15.1%) in the remaining United States.

Conclusions.—Between 1965 and 2007, the prevalence of high-intensity smoking decreased greatly in the United States. The greater decline in high-intensity smoking prevalence in California was related to reduced smoking initiation and a probable increase in smoking cessation.

▶ Tobacco is still the leading cause of preventable deaths and disabilities in the United States, and it is one of the leading causes of job discompetitiveness of the United States. That's right, the costs don't just affect the person who smokes. If that person simply died, it would all be easy, but that person gets disability, medical illness, and increases costs for the rest of us—especially for corporations, which make smokers less competitive for jobs. Although the United States has had reduced intensity in cigarette usage—that is, fewer packs of cigarettes smoked per year per person who smokes—California has done even better. This is a record devotedly to be continued, and hopefully we can wipe out smoking in the United States and the job discompetitiveness it causes over the next 2 decades. If state governments would just ban smoking as a criteria for job hiring—that is, would not hire smokers—and if the federal government would do likewise, a great reduction in smoking would occur. Probably the most important thing a politician could do is advocate for the federal and state governments not to hire smokers.

M. F. Roizen, MD

9 Patient Safety, Complications, and Mishaps in Anesthesia

Correlations Between Controlled Endotracheal Tube Cuff Pressure and Postprocedural Complications: A Multicenter Study
Liu J, Zhang X, Gong W, et al (Tongji Univ School of Medicine, Shanghai, China; Jiaotong Univ School of Medicine, Shanghai, China; et al)
Anesth Analg 111:1133-1137, 2010

Background.—Postoperative respiratory complications related to endotracheal intubation usually present as cough, sore throat, hoarseness, and blood-streaked expectorant. In this study, we investigated the short-term (hours) impact of measuring and controlling endotracheal tube cuff (ETTc) pressure on postprocedural complications.

Methods.—Five hundred nine patients from 4 tertiary care university hospitals in Shanghai, China scheduled for elective surgery under general anesthesia were assigned to a control group without measuring ETTc pressure, and a study group with ETTc pressure measured and adjusted. The duration of the procedure and duration of endotracheal intubation were recorded. Twenty patients whose duration of endotracheal intubation was between 120 and 180 minutes were selected from each group and examined by fiberoptic bronchoscopy immediately after removing the endotracheal tube. Endotracheal intubation-related complications including cough, sore throat, hoarseness, and blood-streaked expectorant were recorded at 24 hours postextubation.

Results.—There was no significant difference in sex, age, height, weight, procedure duration, and duration of endotracheal intubation between the 2 groups. The mean ETTc pressure measured after estimation by palpation of the pilot balloon of the study group was 43 ± 23.3 mm Hg before adjustment (the highest was 210 mm Hg), and 20 ± 3.1 mm Hg after adjustment ($P < 0.001$). The incidence of postprocedural sore throat, hoarseness, and blood-streaked expectoration in the control group was significantly higher than in the study group. As the duration of endotracheal intubation increased, the incidence of sore throat and blood-streaked expectoration in the control group increased. The incidence of sore throat in the study group also increased with increasing duration of endotracheal intubation.

Fiberoptic bronchoscopy in the 20 patients showed that the tracheal mucosa was injured in varying degrees in both groups, but the injury was more severe in the control group than in the study group.

Conclusions.—ETTc pressure estimated by palpation with personal experience is often much higher than measured or what may be optimal. Proper control of ETTc pressure by a manometer helped reduce ETT-related postprocedural respiratory complications such as cough, sore throat, hoarseness, and blood-streaked expectoration even in procedures of short duration (1-3 hours).

▶ This study is important in that it emphasizes the import of small things done daily in managing a patient's airway. Long-term endotracheal intubation may result in a number of airway complications,[1-4] and is an indication for tracheostomy. The use of endotracheal tubes with high-volume, low-pressure cuffs does not eliminate these problems. As shown in this study, even short-term intubation can result in damage to the tracheal mucosa.

Clinicians do not measure the pressure in the cuff of an endotracheal tube.[5,6] Typically, they inflate the cuff of the endotracheal tube in one of 3 ways: (1) with a predetermined volume of air, (2) until there is no air leak with positive pressure ventilation, and (3) until they feel that the pressure in the pilot balloon is adequate. As demonstrated in previous studies, pressure in the cuff of the endotracheal tube cannot be determined by palpation of the pilot balloon.[6] As found in this study, maintaining cuff pressure < 25 mm Hg reduced the incidence of hoarseness, sore throat, and blood-streaked sputum. Fiber-optic examination found that damage to the tracheal mucosa was less severe in patients in whom cuff pressure was monitored and maintained between 15 and 25 mm Hg. Not surprisingly, in both groups, the incidence of symptoms increased with the duration of intubation. As noted by the authors, determining the cuff pressure prior to extubation in the control patients would have further supported their conclusions. Until that study is done, however, minimizing the volume of air used to inflate the cuff of an endotracheal tube to only what is required to allow positive pressure ventilation should decrease damage done to the tracheal mucosa, even in patients intubated for 2 to 3 hours.

C. Lien, MD

References

1. Guyton DC, Barlow MR, Besselievre TR. Influence of airway pressure on minimum occlusive endotracheal tube cuff pressure. *Crit Care Med.* 1997;25:91-94.
2. Fan CM, Ko PC, Tsai K, et al. Tracheal rupture complicating emergent endotracheal intubation. *Am J Emerg Med.* 2004;22:289-293.
3. Deslee G, Brichet A, Lebuffe G, Copin MC, Ramon P, Marquette CH. Obstructive fibrinous tracheal pseudomembrane. A potentially fatal complication of tracheal intubation. *Am J Respir Crit Care Med.* 2000;162:1169-1171.
4. Harris R, Joseph A. Acute tracheal rupture related to endotracheal intubation: case report. *J Emerg Med.* 2000;18:35-39.
5. Ganner C. The accurate measurement of endotracheal tube cuff pressures. *Br J Nurs.* 2001;10:1127-1134.
6. Fernandez R, Blanch L, Mancebo J, et al. Endotracheal tube cuff pressure assessment: pitfalls of finger estimation and need for objective measurement. *Crit Care Med.* 1990;18:1423-1426.

Kinked Endotracheal Tube: Possible Complication of Softening in Warm Water

Busaidy KF, Seabold C, Khalil S (Univ of Texas Health Science Ctr at Houston)
J Oral Maxillofac Surg 69:1329-1330, 2011

Background.—Endotracheal tube (ETT) kinking during intubation is reported infrequently. Significant kinking complicated the intubation of a patient in preparation for an elective temporomandibular joint (TMJ) arthroscopic procedure. The case and possible risk factors for kinking were discussed.

Case Report.—Woman, 53, came for elective bilateral TMJ arthroscopic surgery with lysis of the intra-articular adhesions. She reported no previous problems with intubation or anesthesia. Her range of mouth opening was restricted to about 30 mm secondary to severe TMJ osteoarthritis, and she had a Class 2 Mallampati classification and a diminished range of neck motion because of pain secondary to the radiculopathy. Size 7.0 and 6.5 nasotracheal RAE tubes were softened preoperatively by placing them in a sterile saline solution prewarmed to about 147°F. Midazolam was used to achieve sedation, preoxygenation was accomplished, and the patient was induced with fentanyl, propofol, and rocuronium. Direct laryngoscopy was used, but the 7.0-mm nasal RAE ETT met resistance when intubation was attempted. The resistance appeared to be at the level of the vocal cords and was initially thought to result from too large an ETT. The anterior presentation of the larynx further complicated ETT passage. The 6.5-mm ETT was substituted but it also met resistance, although it was eventually passed with difficulty and without direct visualization of the tube passing through the vocal cords. Capnography and positive auscultation of breath sounds in both lung fields were used to confirm ETT placement in the trachea. The patient's oxygen saturation remained at 100% and her end-tidal carbon dioxide was 34 to 38 mm Hg. When positive pressure ventilation was instituted, an audible cuff leak was noted that did not resolve when more air was instilled into the cuff. Partial airway obstruction was confirmed on capnography waveform. Neither a suction catheter nor a pediatric bougie could be passed through the ETT, both meeting resistance at about 35 cm. A fiberoptic scope found an acute bend of the ETT at 35 cm, about 7 cm from the tube tip. A 7.0-mm oral RAE ETT was used and airway pressures normalized, allowing successful completion of the case.

Conclusions.—ETTs are commonly softened by soaking them in warm saline solution before nasal intubation. This reduces the incidence of nasal trauma and epistaxis. However, the combination of a softened ETT, a limited mouth opening, an anteriorly positioned larynx, and the use of Magill's forceps probably resulted in kinking of the tube. Other causes of kinking include mechanical failure of the ETT, patient positioning, and impingement by retractors during surgery. To avoid more complications, the kinking must be recognized and the patency of the tube secured. The patient's oxygen saturation and end-tidal carbon dioxide levels were maintained within acceptable ranges by ensuring adequate air flow through the partially obstructed ETT and because the problem did not last a long time. Warning signs of obstruction included increased peak inspiratory pressure and the capnograph waveform shape. Alternatives to softening ETTs include use of adequate lubrication, mechanical dilation of the nasal passage, alternative ETT tip design, and use of a red rubber catheter to guide intubation.

▶ This is an interesting report of an infrequent event. It does not, however, provide information regarding the perianesthetic management of this complication.

There is no description of whether damage had been done to the laryngeal structures with the initial intubation attempt, nor is there mention of subsequent airway management with the exception of their intubating successfully with an oral RAE tube. The presence or absence of laryngeal edema, hoarseness, arytenoids dislocation, and other potential complications from this event should have been noted as having occurred or not. Additionally, it would have been important to note how the authors approached extubation of this patient's trachea following surgery.

This case report does highlight 2 important points. An endotracheal tube should not be blindly forced, especially in a nonurgent situation, into the trachea. Endotracheal intubations that are accomplished easily may result in laryngeal damage. With a traumatic intubation, damage is more likely. Second, airway adjuncts, such as a fiberoptic bronchoscope, should be used early in the event of a difficult intubation. Early use in this case would have avoided the trauma caused by a kinked endotracheal tube.

C. Lien, MD

Laryngeal Injury From Prolonged Intubation: A Prospective Analysis of Contributing Factors
House JC, Noordzij JP, Murgia B, et al (Boston Univ Med Ctr, MA)
Laryngoscope 121:596-600, 2011

Objectives/Hypothesis.—The factors leading to laryngeal injury due to intubation are not fully understood. This study sought to determine if duration of intubation, size of endotracheal tube, and/or type of endotracheal tube impact the degree of vocal fold immobility and other laryngeal injury upon extubation.

Study Design.—Prospective study.

Methods.—Sixty-one adult patients intubated for more than 48 hours were examined by recorded flexible nasolaryngoscopy shortly after extubation.

Results.—Forty-one percent of patients had some degree of vocal fold immobility. However, neither the duration of intubation (range, 2–28 days;

mean, 9.1 days), the size of endotracheal tube (range, 6 to 8), nor the type of endotracheal tube significantly affected the degree of laryngeal injury including vocal fold immobility. Additionally, none of the collected demographic information (age, gender, height, weight) significantly affected the degree of laryngeal injury.

Conclusions.—In this cohort, duration of intubation, type of endotracheal tube, and size of endotracheal tube do not significantly correlate to the incidence of vocal fold immobility and degree of laryngeal injury noted after prolonged intubation.

▶ This interesting trial documents that laryngeal injury was found to be extremely common in patients intubated for 2 days or more. Arytenoid and interarytenoid edema and arytenoid erythema, the most commonly identified laryngeal insults, were found in 95% to 97% of patients studied. Interestingly, the authors found that neither the duration of intubation nor the size of the endotracheal tube were significant factors in the injury that was documented. This may have been because of an inadequately sized study population. With duration of intubation, there was a trend toward a worsened laryngeal injury score. With larger endotracheal tubes (the authors studied sizes 6—8), there was a trend toward worsening vocal fold immobility. In both of these findings, however, the P value was ≥ 0.18 and did not approach significance.

The authors found a 41% incidence of vocal cord immobility with prolonged intubation. This was greater than has been reported in other studies (20%). The authors attribute this difference from other work to their ability to review recorded laryngoscopies and look for subtle degrees of injury. One wonders how use of this technology may have influenced other results. Did it allow greater detection of other forms of laryngeal injury? Did it detect injury that was of no clinical significance?

The etiology of the significantly greater incidence of left-sided granulation compared with right-sided granulation that was documented in this study is unknown. Had greater detail been provided regarding how the endotracheal tube was secured and whether it was secured in the same way in all patients, there may have been a rational explanation for the finding. Granuloma formation is due to pressure on and physical irritation of tissue. It is possible that if all endotracheal tubes were secured in the same fashion, the curve in the endotracheal tube as it passed through the vocal cords may have resulted in a consistently greater pressure being applied to the left vocal cord, increasing the risk of granulation. Without knowing the details of endotracheal tube management, however, this is purely speculation.

C. Lien, MD

What Rules of Thumb Do Clinicians Use to Decide Whether to Antagonize Nondepolarizing Neuromuscular Blocking Drugs?

Videira RLR, Vieira JE (Hospital das Clinicas da Faculdade de Medicina da Universidade de Sao Paulo (HC-FMUSP), Brazil)
Anesth Analg 113:1192-1196, 2011

Background.—In anesthesia practice, inadequate antagonism of neuromuscular blocking drugs (NMBD) may lead to frequent prevalence of residual neuromuscular block that is associated with morbidity and death. In this study we analyzed the clinical decision on antagonizing NMBD to generate hypotheses about barriers to the introduction of experts' recommendations into clinical practice.

Methods.—Sequential surveys were conducted among 108 clinical anesthesiologists to elicit the rules of thumb (heuristics) that support their decisions and provide a measurement of the confidence the clinicians have in their own decisions in comparison with their peers' decisions.

Results.—The 2 most frequently used heuristics for administering reversal were "the interval since the last NMBD dose was short" and "the breathing pattern is inadequate," chosen by 73% and 71% of the clinicians, respectively. Clinicians considered that the prevalence of clinically significant residual block is higher in their colleagues' practices than in their own practice (60% vs 16%, odds ratio = 7.8, 95% confidence interval, 3.8 to 16.2, $P = 0.0001$). The clinicians were less likely to use antagonists if >60 minutes had elapsed after a single dose of atracurium (0.5 mg/kg) (31%) in comparison with after rocuronium 0.6 mg/kg (53%) ($P = 0.0035$).

Conclusions.—In our institution, the clinical decision to antagonize NMBD is mainly based on the pharmacological forecast and a qualitative judgment of the adequacy of the breathing pattern. Clinicians judge themselves as better skilled at avoiding residual block than they do their colleagues, making them overconfident in their capacity to estimate the duration of action of intermediate-acting NMBD. Awareness of these systematic errors related to clinical intuition may facilitate the adoption of experts' recommendations into clinical practice.

▶ This article documents that attitudes toward antagonism of residual neuromuscular blockade in a large tertiary care center in Brazil are no different than those in other parts of the world. Clinicians do not routinely antagonize residual neuromuscular block; they overestimate their ability to detect residual neuromuscular block and they feel that they are better at detecting residual neuromuscular block than their colleagues.

The authors documented that residual paralysis in their hospital occurred in 41% of patients. More than one-third of these patients had received neostigmine. Doses, however, were small, 1 to 2 mg. Most commonly, clinicians used the time from last dose of either atracurium of rocuronium and the patient's breathing pattern as the most common means to determine whether to antagonize neuromuscular block. Neither of these parameters is an adequate indicator of degree of residual paralysis or the need for pharmacologic antagonism of residual neuro-muscular block.

Evidence-based practice with regard to monitoring of neuromuscular blockade and dosing of neuromuscular blocking agents and antagonists is not routinely used. The reasons for this remain unclear and may include that few patients with residual neuromuscular block have a more complicated clinical course than those who are fully recovered.[1] As patient surveys and patient satisfaction become increasingly important in assessment of our practice as anesthesiologists, patients' discomfort with residual neuromuscular block may finally be recognized.[2] Acknowledgement of this, as well as continued education about the frequency of postoperative residual neuromuscular block and ways to avoid it may, as has occurred in some countries,[3] lead to improved monitoring of depth of neuromuscular block and a decreased frequency of unacceptable levels of recovery of neuromuscular function in the postoperative period.

C. Lien, MD

References

1. Murphy GS, Szokol JW, Marymont JH, Greenberg SB, Avram MJ, Vender JS. Residual neuromuscular blockade and critical respiratory events in the postanesthesia care unit. *Anesth Analg.* 2008;107:130-137.
2. Murphy GS, Szokol JW, Avram MJ, et al. Intraoperative acceleromyography monitoring reduces symptoms of muscle weakness and improves quality of recovery in the early postoperative period. *Anesthesiology.* 2011;115:946-954.
3. Sorgenfrei IF, Viby-Mogensen J, Swiatek FA. Does evidence lead to a change in clinical practice? Danish anaesthetists' and nurse anesthetists' clinical practice and knowledge of postoperative residual curarization. *Ugeskr Laeger.* 2005;167: 3878-3882.

10 Obstetric Anesthesia

Analgesia for Labor

A Comparison Between Remifentanil and Meperidine for Labor Analgesia: A Systematic Review

Leong WL, Sng BL, Sia ATH (KK Women's and Children's Hosp, Singapore)
Anesth Analg 113:818-825, 2011

Background.—Remifentanil is an ultrashort-acting opioid with favorable pharmacokinetic properties that make it suitable as a labor analgesic. Although it crosses the placenta freely, it is eliminated quickly in the neonate by rapid metabolism and redistribution. We aimed to determine whether remifentanil compared with meperidine is effective in reducing pain scores in laboring parturients. Other effects on the mother, the labor process, and the neonate were also examined.

Methods.—MEDLINE, CINAHL, Embase, Cochrane CENTRAL, and Maternity and Infant Care databases were searched without language restriction using multiple keywords for labor analgesia, remifentanil, and meperidine. Published abstracts from 5 key research meetings and references from retrieved articles were examined for additional studies. Randomized controlled trials in laboring parturients comparing remifentanil with meperidine were selected. Risk of bias was assessed using criteria outlined in the *Cochrane Handbook for Systematic Reviews of Interventions*. We assessed for adequacy of sequence generation, allocation concealment, blinding, and completeness of follow-up. Data were extracted from each study using a standardized data collection form. The primary outcome was reduction in pain scores (visual analog scale [VAS], 0–100 mm). We also evaluated maternal side effects (sedation, oxygen desaturation, and bradypnea) and effects on the neonate (Apgar scores, umbilical cord pH, and Neurologic and Adaptive Capacity Scores).

Results.—Seven studies (349 patients) were identified for inclusion; only 3 studies were suitable for quantitative synthesis in a meta-analysis (233 patients). We found that remifentanil reduces the mean VAS score at 1 hour by 25 mm more than meperidine ($P < 0.001$) (95% confidence interval = 19–31 mm). Limited conclusions can be made regarding the side-effect profile of remifentanil because of insufficient data.

Conclusion.—Compared with meperidine, remifentanil is superior in reducing mean VAS scores for labor pain after 1 hour.

▶ Neuraxial analgesic techniques are the most effective forms of pain relief during labor. Unfortunately, some maternal conditions (eg, coagulopathy) contraindicate the administration of neuraxial analgesia. Many parturients do not have access to neuraxial analgesia, and others do not want it. Systemic opioid administration remains a popular alternative to neuraxial analgesia. Historically, meperidine has been the opioid most often administered systemically during labor, despite evidence of its limited efficacy and various side effects. Enthusiasm for the use of patient-controlled intravenous remifentanil analgesia seems to be growing. This systematic review suggests that remifentanil is more effective than meperidine in reducing maternal pain scores during labor. Of interest, the authors noted that most studies reported high maternal satisfaction scores, despite a modest reduction in pain scores, which suggests that the analgesia was clinically relevant. The authors also noted that the relationship between maternal pain scores and satisfaction scores is not necessarily linear and that the patient-controlled component likely improves maternal satisfaction. The authors recommended that "appropriate supervision (1-to-1 midwifery), supplemental oxygen, and respiratory and oxygen saturation monitoring should … be made available so that patients can be safely monitored and adverse consequences avoided."

D. H. Chestnut, MD

Influence of epidural dexamethasone on maternal temperature and serum cytokine concentration after labor epidural analgesia

Wang L-Z, Hu X-X, Liu X, et al (Jiaxing Maternity and Child Health Care Hosp, China)
Int J Gynaecol Obstet 113:40-43, 2011

Objective.—To evaluate the effects of epidural dexamethasone on maternal temperature and serum cytokine levels after labor epidural analgesia.

Methods.—Sixty healthy term nulliparas in spontaneous labor were randomized to receive epidural analgesia alone using bupivacaine 0.125% and fentanyl 1 µg/mL (group I) or epidural analgesia combined with dexamethasone 0.2 mg/mL (group II) (n = 30 per group). Maternal tympanic temperature was measured before epidural analgesia and hourly thereafter until delivery. Maternal and cord venous blood were sampled for analysis of interleukin-6 (IL-6), tumor necrosis factor-α, and interleukin-10 levels.

Results.—There was no difference in the incidence of intrapartum fever (38°C or more) between the 2 groups (3/30 versus 1/30, $P = 0.612$). The mean maternal temperature increased with time in group I, with the elevation reaching statistical significance at 4 hours post analgesia and at delivery compared with baseline ($P = 0.012$ and $P = 0.043$, respectively). A similar trend was observed with maternal serum IL-6 levels in group I. In group II, maternal temperature and IL-6 levels did not differ from baseline at any time point during labor.

Conclusion.—Epidural dexamethasone alleviates maternal temperature elevation after epidural analgesia. This effect can be attributed to the decrease in IL-6 levels.

▶ The authors concluded that this study provides further support for the hypothesis that increased intrapartum maternal temperature associated with epidural analgesia may be associated with "an underlying maternal inflammatory process." The incidence of frank maternal fever (temperature of 38° Celsius or more) was low in both groups, and the authors acknowledged that the small sample size and a possible type II statistical error may explain the lack of a significant difference between the 2 groups in the incidence of maternal fever. The authors acknowledged several potential risks of epidural administration of dexamethasone, particularly in patients with diabetes mellitus or immunosuppression. Additional (and larger) studies of efficacy, dose response, risks, and benefits are needed.

D. H. Chestnut, MD

Labour analgesia and the baby: good news is no news
Reynolds F (St Thomas' Hosp, London, UK)
Int J Obstet Anesth 20:38-50, 2011

When investigating different methods of maternal pain relief in labour, neonatal outcome has not always been at the forefront, or else maternal changes, such as haemodynamics, fever, length of labour, need for oxytocin or type of delivery, are taken as surrogates for neonatal outcome. It is essential to examine the actual baby and to appreciate that labour pain itself has adverse consequences for the baby. For systemic analgesia, pethidine has been most extensively studied and compared with neuraxial analgesia. It depresses fetal muscular activity, aortic blood flow, short-term heart rate variability and oxygen saturation. In the newborn it exacerbates acidosis, depresses Apgar scores, respiration, neurobehavioural score, muscle tone and suckling. Alternatives have few advantages, remifentanil being the most promising. Neuraxial analgesia is associated with better Apgar scores and variable neurobehavioural changes. Neonatal acid-base status is not only better with epidural than with systemic opioid analgesia, it is also better than with no analgesia. The effect on breast feeding has yet to be established, though it is certainly no worse than that of systemic opioid analgesia. Variations in neuraxial technique have little impact on the newborn. Widespread ignorance of the benefit to the newborn of neuraxial labour analgesia in the UK among non-anaesthetists needs to be combated.

▶ The author acknowledged that intrapartum neuraxial analgesia may cause maternal hypotension and fever, may prolong the second stage of labor, and may increase the need for intravenous oxytocin or instrumental vaginal delivery. However, she emphasized that these known maternal complications of neuraxial analgesia are not valid surrogates for neonatal outcome. Further, she noted that "neonatal acid-base status is not only better with epidural than with systemic opioid analgesia, it is also better than with no analgesia." She acknowledged studies that suggest that "larger doses of [epidural] fentanyl may be associated with slightly impaired breast feeding." However, she noted that "any neonatal effects of epidural fentanyl are mild and outweighed by the outstanding maternal benefit and increased safety of the low-dose combination" of local anesthetic and fentanyl.

D. H. Chestnut, MD

Programmed Intermittent Epidural Bolus Versus Continuous Epidural Infusion for Labor Analgesia: The Effects on Maternal Motor Function and Labor Outcome. A Randomized Double-Blind Study in Nulliparous Women
Capogna G, Camorcia M, Stirparo S, et al (Città di Roma Hospital, Via Maidalchini, Italy)
Anesth Analg 113:826-831, 2011

Background.—Programmed intermittent epidural anesthetic bolus (PIEB) technique may result in reduced total local anesthetic consumption, fewer manual boluses, and greater patient satisfaction compared with continuous epidural infusion (CEI). In this randomized, double-blind study, we compared the incidence of motor block and labor outcome in women who received PIEB or CEI for maintenance of labor analgesia. The primary outcome variable was maternal motor function and the secondary outcome was mode of delivery.

Methods.—Nulliparous, term women with spontaneous labor and cervical dilation <4 cm were eligible to participate in the study. Epidural analgesia was initiated and maintained with a solution of levobupivacaine 0.0625% with sufentanil 0.5 μg/mL. After an initial epidural loading dose of 20 mL, patients were randomly assigned to receive PIEB (10 mL every hour beginning 60 minutes after the initial dose) or CEI (10 mL/h, beginning immediately after the initial dose) for the maintenance of analgesia. Patient-controlled epidural analgesia (PCEA) using a second infusion pump with levobupivacaine 0.125% was used to treat breakthrough pain. The degree of motor block was assessed in both lower extremities using the modified Bromage score at regular intervals throughout labor; the end point was any motor block in either limb. We also evaluated PCEA bolus doses and total analgesic solution consumption.

Results.—We studied 145 subjects (PIEB = 75; CEI = 70). Motor block was reported in 37% in the CEI group and in 2.7% in the PIEB group ($P < 0.001$; odds ratio = 21.2; 95% CI: 4.9−129.3); it occurred earlier ($P = 0.008$) (hazard ratio = 7.8; 95% CI: 1.9−30.8; $P = 0.003$) and was more frequent at full cervical dilation in the CEI group ($P < 0.001$). The incidence of instrumental delivery was 20% for the CEI group and 7% for the PIEB group ($P = 0.03$). Total levobupivacaine consumption, number of patients requiring additional PCEA boluses, and mean number

TABLE 2.—Labor Analgesia

	CEI ($n = 70$)	PIEB ($n = 75$)	P Value
Total dose of levobupivacaine (mg)	37 (31—44)	31 (25—38)	0.001
Total dose of sufentanil (μg)	28 (24—34)	25 (20—30)	0.009
Patients requiring PCEA boluses (n)	28	6	<0.001
PCEA boluses for each patient (n)	1 (1—2)	1 (1—1)	<0.001

Data are presented as median (interquartile range) or number.

CEI = continuous epidural infusion; PCEA = patient-controlled epidural analgesia; PIEB = programmed intermittent epidural bolus.

of PCEA boluses per patient were lower in the PIEB group ($P < 0.001$). No differences in pain scores and duration of labor analgesia were observed.

Conclusions.—Maintenance of epidural analgesia with PIEB compared with CEI resulted in a lower incidence of maternal motor block and instrumental vaginal delivery (Table 2).

▶ Despite the difference in motor block between the continuous epidural infusion (CEI) and programmed intermittent epidural anesthetic bolus (PIEB) groups, the difference in total local anesthetic dose between groups was modest (median total dose of levobupivacaine of 37 mg in the CEI group vs 31 mg in the PIEB group; Table 2). Thus the authors suggested that the greater prevalence of motor block in the CEI group cannot be explained merely by the larger total dose of local anesthetic in that group. The authors hypothesized that "the reason for the analgesic success of intermittent boluses compared with continuous administration may be related to differences in the dispersion of solutions in the epidural space." The authors acknowledged that the decision to perform instrumental vaginal delivery was made by "individual obstetricians, whose practices may vary." However, they noted that obstetrician bias was unlikely, given that both the obstetricians and the study subjects were blinded to the study group assignment.

D. H. Chestnut, MD

Racial and Ethnic Disparities in Neuraxial Labor Analgesia
Toledo P, Sun J, Grobman WA, et al (Northwestern Univ, Chicago, IL)
Anesth Analg 114:172-178, 2012

Background.—Racial and ethnic disparities in the treatment of pain have been well documented, and there is evidence of such disparities in neuraxial analgesia use. Our objectives of this study were to analyze racial/ethnic disparities in neuraxial analgesia use, as well as anticipated use, among laboring Hispanic, African-American, and Caucasian women, and to evaluate sociodemographic, clinical, and decision-making predictors of actual and anticipated neuraxial analgesia use among these women.

Methods.—Laboring women, in a large urban academic hospital, were interviewed using a face-to-face survey to determine individual factors that may influence choice of labor analgesia. After delivery, the type of labor analgesia used was recorded. The primary outcome was use of neuraxial analgesia. Multivariable logistic regression models were estimated to test the likelihood that race and ethnicity were significantly associated with neuraxial analgesia use, anticipated neuraxial analgesia use, and the intrapartum decision to use neuraxial analgesia.

Results.—There was a univariate association between race/ethnicity and anticipated as well as actual use of neuraxial analgesia. However, there was no association between race/ethnicity and the intrapartum decision to use neuraxial analgesia. After controlling for confounders, the association between race/ethnicity and actual use of neuraxial analgesia no longer remained significant (adjusted odds ratio: Hispanic versus Caucasian women 0.66, 95% confidence interval [CI]: 0.24 to 1.80; African-American versus Caucasian women 0.93, 95% CI: 0.31 to 2.77). In contrast, Hispanic women were less likely than Caucasian women to anticipate using neuraxial analgesia even after controlling for confounders (adjusted odds ratio 0.40, 95% CI: 0.20 to 0.82).

Conclusions.—After controlling for confounding variables, Hispanic women anticipated using neuraxial analgesia at a lower rate than other racial/ethnic groups; however, actual use was similar among groups.

▶ The results of this study differ from the results of earlier studies that observed that Hispanic and/or African American women were less likely to use neuraxial analgesia during labor than Caucasian women. The authors suggested that the retrospective design of those earlier studies may have limited the investigators' ability to identify information that is important in the decision-making process. The authors also suggested that interhospital variation in approaches to labor analgesia education and delivery may affect racial and ethnic disparities. In the authors' hospital, an anesthesia provider discusses labor analgesia with every parturient shortly after admission. In contrast, in some hospitals, an anesthesia provider may not see a parturient until she requests neuraxial analgesia; therefore, if a parturient did not have antepartum education regarding neuraxial analgesia, then "she would not know or be motivated to request it." The authors stated that their "most consistent finding was the association between income and actual and anticipated neuraxial analgesia use." They speculated that their study's results likely underestimated overall racial and ethnic disparities in the use of intrapartum neuraxial analgesia in the United States. They noted that their institution is located in a nondepressed urban environment, and approximately half of the study subjects were college educated and had an annual income greater than $50 000. Further, all of the parturients in this study had an obstetrician or midwife from whom they received prenatal care, and the authors' findings might not reflect outcomes for women without adequate prenatal care or who receive prenatal care from other providers such as family physicians. Altogether, the authors acknowledged that their patient population and obstetric practice style might not reflect the general population in the United States.

D. H. Chestnut, MD

The Effect of Manipulation of the Programmed Intermittent Bolus Time Interval and Injection Volume on Total Drug Use for Labor Epidural Analgesia: A Randomized Controlled Trial
Wong CA, McCarthy RJ, Hewlett B (Northwestern Univ Feinberg School of Medicine, Chicago, IL)
Anesth Analg 112:904-911, 2011

Background.—Programmed intermittent bolus administration of epidural anesthetic solution compared with continuous infusion results in decreased anesthetic consumption and increased patient satisfaction. In this randomized and blinded study, we evaluated bupivacaine consumption and other analgesic outcomes when the programmed intermittent bolus time interval and volume were manipulated during the maintenance of epidural labor analgesia.

Methods.—Healthy, term, nulliparous women in spontaneous labor had combined spinal-epidural labor analgesia initiated with intrathecal bupivacaine 1.25 mg and fentanyl 15 µg, followed by an epidural test dose (lidocaine 45 mg with epinephrine 15 µg). Subjects were randomized to 1 of 3 programmed intermittent bolus dose regimens for maintenance of analgesia: 2.5 mL every 15 minutes (2.5/15), 5 mL every 30 minutes (5/30), or 10 mL every 60 minutes (10/60). The maintenance epidural solution consisted of bupivacaine 0.625 mg/mL with fentanyl 1.95 µg/mL. Breakthrough pain was treated initially with patient-administered epidural bolus doses, followed by manual boluses administered by the anesthesiologist if necessary. The primary outcome was total bupivacaine consumption per hour of labor. A linear mixed-effects model was used to model each patient's overall bupivacaine consumption per hour; the fixed effect was basal bupivacaine administration rate and the random effect was the area under the pain score versus time curve.

Results.—One hundred ninety women were studied. The median (interquartile range) adjusted bupivacaine consumption per hour of labor was 8.8 mg (8.0–9.7 mg) in group 10/60 compared with 10.0 mg (9.3–10.8 mg) in group 5/30 and 10.4 mg (9.6–11.2 mg) in group 2.5/15 ($P = 0.005$). There were no differences in area under the pain score versus time curve, pain scores at delivery, patient-controlled epidural analgesia requests or administrations, number of manual bolus doses for breakthrough pain, time to first patient-controlled epidural analgesia or manual bolus dose, or patient satisfaction with labor analgesia.

Conclusions.—Extending the programmed intermittent bolus interval and volume from 15 minutes to 60 minutes, and 2.5 mL to 10 mL, respectively, decreased bupivacaine consumption without decreasing patient comfort or satisfaction.

▶ The authors cited studies suggesting that administration of maintenance epidural solutions as programmed or automated intermittent bolus injections results in a smaller total dose of bupivacaine, decreased need for manual bolus injection by the anesthesiologist, and greater patient satisfaction in laboring women than does continuous epidural infusion. Given that there is no commercial pump that can be programmed to administer both intermittent bolus and patient-controlled bolus injections, the authors prepared and used 2 pumps with the same epidural solution for each patient. The authors concluded that "although the programmed intermittent epidural bolus technique clearly provides equal or better analgesia with less drug, the mechanism of this finding has not been fully elucidated." The authors acknowledged that although they "have shown that a larger volume administered at a longer interval results in less bupivacaine consumption than smaller volumes at shorter intervals, the difference in bupivacaine consumption is unlikely to be clinically relevant when using low-concentration solutions that result in minimal or no motor blockade." The authors noted that "current epidural pump technology supports continuous epidural infusion, patient-controlled epidural analgesia (PCEA) without a background infusion, and PCEA with a background infusion, but not programmed intermittent epidural bolus regimens, with or without supplemental PCEA."

D. H. Chestnut, MD

Analgesia for Labor: Obstetric Outcome and Economic Issues

Neuraxial Labor Analgesia for Vaginal Delivery and Its Effects on Childhood Learning Disabilities
Flick RP, Lee KM, Hofer RE, et al (Mayo Clinic, Rochester, MN)
Anesth Analg 112:1424-1431, 2011

Background.—In prior work, children born to mothers who received neuraxial anesthesia for cesarean delivery had a lower incidence of subsequent learning disabilities compared with vaginal delivery. The authors speculated that neuraxial anesthesia may reduce stress responses to delivery, which could affect subsequent neurodevelopmental outcomes. To further explore this possibility, we examined the association between the use of neuraxial labor analgesia and development of childhood learning disabilities in a population-based birth cohort of children delivered vaginally.

Methods.—The educational and medical records of all children born to mothers residing in the area of 5 townships of Olmsted County, Minnesota from 1976 to 1982 and remaining in the community at age 5 years were reviewed to identify those with learning disabilities. Cox proportional hazards regression was used to compare the incidence of learning disabilities between children delivered vaginally with and without neuraxial labor analgesia, including analyses adjusted for factors of either potential clinical relevance or that differed between the 2 groups in univariate analysis.

Results.—Of the study cohort, 4684 mothers delivered children vaginally, with 1495 receiving neuraxial labor analgesia. The presence of childhood learning disabilities in the cohort was not associated with use of labor neuraxial analgesia (adjusted hazard ratio, 1.05; 95% confidence interval, 0.85–1.31; $P = 0.63$).

Conclusion.—The use of neuraxial analgesia during labor and vaginal delivery was not independently associated with learning disabilities diagnosed before age 19 years. Future studies are needed to evaluate potential mechanisms of the previous finding indicating that the incidence of learning disabilities is lower in children born to mothers via cesarean delivery under neuraxial anesthesia compared with vaginal delivery.

▶ The authors noted that human neurodevelopment is especially vulnerable to pharmacologic and environmental insults that occur between the third trimester of pregnancy and several (3-4) years after birth. The authors cited animal studies demonstrating that exposure to sedative and anesthetic drugs during the critical periods of rapid neural development may cause accelerated neuroapoptosis that is associated with impaired learning and memory. In an earlier study, this group of investigators observed that "exposure to anesthesia before age 4 years was a risk factor for the development of learning disabilities in children receiving multiple, but not single, anesthetics."[1] In a subsequent study, this group of investigators observed that children exposed to general anesthesia for cesarean delivery were not more likely to develop learning disabilities than children who were delivered vaginally.[2] However, these investigators unexpectedly observed that the adjusted risk of learning disabilities was lower in children who were delivered via cesarean delivery with neuraxial anesthesia than in children who were delivered vaginally or who were exposed to general anesthesia for cesarean delivery.[2] The authors speculated that if this apparent protective effect resulted from the reduction in stress mediated by neuraxial anesthesia for cesarean delivery, then neuraxial analgesia during labor might have a similar beneficial effect in children delivered vaginally. However, in this study, the use of neuraxial analgesia during labor did not have a protective effect on the development of learning disabilities. The authors speculated that the high frequency of instrumental vaginal deliveries in the neuraxial analgesia group may have increased fetal stress, "counterbalancing any beneficial stress-reducing effects of neuraxial analgesia that the mother might experience."

D. H. Chestnut, MD

References

1. Wilder RT, Flick RP, Sprung J, et al. Early exposure to anesthesia and learning disabilities in a population-based birth cohort. *Anesthesiology.* 2009;110:796-804.
2. Sprung J, Flick RP, Wilder RT, et al. Anesthesia for cesarean delivery and learning disabilities in a population-based birth cohort. *Anesthesiology.* 2009;111:302-310.

β2-Adrenergic Receptor Genotype and Other Variables that Contribute to Labor Pain and Progress

Reitman E, Conell-Price J, Evansmith J, et al (Columbia Univ, NY)
Anesthesiology 114:927-939, 2011

Background.—β2-Adrenergic receptor (β2AR) activity influences labor. Its genotype affects the incidence of preterm delivery. We determined the effect of β2AR genotype on term labor progress and maternal pain.

Methods.—We prospectively enrolled 150 nulliparous parturients in the third trimester and obtained sensory thresholds, demographic information, and DNA. Cervical dilation, pain scores, and labor management data were extracted with associated times. The association of genetic and demographic factors with labor was tested using mixed effects models.

Results.—Parturients who express Gln at the 27 position of the β2AR had slower labor ($P < 0.03$). They progressed from $1-10$ cm dilation in approximately 21 h compared with 14 h among other patients. Asian ethnicity, previously associated with slower labor, is highly associated with this polymorphism ($P < 0.0001$). Heavier and black patients had slower latent labor ($P < 0.01$, 0.01). Neuraxial analgesia was associated with slower labor progress ($P < 0.0001$). It could take up to 36 h for parturients who were black and/or more than median weight (165 lb) to transition from 1 cm cervical dilation to active labor. However, after this active phase began, labor rates among these patients were similar to that of other parturients.

Conclusions.—We detected a strong association between β2AR genotype and slower labor. Asian ethnicity may be a proxy for β2AR genotype. Black women and those of higher than average weight have slower latent labor. These results confirm many of the associations found when this mathematical model was applied to a large retrospective cohort, further validating this approach to description and analysis of labor progress.

▶ Of interest, the authors observed that parturients who underwent instrumental vaginal delivery had significantly higher pain scores in early labor compared with the initial pain scores among parturients who had a normal spontaneous vaginal delivery. Other studies have suggested that more severe pain in early labor may be a marker for an increased risk for operative delivery. The authors also noted that "women often come to the labor room because of pain and are more likely to request neuraxial analgesia earlier if they have more pain." The authors stated that the use of their pain model in a patient population in which the use of neuraxial analgesia is less prevalent will allow assessment of factors that affect pain in later labor. Undoubtedly, future studies will enhance our understanding of genetic effects on labor pain and the progress of labor.

D. H. Chestnut, MD

Anesthesia for Cesarean Delivery

Committee Opinion No. 465: Antimicrobial Prophylaxis for Cesarean Delivery: Timing of Administration

()
Obstet Gynecol 116:791-792, 2010

Antimicrobial prophylaxis for cesarean delivery has been a general practice for cesarean deliveries because it significantly reduces postoperative maternal infectious morbidity. Recently, several randomized clinical trials investigated the timing of antimicrobial prophylaxis for cesarean delivery. The Committee on Obstetric Practice recommends antimicrobial prophylaxis for all cesarean deliveries unless the patient is already receiving appropriate antibiotics (eg, for chorioamnionitis) and that prophylaxis should be administered within 60 minutes of the start of the cesarean delivery.

▶ The American College of Obstetricians and Gynecologists (ACOG) Committee on Obstetric Practice called attention to 2 randomized controlled trials demonstrating that preoperative administration of a prophylactic antibiotic (ie, cefazolin) significantly reduced the occurrence of postcesarean endometritis and total maternal infectious morbidity compared with administration of the antibiotic after clamping of the umbilical cord. These studies also suggested that preoperative administration of prophylactic cefazolin was "not associated with an increase in neonatal infectious morbidity or the selection of antimicrobial resistant bacteria causing neonatal sepsis." However, the authors acknowledged that the aforementioned studies "were not powered to analyze those outcomes," and they suggested that additional prospective studies are needed to evaluate neonatal outcome.

D. H. Chestnut, MD

Continuous Subcutaneous Instillation of Bupivacaine Compared to Saline Reduces Interleukin 10 and Increases Substance P in Surgical Wounds After Cesarean Delivery

Carvalho B, Clark DJ, Yeomans DC, et al (Stanford Univ School of Medicine, CA)
Anesth Analg 111:1452-1459, 2010

Background.—Recent evidence suggests that locally delivered local anesthetics may exert tissue-damaging effects such as chondrolysis after intraarticular injection. Alteration of the inflammatory response is a potential mechanism for local anesthetic-induced tissue toxicity. In this study, we tested the effects of continuous local anesthetic infiltration on the release of inflammatory and nociceptive mediators in skin wounds after cesarean delivery.

Methods.—Thirty-eight healthy women undergoing cesarean delivery with spinal anesthesia were enrolled in this study, and were randomized to receive subcutaneous surgical wound infiltration with bupivacaine 5 mg/mL or saline at 2 mL/h for 24 hours after cesarean delivery. Wound exudate was sampled at 1, 3, 5, 7, and 24 hours after cesarean delivery using a subcutaneous wound drain technique. Cytokines, chemokines, substance P, prostaglandin E_2, and nerve growth factor were assayed using multiplex Bio-Plex® (Bio-Rad, Hercules, CA) and enzyme-linked immunosorbent assays.

Results.—Bupivacaine wound infusion resulted in a significant decrease of interleukin 10 and increase of substance P in wounds compared with saline infusion (area under the 24-hour concentration-time curve; $P < 0.001$). No statistically significant differences were detected for other cytokines, nerve growth factor, and prostaglandin E_2.

Conclusions.—This study demonstrates that the continuous administration of clinically used doses of bupivacaine into wounds affects the local composition of wound mediators. Observed changes in interleukin 10 are compatible with a disruption of antiinflammatory mechanisms. Whether such modulation combined with the release of the proinflammatory mediator substance P results in an overall proinflammatory wound response will require future studies of wound healing.

▶ The authors reported "the novel and somewhat unexpected finding that continuous instillation of the local anesthetic bupivacaine at clinically used doses markedly decreased interleukin-10 (IL-10) and increased substance P (SP) in wound exudates of women after cesarean delivery." The authors stated that, "the change in IL-10 is compatible with a disruption of antiinflammatory mechanisms, and this result, combined with the release of the proinflammatory mediator SP, may indicate an overall proinflammatory wound response." The authors suggested that continuous subcutaneous instillation of bupivacaine in women "may exert a net proinflammatory effect by altering the composition of wound inflammatory mediators and triggering the release of proinflammatory neuropeptides." Additional studies are needed to assess the risk-benefit ratio of continuous postcesarean instillation of local anesthetic, especially in light of the fact that in this study, continuous instillation of bupivacaine did not decrease postoperative pain scores and analgesic drug consumption.

D. H. Chestnut, MD

ED_{50} and ED_{95} of Intrathecal Bupivacaine in Morbidly Obese Patients Undergoing Cesarean Delivery
Carvalho B, Collins J, Drover DR, et al (Stanford Univ School of Medicine, CA)
Anesthesiology 114:529-535, 2011

Background.—It has been suggested that morbidly obese parturients may require less local anesthetic for spinal anesthesia. The aim of this study was to determine the effective dose (ED_{50}/ED_{95}) of intrathecal bupivacaine for cesarean delivery in morbidly obese patients.

Methods.—Morbidly obese parturients (body mass index equal to or more than 40) undergoing elective cesarean delivery were enrolled in this double-blinded study. Forty-two patients were randomly assigned to receive intrathecal hyperbaric bupivacaine in doses of 5, 6, 7, 8, 9, 10, or 11 mg (n = 6 per group) coadministered with 200 μg morphine and 10 μg fentanyl. Success (induction) was defined as block height to pinprick equal to or more than T6 and success (operation) as success (induction) plus no requirement for epidural supplementation throughout surgery. The ED_{50}/ED_{95} values were determined using a logistic regression model.

Results.—ED_{50} and ED_{95} (with 95% confidence intervals) for success (operation) were 9.8 (8.6—11.0) and 15.0 (10.0—20.0), respectively, and were similar to corresponding values of a nonobese population determined previously using similar methodology. We were unable to measure ED_{50}/ED_{95} values for success (induction) because so few blocks failed initially, even at the low-dose range. There were no differences with regard to secondary outcomes (*i.e.*, hypotension, vasopressor use, nausea, and vomiting).

Conclusions.—Obese and nonobese patients undergoing cesarean delivery do not appear to respond differently to modest doses of intrathecal bupivacaine. This dose-response study suggests that doses of intrathecal bupivacaine less than 10 mg may not adequately ensure successful intraoperative anesthesia. Even when the initial block obtained with a low dose is satisfactory, it will not guarantee adequate anesthesia throughout surgery.

▶ The authors called attention to their observation that a T6 block to pinprick did not always predict intraoperative success of the spinal anesthetic. The authors noted that their study highlights the difficulty of predicting the ideal dose of intrathecal hyperbaric bupivacaine in morbidly obese women undergoing cesarean delivery. They observed that morbidly obese patients seem to have a "much more variable response to intrathecal dosing, compared with leaner patients." They concluded that "determining the optimal dose for every [morbidly obese] patient is impossible due to the large variations in individual response to intrathecal local anesthetics." They noted that failure of neuraxial anesthesia is more problematic in morbidly obese patients, given the potential for difficult airway management. Thus, the authors concluded that morbidly obese women undergoing cesarean delivery are "ill-suited for a single-shot [anesthetic] technique." They suggested that it is advantageous to use a continuous catheter-based anesthetic technique, such as a combined spinal-epidural, continuous spinal, or epidural technique in morbidly obese women undergoing cesarean delivery.

D. H. Chestnut, MD

Efficacy of low-dose bupivacaine in spinal anaesthesia for Caesarean delivery: systematic review and meta-analysis

Arzola C, Wieczorek PM (Mount Sinai Hosp and Univ of Toronto, Ontario, Canada; SMBD-Jewish General Hosp and McGill Univ, Montreal, Quebec, Canada)
Br J Anaesth 107:308-318, 2011

Spinal anaesthesia is the preferred anaesthetic technique for elective Caesarean deliveries. Hypotension is the most common side-effect and has both maternal and neonatal consequences. Different strategies have been attempted to prevent spinal-induced hypotension, including the use of low-dose bupivacaine. We conducted a systematic search for randomized controlled trials comparing the efficacy of spinal bupivacaine in low dose (LD ≤8 mg) with conventional dose (CD > 8 mg) for elective Caesarean delivery. Thirty-five trials were identified for eligibility assessment, 15 were selected for data extraction, and 12 were finally included in the meta-analysis. We investigated sources of heterogeneity, subgroup analysis, and meta-regression for confounding variables (baricity, intrathecal opioids, lateral vs sitting position, uterine exteriorization, and study population). Sensitivity analysis was performed to test the robustness of the results. In the LD group, the need for analgesic supplementation during surgery was significantly higher [risk ratio (RR)=3.76, 95% confidence interval (95% CI)=2.38−5.92] and the number needed to treat for an additional harmful outcome (NNTH) was 4 (95% CI=2−7). Furthermore, the LD group exhibited a lower risk of hypotension (RR=0.78, 95% CI=0.65−0.93) and nausea/vomiting (RR=0.71, 95% CI=0.55−0.93). Conversion to general anaesthesia occurred only in the LD group (two events). Neonatal outcomes (Apgar score, acid-base status) and clinical quality variables (patient satisfaction, surgical conditions) showed non-significant differences between LD and CD. This meta-analysis demonstrates that low-dose bupivacaine in spinal anaesthesia compromises anaesthetic efficacy (risk of analgesic supplementation: high grade of evidence), despite the benefit of lower maternal side-effects (hypotension, nausea/vomiting: moderate grade of evidence).

▶ The authors concluded that for women receiving spinal anesthesia for cesarean delivery, lower doses of intrathecal bupivacaine "cannot be recommended unless an epidural catheter is in place ... to rescue the block if anaesthesia is inadequate or becomes inadequate during surgery."

D. H. Chestnut, MD

Extending epidural analgesia for emergency Caesarean section: a meta-analysis

Hillyard SG, Bate TE, Corcoran TB, et al (Royal Perth Hosp, Western Australia, Australia; Guy's and St Thomas' NHS Foundation Trust, London, UK; et al)
Br J Anaesth 107:668-678, 2011

There is no high-level evidence supporting an optimal top-up solution to convert labour epidural analgesia to surgical anaesthesia for Caesarean section. The aim of this meta-analysis was to identify the best epidural solutions for emergency Caesarean section anaesthesia, with respect to rapid onset and low supplementation of intraoperative block. Eleven randomized controlled trials, involving 779 parturients, were identified for inclusion after a systematic literature search and risk of bias assessment. 'Top-up' boluses were classified into three groups: 0.5% bupivacaine or levobupivacaine (Bup/Levo); lidocaine and epinephrine, with or without fentanyl (LE ± F); and 0.75% ropivacaine (Ropi). Pooled analysis using the fixed-effects method was used to calculate the mean difference (MD) for continuous outcomes and risk ratio (RR) for dichotomous outcomes. Lidocaine and epinephrine, with or without fentanyl, resulted in a significantly faster onset of sensory block [MD -4.51 min, 95% confidence interval (CI) -5.89 to -3.13 min, $P<0.00001$]. Bup/Levo was associated with a significantly increased risk of intraoperative supplementation compared with the other groups (RR 2.03; 95% CI 1.22–3.39; $P=0.007$), especially compared with Ropi (RR 3.24, 95% CI 1.26–8.33, $P=0.01$). Adding fentanyl to a local anaesthetic resulted in a significantly faster onset but did not affect the need for intraoperative supplementation. Bupivacaine or levobupivacaine 0.5% was the least effective solution. If the speed of onset is important, then a lidocaine and epinephrine solution, with or without fentanyl, appears optimal. If the quality of epidural block is paramount, then 0.75% ropivacaine is suggested.

▶ The authors observed that in all the clinical trials included in this meta-analysis, epidural administration of a solution of lidocaine and epinephrine, with or without fentanyl, resulted in a median onset time of less than 15 minutes. The authors stated that there were insufficient trials to assess the effect of adding bicarbonate to the lidocaine-epinephrine solution in this meta-analysis. They also noted that although the addition of bicarbonate to the lidocaine-epinephrine solution appears to hasten the onset time, "some of the time-saving might … be offset by drug preparation time, and there are safety implications when mixing drugs in an emergency situation." The authors acknowledged that this meta-analysis did not include trials that evaluated epidural administration of 3% 2-chloroprocaine, a local anesthetic with a rapid onset but short duration of action. The authors acknowledged that 3% 2-chloroprocaine is widely used for extension of epidural anesthesia for emergency cesarean delivery in North America, but it is not available in the United Kingdom.

D. H. Chestnut, MD

Five Unit Bolus Oxytocin at Cesarean Delivery in Women at Risk of Atony: A Randomized, Double-Blind, Controlled Trial

King KJ, Douglas MJ, Unger W, et al (John Hunter Hosp, New South Wales, Australia; British Columbia Women's Hosp, Vancouver, Canada; et al)
Anesth Analg 111:1460-1466, 2010

Background.—IV bolus oxytocin is used routinely during cesarean delivery to prevent postpartum hemorrhage. Its adverse hemodynamic effects are well known, resulting in a recent change in dose from 10 IU to 5. Whether a 5 IU bolus has any advantages over infusion alone is unclear. We tested the hypothesis that a 5 IU IV bolus of oxytocin before the initiation of a continuous infusion decreases the need for additional uterotonic drugs in the first 24 hours after delivery in women with risk factors for uterine atony undergoing cesarean delivery, compared with infusion alone.

Methods.—A prospective, randomized, double-blind, controlled trial was conducted in 143 subjects undergoing cesarean delivery with at least 1 risk factor for uterine atony. Subjects received 5 IU bolus of oxytocin or normal saline IV over 30 seconds after umbilical cord clamping. All subjects received an infusion of 40 IU oxytocin in 500 mL normal saline over 30 minutes, followed by 20 IU in 1 L over 8 hours. The primary outcome was the need for additional uterotonics in the first 24 hours after delivery. Secondary outcomes included uterine tone as assessed by the surgeon (5-point Likert scale: 0 = "floppy," 4 = "rock hard"), estimated blood loss, side effects of bolus administration, and the oxytocin bolus-placental delivery interval.

Results.—There was no difference in the need for additional uterotonic drugs in the first 24 hours between groups. There was a significant difference in uterine tone immediately after placental delivery ($P < 0.01$) (2.8 in the oxytocin group [95% confidence interval 2.6–3.0] vs 2.2 in the saline group [95% confidence interval 1.8–2.5]), which disappeared after 5 minutes. There were no differences in observed or reported side effects between groups.

Conclusions.—We found that a 5 IU IV bolus of oxytocin added to an infusion did not alter the need for additional uterotonic drugs to prevent or treat postpartum hemorrhage in the first 24 hours in women undergoing cesarean delivery with risk factors for uterine atony, despite causing an initial stronger uterine contraction. Our study was not powered to find a difference in side effects between groups. These results suggest that an oxytocin infusion may be adequate without the need for a bolus, even in high-risk patients.

▶ This study was unique in that all patients had at least 1 risk factor for postpartum hemorrhage caused by uterine atony. The administration of a 5-IU intravenous bolus of oxytocin (before initiation of a continuous intravenous infusion of oxytocin) did not reduce the need for administration of additional uterotonic drugs over the next 24 hours, and it did not result in a reduction in estimated blood loss. The authors called attention to published reports of serious maternal side effects (eg, hypotension) following intravenous bolus administration of oxytocin at cesarean delivery. The authors noted that these side effects seem to be related to both the dose and speed of injection of the oxytocin. The authors emphasized that they gave a high-dose intravenous infusion of oxytocin to every patient after the intravenous bolus of either oxytocin or placebo, which likely explains the lack of difference between groups in outcome.

D. H. Chestnut, MD

General anesthesia for cesarean delivery at a tertiary care hospital from 2000 to 2005: a retrospective analysis and 10-year update
Palanisamy A, Mitani AA, Tsen LC (Brigham and Women's Hosp, Boston, MA)
Int J Obstet Anesth 20:10-16, 2011

Background.—Complications from general anesthesia for cesarean delivery are a leading cause of anesthesia-related mortality. As a consequence, the overall use of general anesthesia in this setting is becoming less common. The impact and implications of this trend are considered in relation to a similar study performed at our institution 10 years ago.

Methods.—The hospital database for all cesarean deliveries performed during six calendar years (January 1, 2000 through December 31, 2005) was reviewed. The medical records of all parturients who received general anesthesia were examined to collect personal details and data pertinent to the indications for cesarean delivery and general anesthesia, mode of airway management and associated anesthetic complications.

Results.—Cesarean deliveries accounted for 23.65% to 31.51% of an annual total ranging from 8543 to 10091 deliveries. The percentage of cases performed under general anesthesia ranged from 0.5% to 1%. A perceived lack of time for neuraxial anesthesia accounted for more than half of the general anesthesia cases each year, with maternal factors accounting for 11.1% to 42.9%. Failures of neuraxial techniques accounted for less than 4% of the general anesthesia cases. There was only one case of difficult intubation and no anesthesia-related mortality was recorded.

Conclusion.—The use of general anesthesia for cesarean delivery is low and declining. These trends may reflect the early and increasing use of neuraxial techniques, particularly in parturients with co-existing morbidities. A significant reduction in exposure of trainees to obstetric general anesthesia has been observed.

▶ Despite the increased cesarean delivery rate, the authors attributed the steady decline in the use of general anesthesia for cesarean delivery at their institution to several factors. First, during the last decade, an increasing number of high-risk obstetric patients have been evaluated by their antenatal anesthesia consult service, which has allowed optimization of patients' medical conditions, initiation of multidisciplinary discussions, and planning of anesthetic management. Second, the authors and their colleagues have emphasized prophylactic placement of an epidural catheter in high-risk patients (eg, obesity, difficult airway) in early labor; the correct placement of the epidural catheter is confirmed with small doses of local anesthetic (in some cases before the first request for analgesia), and the epidural catheter subsequently provides a readily available route for providing neuraxial anesthesia if necessary to perform an emergency cesarean delivery. Third, the authors and their colleagues have adopted a more aggressive approach toward management of inadequate neuraxial block (eg, prompt replacement of an epidural catheter that is providing suboptimal labor analgesia, administration of supplemental intravenous analgesia during cesarean delivery), and they speculated that this practice may have reduced the incidence of intraoperative conversion to general anesthesia. And fourth, the authors and their colleagues have demonstrated an increased willingness to administer spinal anesthesia for emergency cesarean delivery, and in some high-risk patients (eg, morbid obesity) they have intentionally used a continuous spinal anesthetic technique. The authors lamented the fact that the dramatic increase in the use of neuraxial anesthetic techniques for cesarean delivery has resulted in a worrying decrease in residents' exposure to general anesthesia for cesarean delivery.

D. H. Chestnut, MD

Maternal Cardiac Output Changes After Crystalloid or Colloid Coload Following Spinal Anesthesia for Elective Cesarean Delivery: A Randomized Controlled Trial

McDonald S, Fernando R, Ashpole K, et al (Royal Free Hosp NHS Trust, London, UK; Univ Hosp of South Manchester NHS Foundation Trust, Wythenshawe, Manchester, UK)
Anesth Analg 113:803-810, 2011

Background.—Minimizing hypotension associated with spinal anesthesia for cesarean delivery by administration of IV fluids and vasopressors reduces fetal and maternal morbidity. Most studies have concentrated on noninvasive systolic blood pressure (SBP) measurements to evaluate the effect of such regimens. We used a suprasternal Doppler flow technique to measure maternal cardiac output (CO) variables in parturients receiving a phenylephrine infusion combined with the rapid administration of crystalloid or colloid solution at the time of initiation of anesthesia (coload). We hypothesized that a colloid coload compared with a crystalloid coload would produce a larger sustained increase in CO and therefore reduce vasopressor requirements.

Methods.—We recruited 60 healthy term women scheduled for elective cesarean delivery under spinal anesthesia for this randomized double-blind study. Baseline heart rate, baseline SBP, and CO variables including stroke volume, corrected flow time, and contractility were recorded in the left lateral tilt position. At the time of spinal injection, subjects were allocated to receive a rapid 1-L coload of either 6% w/v hydroxyethyl starch solution (HES) or Hartmann (crystalloid) solution (HS). A phenylephrine infusion was titrated to maintain maternal baseline SBP. CO was measured at 5-minute intervals for 20 minutes after initiation of spinal anesthesia. The primary outcome, CO, was compared between groups, as were secondary outcomes: phenylephrine dose and maternal hemodynamic and fetal outcome data.

Results.—Maternal demographics, surgical times, and fetal outcome data were similar between groups. There were no significant differences between groups in any measured CO variable at any time point. CO was transiently higher than baseline at 5 minutes in the HS group and at 5 and 10 minutes in the HES group (range, 0.13–1.74 L/min); the overall mean difference in CO between crystalloid and colloid over the study period was 0.06 L/min (95% confidence interval: −0.46 to 0.58). Stroke volume was higher than baseline in both groups throughout; peak velocity was consistently higher than baseline only in the HES group; and corrected flow time increased in both groups; the effect was transient in the HS but sustained in the HES group. Heart rate was not different at any time point within or between groups but did decrease over time. The total phenylephrine dose from time of spinal anesthesia to delivery was similar between groups.

Conclusion.—We found no difference in CO in women randomized to colloid or crystalloid coload. In addition, there were no differences in vasopressor requirements or hemodynamic stability. We conclude that there is no advantage in using colloid over crystalloid when used in combination with a phenylephrine infusion during spinal anesthesia for elective cesarean delivery.

▶ This study was the first published comparison of crystalloid and colloid administered as a coload (ie, at the time of induction of spinal anesthesia for cesarean delivery). This article was accompanied by an excellent and comprehensive editorial by Mercier.[1] On the basis of his review of published studies, Mercier[1] made the following conclusions: first, it is useful to include a fluid loading technique with vasopressor prophylaxis to "prevent or mitigate" hypotension during administration of spinal anesthesia for cesarean delivery. Second, "crystalloid preloading is ineffective or poorly effective and should be replaced by one of the three other available fluid loading techniques" (ie, colloid preload, crystalloid coload, or colloid coload). Third, fluid loading should be avoided in some specific situations when the mother is at risk for fluid overload (eg, multiple gestation, severe preeclampsia, some cardiovascular diseases). Fourth, in emergency cases in which severe hypotension is less likely to occur and there is little time for administration of a fluid preload, a fluid coload seems preferable. Fifth, no fluid loading technique is completely effective in preventing maternal hypotension, and therefore "use of some sort of vasopressor regimen should always be considered."

D. H. Chestnut, MD

Reference

1. Mercier FJ. Fluid loading for cesarean delivery under spinal anesthesia: have we studied all the options? *Anesth Analg.* 2011;113:677-680.

Prior Epidural Lidocaine Alters the Pharmacokinetics and Drug Effects of Extended-Release Epidural Morphine (DepoDur®) After Cesarean Delivery

Atkinson Ralls L, Drover DR, Clavijo CF, et al (Stanford Univ School of Medicine, CA; Univ of Colorado, Denver)
Anesth Analg 113:251-258, 2011

Background.—A potential physicochemical interaction between epidural local anesthetics and extended-release epidural morphine (EREM) could negate the sustained release. In this study, we sought to determine the pharmacokinetic and drug effects of prior epidural lidocaine administration on EREM.

Methods.—Thirty healthy women undergoing cesarean delivery were enrolled in this randomized study. Patients received 8 mg EREM 1 hour after either a combined spinal-epidural (intrathecal bupivacaine and fentanyl 20 μg with no epidural medication; group SE) or an epidural anesthetic (epidural 2% lidocaine with fentanyl 100 μg; group E). Maximal concentration (Cmax), time to Cmax (Tmax), and AUC_{0-last} (area under the concentration-time curve until the last plasma concentration that was below the limit of quantitation) for morphine levels were determined from a plasma sample at 0, 5, 10, 15, and 30 minutes, and 1, 4, 8, 12, 24, 36, 48, and 72 hours. Drug effects including pain, analgesic use, and side effects were measured for 72 hours after cesarean delivery.

Results.—Epidural lidocaine administration (20—35 mL) 1 hour before epidural EREM administration increased the Cmax in group E (11.1 ± 4.9) compared with group SE (8.3 ± 7.1 ng/mL) ($P = 0.038$). There were no significant effects on Tmax and AUC_{0-last} of venous morphine between the groups ($P > 0.05$). There was an increased incidence in vomiting, oxygen use, and hypotension in group E (patients who received lidocaine before EREM).

Conclusion.—A large dose of epidural lidocaine 1 hour before EREM administration alters the pharmacokinetics and drug effects of EREM. Clinicians must apply caution when EREM is administered even 1 hour after an epidural lidocaine "top-up" for cesarean delivery.

▶ The authors of this study cited a pooled analysis of 6 earlier studies, which demonstrated a higher maximal concentration when a 3-mL lidocaine-epinephrine test dose was administered less than 15 minutes before administration of extended-release epidural morphine (EREM).[1] However, the pharmacokinetics were similar when EREM was administered at least 15 minutes after administration of the lidocaine-epinephrine test dose.[1] The authors of this study concluded that administration of a large dose (ie, 20-35 mL) of epidural lidocaine 1 hour before administration of EREM alters the pharmacokinetics and drug effects of EREM. Thus, the authors concluded that EREM should be avoided, administered at a reduced dose, or given at a dosing interval of more than 1 hour after epidural administration of a large volume of epidural lidocaine. The authors stated that "preferably, EREM should be used for elective cesarean delivery using a combined spinal-epidural technique, whereby EREM is placed in the epidural space without any concomitant lidocaine."

D. H. Chestnut, MD

Reference

1. Viscusi ER, Gambling DR, Hughes TL, Manvelian GZ. Pharmacokinetics of extended-release epidural morphine sulfate: pooled analysis of six clinical studies. *Am J Health Syst Pharm.* 2009;66:1020-1030.

The effect of labor on sevoflurane requirements during cesarean delivery

Erden V, Erkalp K, Yangin Z, et al (Vakif Gureba Educational Hosp, İstanbul, Turkey)
Int J Obstet Anesth 20:17-21, 2011

Background.—Labor results in the release of sensitizing substances such as progesterone, prostaglandins, cytokines and cortisol, some of which have been observed to participate in sleep regulation. We hypothesized that these substances could affect sleep regulation and therefore the amount of volatile agent required to provide general anesthesia for cesarean delivery.

Methods.—A total of 50 patients were enrolled, of whom 25 had uterine activity less than 30 Montevideo units (Prelabor group) and 25 had uterine activity greater than 80 Montevideo units (Labor group). Anesthesia was maintained with 50% oxygen in nitrous oxide with sevoflurane. Sevoflurane concentration was adjusted to sustain a constant Bispectral Index (BIS) value of 40—55. Prolactin, progesterone and cortisol levels were evaluated immediately before cesarean delivery.

Results.—End-tidal concentrations of sevoflurane in the Prelabor group were higher than in the Labor group with similar Bispectral Index values. No significant differences were found in prolactin, progesterone and cortisol levels between the two groups.

Conclusion.—Anesthetic requirements for sevoflurane, as measured by Bispectral Index, decrease in laboring versus non-laboring parturients undergoing cesarean delivery. Prolactin, progesterone and cortisol do not appear to be responsible for this observation.

▶ In an earlier study, Yoo et al.[1] observed that prior labor was associated with lower intraoperative bispectral index measurements during general anesthesia (with sevoflurane and nitrous oxide) and reduced postoperative analgesic drug consumption in women undergoing cesarean delivery when compared with similar women who underwent cesarean delivery without prior labor.

D. H. Chestnut, MD

Reference

1. Yoo KY, Jeong CW, Kang MW, et al. Bispectral index values during sevoflurane-nitrous oxide general anesthesia in women undergoing cesarean delivery: a comparison between women with and without prior labor. *Anesth Analg.* 2008;106:1827-1832.

The Effect of Maternal and Fetal β2-Adrenoceptor and Nitric Oxide Synthase Genotype on Vasopressor Requirement and Fetal Acid-Base Status During Spinal Anesthesia for Cesarean Delivery

Landau R, Liu S-K, Blouin J-L, et al (Univ of Washington, Seattle; Univ Hosps of Geneva, Switzerland; et al)

Anesth Analg 112:1432-1437, 2011

Background.—Previous work demonstrated that maternal haplotypes of the β_2-adrenoceptor gene (*ADRB2*) influence ephedrine requirements during cesarean delivery. The use of ephedrine versus a pure α-adrenergic agonist such as phenylephrine has been associated with lower umbilical artery (UA) pH, thought to be secondary to increased fetal metabolism. There are no data evaluating the effect of fetal/neonatal genotypes on the metabolic response to maternally administered vasopressors. We hypothesized that neonatal *ADRB2* genotype would affect the extent of neonatal acidemia. We also examined the effect of maternal *ADRB2* and the endothelial nitric oxide synthase gene (*NOS3*) on ephedrine and phenylephrine requirements for treatment of maternal hypotension.

Methods.—The study was performed on 104 Chinese women scheduled for cesarean delivery under spinal anesthesia who were participating in a double-blind randomized clinical trial evaluating the maternal and neonatal effects of ephedrine versus phenylephrine infusions. Blood samples were drawn from the UA, umbilical vein, and maternal radial artery to measure blood gas values and lactate, ephedrine, and phenylephrine concentrations, and to determine maternal and neonatal genotype at nonsynonymous single nucleotide polymorphisms at codons 16 (rs1042713) and 27 (rs1042714) of *ADRB2* and codon 298 (rs1799983) of *NOS*. Clinical variables (UA pH, UA lactate, and dose of vasopressors) among genotypes were compared, and regression models were created to assess the effect of genotype on vasopressor dose and fetal acid-base status.

Results.—Maternal *ADRB2* genotype did not affect the ephedrine dose. Neonatal genotype at codon 16 influenced fetal acid-base status. UA pH was higher in Arg16 homozygous neonates (7.31 ± 0.03 in p.16Arg/Arg vs. 7.25 ± 0.11 in p.16 Arg/Gly and p.16 Gly/Gly; $P < 0.001$, 95% confidence interval (CI) of difference 0.03 ~ 0.09) and UA lactate was lower (2.67 mmol/L ± 0.99 in p.16Arg/Arg vs 4.28 mmol/L ± 2.79 in. p.16 Arg/Gly and p.16 Gly/Gly; $P < 0.001$, 95% CI of difference −2.40 ~ −0.82). In neonates born to mothers receiving ephedrine, the magnitude of the difference among genotypes was even greater (pH 7.30 ± 0.02 in p.16Arg/Arg vs. 7.19 ± 0.10 in p.16 Arg/Gly and p.16 Gly/Gly; $P < 0.001$, 95% CI of difference 0.07 ~ 0.14) and UA lactate was lower (3.66 mmol/L ± 1.30 in p.16Arg/Arg vs. 5.79 mmol/L ± 2.88 in p.16 Arg/Gly and p.16 Gly/Gly; $P = 0.003$, 95% CI of difference −3.48 ~ −0.80). In a multiple linear regression model ($R^2 = 63.6\%$; $P = 0.03$), neonatal *ADRB2* genotypes (p.16Arg/Arg and p.27Gln/Glu) and lower neonatal birth weight predicted lower UA lactate concentrations. Phenylephrine dose was not affected by maternal

ADRB2 or *NOS3* genotypes, and neonatal *NOS3* genotype did not affect UA pH or UA lactate.

Conclusion.—In contrast to previous findings in a North American cohort, maternal *ADRB2* genotype did not affect ephedrine requirements during elective cesarean delivery in a Chinese cohort. However, our findings suggest that neonatal *ADRB2* p.Arg16 homozygosity confers a protective effect against developing ephedrine-induced fetal acidemia.

▶ The authors concluded that the most important finding in this study was that umbilical artery (UA) pH was higher and UA lactate was lower in neonates that were Arg16 homozygous than in neonates with the 2 other genotypes of *ADRB2*. Further, among neonates whose mothers had received ephedrine, the dose of ephedrine was associated with neonatal acidemia (ie, decreased UA pH) only in those neonates who carried 1 or 2 Gly16 alleles; this association was not observed in neonates who were Arg16 homozygous. These observations should be considered in the context of the contemporary understanding of the mechanism by which ephedrine causes neonatal acidemia, despite laboratory evidence that ephedrine protects or restores uteroplacental perfusion. The authors cited evidence that supports the hypothesis that "the underlying mechanism by which ephedrine causes neonatal acidemia is transfer of ephedrine across the placenta and stimulation of metabolic processes in the fetus."

D. H. Chestnut, MD

The Rising Cesarean Delivery Rate in America: What Are the Consequences?
Blanchette H (New York Med College, Valhalla)
Obstet Gynecol 118:687-690, 2011

Cesarean delivery is now the most common operation in the United States, and it has increased dramatically from 5.8% in 1970 to 32.3% in 2008. This rise has not resulted in significant improvement in neonatal morbidity or maternal health. Three recent studies of elective repeat cesarean deliveries performed before 39 completed weeks of gestation have demonstrated increased respiratory and other adverse neonatal outcomes. Maternal mortality in the United States has increased from 10 per 100,000 to 14 per 100,000 from 1998 to 2004. Contributing to this is an increasing incidence of placenta accreta associated with multiple uterine scars requiring the need for emergency cesarean hysterectomy, blood transfusion, and maternal mortality due to obstetric hemorrhage. To reverse the trend of the rising cesarean delivery rate, obstetricians must reduce the primary rate and avoid the performance of a uterine incision unless absolutely necessary for fetal or maternal indications. For women with one previous low transverse cesarean delivery, obstetricians should promote a trial of labor after previous cesarean delivery in those women who desire three or more children.

▶ The author noted that between 1998 and 2004, the maternal mortality rate in the United States increased from 10 per 100 000 to 14 per 100 000. The author acknowledged that contributing factors include advanced maternal age, a significant increase in the prevalence and severity of maternal obesity, an increased incidence of other comorbidities, and an increased incidence of multiple gestation, which often necessitates operative delivery. However, he called attention to the "alarming concern of an increased incidence of placenta accreta associated with multiple uterine scars, requiring the need for emergency cesarean hysterectomy, blood transfusion, and maternal mortality due to obstetrical hemorrhage." The author correctly stated that "patients requesting an elective primary cesarean delivery on maternal request should be extensively counseled regarding the risk of this procedure, particularly if they are planning to have several children."

D. H. Chestnut, MD

The Unanticipated Difficult Intubation in Obstetrics
Mhyre JM, Healy D (The Univ of Michigan Health System, Ann Arbor)
Anesth Analg 112:648-652, 2011

In this focused review, we discuss an algorithm specifically for the unanticipated difficult intubation in obstetrics. This generic algorithm emphasizes a standardized and prespecified sequence of interventions to provide safe, efficient, and effective airway management for the emergency obstetric surgical patient. Individual institutions and anesthesia providers are encouraged to use this framework to select specific pieces of equipment for each step, and to create regular opportunities for all obstetric anesthesia providers to become facile with each airway device and to integrate the algorithm under simulated conditions (Fig 1, Table 2).

▶ Failed intubation occurs in approximately 1 in 300 obstetric patients who undergo induction of general anesthesia for cesarean delivery. The authors correctly note that "the most effective strategy to manage the difficult airway in obstetrics is to avoid it." The authors emphasize the importance of proper positioning of the patient. They state that "for most women, particularly those who are obese, the optimal position is ramped with left uterine displacement," and they further state that "the ideal ramp aligns the external auditory meatus with the xiphoid process in a horizontal plane." The authors provide a suggested algorithm for management of cases of unexpected difficult intubation (Fig 1). They also provide a list of secondary intubation equipment options (Table 2). The authors suggest that "videolaryngoscopy is becoming the rescue strategy of choice, and some authors even advocate it as the primary laryngoscopic technique." The availability of videolaryngoscopy and extraglottic airway options (eg, laryngeal mask airway) has likely resulted in a decreased need for invasive airway techniques in obstetric patients. Nonetheless, the authors' algorithm acknowledges that invasive airway access may be needed in some cases of failed intubation and ventilation. Frequent training may be necessary to maintain proficiency in invasive airway techniques. However, the authors state that "review of closed claims data for injuries attributed to invasive airway access suggests that the most serious complication of any emergent invasive

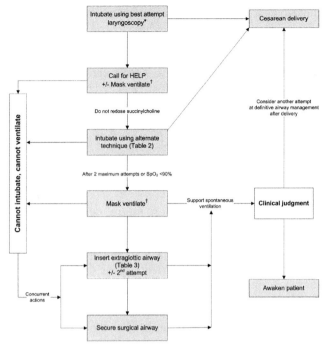

FIGURE 1.—Suggested algorithm. *Adjust cricoid pressure; backward, upward, rightward pressure (BURP); bougie; minor position adjustments. †Oral airway, jaw thrust, adjust cricoid pressure, 2-handed technique. (Reprinted from Mhyre JM, Healy D. The unanticipated difficult intubation in obstetrics. *Anesth Analg.* 2011;112:648-652, with permission from International Anesthesia Research Society.)

TABLE 2.—Options for Secondary Intubation Equipment

	Manufacturer
Direct laryngoscopes	
McCoy blade	
Miller blade inserted by a paramolar approach	
Intubation guides	
LMA FasTrach™ ± fiberoptic bronchoscope	LMA North America, San Diego, CA
Air-Q™ ± fiberoptic bronchoscope	Cookgas, St. Louis, MO
Lighted stylet	
Videolaryngoscopes	
C-Mac®	Karl Storz, Tuttlingen, Germany
GlideScope®	Verathon Medical, Bothell, WA
Airtraq®	Prodol Ltd., Vizcaya, Spain
Pentax-AWS™	Hoya Corp., Tokyo, Japan
Truview EVO2™	Truphatek Holdings Ltd., Netanya, Israel
McGRATH® Series5	Aircraft Medical, Edinburgh, UK
McGRATH® MAC	Aircraft Medical, Edinburgh, UK
Coopdech® C-Scope	Daiken Medical Co., Osaka, Japan
Optical stylets	
Bonfils™	Karl Storz, Tuttlingen, Germany
Levitan™	Clarus Medical, Minneapolis, MN
Shikani SOS™	Clarus Medical, Minneapolis, MN
Video System™ (CVS)	Clarus Medical, Minneapolis, MN
Video RIFL®	AI Medical Devices, Inc., Williamston, MI

airway technique is a failure to apply the technique early enough, before the consequences of significant hypoxia develop."

D. H. Chestnut, MD

Complications in Obstetrics and Obstetric Anesthesia

A Growing Problem: Maternal Death and Peripartum Complications Are Higher in Women With Grown-Up Congenital Heart Disease
Karamlou T, Diggs BS, McCrindle BW, et al (Seattle Children's Hosp, Washington; Oregon Health & Science Univ, Portland; Hosp for Sick Kids, Toronto, Ontario, Canada; et al)
Ann Thorac Surg 92:2193-2199, 2011

Background.—As patients with grown-up congenital heart disease (GUCH) increase, more women with GUCH will become pregnant. Heart surgeons may be involved in maternal GUCH care, yet the prevalence, characteristics, and outcomes for these women are unknown. We determined the national prevalence of GUCH parturients, their diagnostic makeup, and whether they have increased risk of peripartum complications, maternal or fetal death.

Methods.—We searched the Nationwide Inpatient Sample for women undergoing delivery in the United States between 1998 and 2007, with GUCH patients indicated by a code for "congenital cardiac diagnosis complicating pregnancy," Patient and hospital characteristics were compared between women with and without GUCH. National estimates for maternal and fetal mortality, cardiac complications, induction, caesarean or surgically assisted birth, and preterm delivery were derived. Outcomes were compared between women with and without GUCH, and also within diagnostic GUCH subgroups.

Results.—A total of 39.9 million births occurred, 26,973 (0.07%) of which were GUCH. Mean age was 27 years for both groups. Most common congenital diagnoses included ventricular septal defect (VSD) in 15%, aortic stenosis or insufficiency in 13%, atrial septal defect in 13%, pulmonary stenosis in 4%, and tetralogy of Fallot in 2%. Stillborn delivery was equivalent among groups. Maternal mortality was 18-fold higher in GUCH parturients (0.09%) compared with women without GUCH (0.005%; $p < 0.001$). Complications were higher for GUCH parturients compared with age-matched women, including cardiac complications (2.3% vs 0.2%), induction (37% vs 33%), caesarean or surgically assisted birth (45% vs 35%), and preterm delivery (10% vs 7%), $p < 0.001$ for all. A diagnosis of VSD was associated with the highest risk of maternal death and complications ($p < 0.05$ for all). More GUCH women delivered at teaching hospitals (58%) compared with women without GUCH (45%; $p < 0.001$).

Conclusions.—The GUCH parturients, especially those with VSD, have increased risk of mortality and peripartum complications compared with other age-matched women. Despite these risks, nearly 50% of GUCH patients deliver at nonteaching hospitals. Current national practice patterns for GUCH women are inadequate, and outcomes could be improved by education and proper triage of even relatively "simple" GUCH lesions such as atrial septal defect and VSD. Further studies that investigate risk-adjusted outcomes in a variety of care settings are necessary to resolve this complex issue.

▶ The authors reviewed an administrative database that had important limitations; for example, inability to determine whether a grown-up congenital heart disease (GUCH) parturient had undergone a previous surgical repair for congenital heart disease. They suspect that the increased risk associated with ventricular septal defect (VSD) may be attributable to unrepaired VSDs with possible Eisenmenger physiology. Another study is cited in which atrial septal defects were associated with similar risk escalation, perhaps for the same reason. Although maternal mortality was much higher in GUCH parturients than in their non-GUCH counterparts, the absolute risk for mortality (approximately 1 in 1000) was still reassuringly low in view of the possible high frequency of uncorrected congenital heart disease. Differences in peripartum complications were significant but not staggering (eg, preterm birth 10.2% vs 7.2%). There was a trend toward higher mortality in urban teaching hospitals than in nonteaching hospitals, but the database did not permit risk stratification of the GUCH patients among types of hospitals. The data presented are provocative but raise more questions than they answer. It appears that too many GUCH women receive inadequate long-term follow-up per se, inadequate advice about pregnancy, and inadequate prenatal care during pregnancy. These challenges need to be addressed, because the prevalence of pregnancy in women with GUCH is rising steadily.

G. P. Gravlee, MD

Anesthesia-Related Maternal Mortality in the United States: 1979–2002
Hawkins JL, Chang J, Palmer SK, et al (Univ of Colorado School of Medicine, Aurora; Ctrs for Disease Control and Prevention, Atlanta, GA; Oregon Anesthesiology Group, Portland; et al)
Obstet Gynecol 117:69-74, 2011

Objective.—To examine 12 years of anesthesia-related maternal deaths from 1991 to 2002 and compare them with data from 1979 to 1990, to estimate trends in anesthesia-related maternal mortality over time, and to compare the risks of general and regional anesthesia during cesarean delivery.

Methods.—The authors reviewed anesthesia-related maternal deaths that occurred from 1991 to 2002. Type of anesthesia involved, mode of delivery, and cause of death were determined. Pregnancy-related mortality ratios, defined as pregnancy-related deaths due to anesthesia per million live births were calculated. Case fatality rates were estimated by applying a national estimate of the proportion of regional and general anesthetics to the national cesarean delivery rate.

Results.—Eighty-six pregnancy-related deaths were associated with complications of anesthesia, or 1.6% of total pregnancy-related deaths. Pregnancy-related mortality ratios for deaths related to anesthesia is 1.2 per million live births for 1991—2002, a decrease of 59% from 1979—1990. Deaths mostly occurred among younger women, but the percentage of deaths among women aged 35—39 years increased substantially. Delivery method could not be determined in 14%, but the remaining 86% were undergoing cesarean delivery. Case-fatality rates for general anesthesia were 16.8 per million in 1991—1996 and 6.5 per million in 1997—2002, and for regional anesthesia were 2.5 and 3.8 per million, respectively. The resulting risk ratio between the two techniques for 1997—2002 was 1.7 (confidence interval 0.6—4.6, $P = .2$).

Conclusion.—Anesthetic-related maternal mortality decreased nearly 60% when data from 1979—1990 were compared with data from 1991—2002. Although case-fatality rates for general anesthesia are falling, rates for regional anesthesia are rising.

Level of Evidence.—II (Tables 1 and 3).

▶ The authors noted that the anesthesia-related maternal death rate in the United States has stabilized at approximately 1 maternal death per million live births (Table 1). Between 1985 and 1990, almost 17 women died as a result of general anesthesia for cesarean delivery for every 1 woman who died as a result of regional anesthesia for cesarean delivery (Table 3). For the years 1997 through 2002, case fatality rates for general anesthesia for cesarean delivery decreased substantially, whereas those for regional anesthesia for cesarean delivery increased slightly, so that there was no significant difference in maternal mortality rates between general and regional anesthesia for cesarean delivery (Table 3). The authors noted that "improvements in [the] case fatality rate for general anesthesia are especially notable considering it is used for the highest risk patients and most hurried emergencies." The authors cited a closed-claims report of 22 maternal cardiac arrests on labor and delivery units between 1998 and 2006.[1] Maternal outcomes were poor; 10 of the 22 women died, 11 had anoxic brain damage, and only 1 woman survived neurologically intact. Only 1 of these 22 cases

TABLE 1.—Pregnancy-Related Mortality Ratio Due to Anesthesia in the United States and United Kingdom, 1979—2002

Triennium	United States*	United Kingdom†
1979—1981	4.3	8.7
1982—1984	3.3	7.2
1985—1987	2.3	1.9
1988—1990	1.7	1.7
1991—1993	1.4	3.5
1994—1996	1.1	0.5
1997—1999	1.2	1.4
2000—2002	1.0	3.0

*Maternal deaths per million live births.
†Maternal deaths per million maternities (live births, stillbirths, pregnancy terminations, ectopic pregnancies, and abortions).

TABLE 3.—Case Fatality Rates and Rate Ratios of Anesthesia-Related Deaths During Cesarean Delivery by Type of Anesthesia in the United States, 1979–2002

Year of Death	Case Fatality Rates* General Anesthetic	Regional Anesthetic	Rate Ratios
1979–1984	20.0	8.6	2.3 (95% CI 1.9–2.9)
1985–1990	32.3	1.9	16.7 (95% CI 12.9–21.8)
1991–1996	16.8	2.5	6.7 (95% CI 3.0–14.9)
1997–2002	6.5	3.8	1.7 (95% CI 0.6–4.6)

CI, confidence interval.
*Deaths per million general or regional anesthetics.

involved general anesthesia and failed intubation. Thirteen women suffered respiratory arrest during/after administration of neuraxial analgesia/anesthesia; 8 women suffered respiratory arrest as a result of unintentional subarachnoid block during administration of labor epidural analgesia, and 5 women suffered respiratory arrest as a complication of administration of spinal anesthesia for cesarean delivery. Inadequate monitoring, unavailability of airway equipment, and delayed resuscitation were factors that contributed to the poor outcome in some of these cases.[1]

D. H. Chestnut, MD

Reference

1. Lofsky AS. Doctors company reviews maternal arrests cases. *APSF Newsletter.* 2007;22:28-30.

Anesthetic considerations for placenta accreta

Lilker SJ, Meyer RA, Downey KN, et al (Mount Sinai Hosp, Toronto, Ontario, Canada)
Int J Obstet Anesth 20:288-292, 2011

Background.—When diagnosed antenatally placenta accreta has often been managed by cesarean hysterectomy, but recently techniques involving uterine preservation have been developed. Uterine artery embolization has become an adjuvant treatment, although the potential for obstetric hemorrhage still exists. A multidisciplinary approach has permitted the development of anesthetic strategies for these patients.

Methods.—A retrospective case note review of patients with placenta accreta between 2000 and 2008 at our institution was conducted. Anesthetic technique, estimated blood loss, requirement for blood products and disposition of patients postoperatively were recorded.

Results.—A total of 23 cases were identified. In six, epidural anesthesia with progression to general anesthesia was planned. In 17 cases, neuraxial anesthesia was planned and in five of these (29%) excessive blood loss necessitated conversion to general anesthesia. Nine patients (39%) had intraoperative blood loss estimated at >2 L, and six required intraoperative blood transfusion. Eleven patients (48%) required hysterectomy, seven of which were performed on the day of delivery.

Conclusion.—In this case series, the expectation of major blood loss at cesarean delivery in the presence of placenta accreta and attempts at uterine conservation surgery initially prompted a conservative approach using general anesthesia. Greater experience has permitted modification of this approach and neuraxial anesthesia is now employed more frequently. When managed appropriately, most patients are able to tolerate both prolonged surgery and significant blood loss under epidural anesthesia (Fig 1).

▶ The authors describe their institution's management of pregnant women who have a known placenta accreta and who desire to retain their uterus and preserve future reproductive capability. This management plan typically includes femoral arterial insertion of uterine artery balloon-tipped catheters by an interventional radiologist before cesarean delivery. Following delivery of the infant, the adherent placenta is left in situ, and the uterine incision is closed. Attempts to

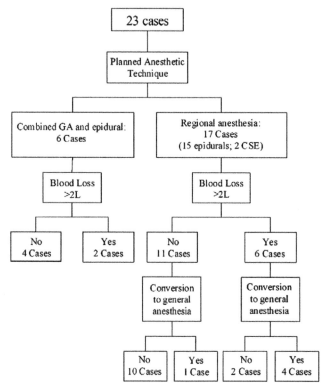

FIGURE 1.—Anesthetic management outcome of 23 cases of placenta accreta. (Reprinted from Lilker SJ, Meyer RA, Downey KN, et al. Anesthetic considerations for placenta accreta. *Int J Obstet Anesth.* 2011;20:288-292, with permission from Elsevier.)

reduce bleeding may include inflation of the uterine artery balloons and uterine artery embolization. In this case series, the authors used neuraxial anesthesia to provide (1) analgesia for the placement of the femoral artery sheaths, (2) intraoperative anesthesia, and (3) postoperative analgesia. In their last 17 cases, excessive blood loss necessitated intraoperative administration of general anesthesia in 5 (29%) patients (Fig 1). The authors stated that planned preoperative administration of general anesthesia may be wise in patients in whom endotracheal intubation is suspected to be difficult. They correctly noted that in such cases, the difficult airway must be managed "in conjunction with ... hemodynamic instability and rapid, large-volume fluid administration that may increase any airway soft tissue edema."

D. H. Chestnut, MD

Antenatal diagnosis of placenta accreta leads to reduced blood loss
Tikkanen M, Paavonen J, Loukovaara M, et al (Univ Central Hosp, Helsinki, Finland)
Acta Obstet Gynecol Scand 90:1140-1146, 2011

Objective.—Placenta accreta is one of the most devastating pregnancy complications. We sought to compare outcomes between women with placenta accreta when diagnosed antenatally or intrapartum, and to define predictors of the antenatal diagnosis.

Design.—Retrospective case—control study.

Setting.—University teaching hospital.

Population.—Twenty-four women with placenta accreta diagnosed antenatally and 20 women discovered intrapartum.

Methods.—Chart review of historical and delivery-associated variables. Rates were compared between the groups.

Main Outcome Measures.—Placenta accreta diagnosed antenatally or intrapartum.

Results.—Women with antenatal diagnosis had a lower estimated blood loss of a median of 4500 ml (range 100—15000 ml) compared with 7800 ml (range 2500—17000 ml, *p*=0.012) and required fewer units of packed red blood cells transfused (median 7; range 0—27 compared with 13.5; range 4—31, *p*=0.026). Nineteen (79%) women diagnosed antenatally had balloon catheter occlusion carried out during the cesarean section. Five (21%) had the entire placenta left in situ. There was no difference in the rate of surgical complications or duration of hospitalization. The clinical diagnosis among women with antenatal diagnosis was more often placenta percreta (*p*=0.013). The risk factor profile of women with antenatal diagnosis of placenta accreta included higher gravidity (*p*=0.014) and parity (*p*<0.0001), history of cesarean section (*p*=0.004), and placenta previa in the current pregnancy (*p*<0.001).

Conclusions.—Antenatal diagnosis of placenta accreta may reduce peripartum blood loss and the need for blood transfusion. Women with antenatal diagnosis more often have placenta previa and history of previous cesarean section, and the clinical diagnosis is more often placenta percreta.

▶ This retrospective study provides further evidence of the value of antepartum diagnosis of placenta accreta, which allows unhurried, multidisciplinary consideration of management options and facilitates the mobilization and availability of valuable resources (eg, skilled personnel, blood and blood products). Higher gravidity and parity, a history of previous cesarean delivery, and the presence of placenta previa in the current pregnancy were factors associated with the antenatal diagnosis of placenta accreta.

D. H. Chestnut, MD

Association of Epidural-Related Fever and Noninfectious Inflammation in Term Labor

Riley LE, Celi AC, Onderdonk AB, et al (Brigham and Women's Hosp and Massachusetts General Hosp, Boston; Massachusetts General Hosp, Boston; Brigham and Women's Hosp, Boston, MA; et al)
Obstet Gynecol 117:588-595, 2011

Objective.—To investigate the role of infection and noninfectious inflammation in epidural analgesia-related fever.

Methods.—This was an observational analysis of placental cultures and serum admission and postpartum cytokine levels obtained from 200 women at low risk recruited during the prenatal period.

Results.—Women receiving labor epidural analgesia had fever develop more frequently (22.7% compared with 6% no epidural; $P=.009$) but were not more likely to have placental infection (4.7% epidural, 4.0% no epidural; $P>.99$). Infection was similar regardless of maternal fever (5.4% febrile, 4.3% afebrile; $P=.7$). Median admission interleukin (IL)-6 levels did not differ according to later epidural (3.2 pg/mL compared with 1.6 pg/mL no epidural; $P=.2$), but admission IL-6 levels greater than 11 pg/mL were associated with an increase in fever among epidural users (36.4% compared with 15.7% for 11 pg/mL or less; $P=.008$). At delivery, both febrile and afebrile women receiving epidural had higher IL-6 levels than women not receiving analgesia.

Conclusion.—Epidural-related fever is rarely attributable to infection but is associated with an inflammatory state.

▶ The authors concluded that this study suggests that "epidural analgesia-related fever results from a noninfectious inflammatory process and women with higher IL-6 levels on admission in labor are at increased risk for developing fever." Of interest, among women without fever, postpartum levels of interleukin (IL)-6 and IL-8 were higher among those women who received epidural analgesia. The authors suggested that this finding provides additional support for the possibility that epidural analgesia plays a role in cytokine activation.

The authors further suggested that epidural analgesia may increase the risk of noninfectious inflammatory fever during labor in women with evidence of an activated immune system on admission.

D. H. Chestnut, MD

Effect of a comprehensive obstetric patient safety program on compensation payments and sentinel events

Grunebaum A, Chervenak F, Skupski D (New York Weill Cornell Med Ctr)
Am J Obstet Gynecol 204:97-105, 2011

Our objective was to describe a comprehensive obstetric patient safety program and its effect on reducing compensation payments and sentinel adverse events. From 2003 to 2009, we implemented a comprehensive obstetric patient safety program at our institution with multiple integrated components. To evaluate its effect on compensation payments and sentinel

---

TABLE 1.—Standardized Protocol for Induction or Augmentation With Oxytocin

Item	Protocol
a.	Only a premixed oxytocin solution is used
b.	The oxytocin infusion is limited to intravenous route via an infusion pump
c.	A buretrol infusion is used with a "smart pump" (a pump that comes with error reduction system and drug library capabilities)
d.	The infusion is piggybacked into the port most proximal to patient
e.	A written attending order (electronic template) is required before the start of oxytocin
f.	Before the start of oxytocin an attending must document the plan of care including indication, fetal presentation and station, cervical status, estimated fetal weight, pelvic adequacy, and fetal heart rate assessment.
g.	An attending must be available on the same floor as labor and delivery floor at all times while the patient is on oxytocin
h.	Before initiation of oxytocin a reassuring fetal heart rate must be present for a minimum of 20 minutes
i.	The oxytocin concentration is a premixed solution of 30 U per 500 mL. No individual mixing of solutions is permitted onsite.
j.	The oxytocin infusion begins at 1 mU per minute.
k.	The infusion is increased by 1 mU per minute no more frequently than every 15 minutes
l.	An attending must evaluate, document, and determine the plan of care if the oxytocin dosage reaches 20 mU per minute
m.	The maximum oxytocin dosage cannot exceed 40 mU per minute
n.	If the oxytocin infusion was discontinued for 20 minutes or less, it may be restarted at a lower rate than before discontinuation. If it was stopped for greater than 20 minutes then it should be restarted at 1 mU per minute
o.	Only a nurse can titrate oxytocin. The nurse can stop or titrate the oxytocin infusion if indicated. The doctor must be notified of this.
p.	The oxytocin infusion must be stopped or titrated for any of the following: uterine hyperstimulation/tachysystole (contractions less than 2 minutes in frequency and/or lasting longer than 90 seconds and/or more than 5 contractions in any 10 minute period); elevated uterine resting tone; nonreassuring fetal heart rate tracing; presumed uterine rupture; water intoxication
q.	The attending physician must be notified of any hyperstimulation/tachystole, abnormal fetal heart rate changes and/or stoppage or down titration of oxytocin.
r.	Terbutaline may be given if stopping oxytocin does not lead to a normalization of fetal heart rate changes in the presence of hyperstimulation
s.	Oxytocin should be discontinued as soon as a cesarean delivery is planned

events, we gathered data on compensation payments and sentinel events retrospectively from 2003, when the program was initiated, through 2009. Average yearly compensation payments decreased from $27,591,610 between 2003-2006 to $2,550,136 between 2007-2009, sentinel events decreased from 5 in 2000 to none in 2008 and 2009. Instituting a comprehensive obstetric patient safety program decreased compensation payments and sentinel events resulting in immediate and significant savings (Table 1).

▶ This article describes a comprehensive obstetric patient safety program in a tertiary academic medical center. Of interest to anesthesiologists, the authors describe their use of interdisciplinary team training programs on the labor and delivery unit. Further, they describe their use of multidisciplinary obstetric emergency drills for situations such as maternal cardiac arrest, shoulder dystocia, emergency cesarean delivery, and maternal hemorrhage. The authors also call attention to their maternal thromboprophylaxis protocol. In addition to administration of pharmacologic anticoagulation prophylaxis for high-risk patients, the authors have implemented the routine use of intermittent lower extremity pneumatic compression devices for all patients undergoing cesarean delivery. The authors' standardized protocol for oxytocin induction or augmentation of labor is also of interest to anesthesiologists (Table 1). The authors use only a premixed oxytocin solution, and the oxytocin infusion is limited to intravenous route via an infusion pump.

D. H. Chestnut, MD

Emergency peripartum hysterectomy: A 10-year review at the Royal Hospital for Women, Sydney
Awan N, Bennett MJ, Walters WAW (Univ of New South Wales, Sydney, Australia; Royal Hosp for Women, Sydney, New South Wales, Australia)
Aust N Z J Obstet Gynaecol 51:210-215, 2011

Background.—There appears to be a rise in the rate of emergency peripartum hysterectomy (EPH) in the developed world.

Aims.—To determine the incidence, indications, risk factors, complications and management of EPH in our tertiary level teaching hospital, the Royal Hospital for Women (RHW) in Sydney, over the last decade.

Methods.—A retrospective analysis was conducted of all cases of EPH performed at the RHW between the years 1999–2008 inclusive. EPH was defined as one performed after 20 weeks gestation for uncontrollable uterine bleeding not responsive to conservative measures occurring at any time after delivery but within the first 6 weeks post-partum. Cases were ascertained via our hospital obstetric database.

Results.—There were 33 EPH among 38 998 births, a rate of 0.85 per 1000 births. Indications for EPH were morbid adherence of the placenta (54.8%), placenta praevia (19.4%), uterine atony (12.9%) and uterine rupture or cervical laceration (9.7%). A significant association between previous caesarean section (CS) and abnormal placentation was confirmed ($P = 0.011$), especially for morbid adherence of the placenta ($P = 0.004$). There was one maternal death. Maternal morbidity was significant, with disseminated intravascular coagulation and urinary tract injury among the most common complications. All women required blood transfusions, and over a quarter were admitted to the intensive care unit.

Conclusions.—In our series, abnormal placentation causing severe haemorrhage was the commonest indication for EPH. Previous CS is a risk factor for abnormal placentation and particularly for morbid adherence of the placenta. The morbidity associated with EPH is considerable.

▶ Abnormal placentation was the indication for 74% of emergency peripartum hysterectomies (EPH) performed in this large retrospective study, and morbid adherence of the placenta (ie, placenta accreta, placenta increta, placenta percreta) was present in most of these cases of abnormal placentation. The authors noted that abnormal placentation has emerged as the leading cause of EPH, not only because of improved management of uterine atony and a reduced incidence of uterine rupture, but also because of an actual increase in the incidence of morbidly adherent placenta, which is likely a result of the increased cesarean delivery rate. Antenatal diagnosis of placenta accreta facilitates planning and preparation for these challenging cases. Unfortunately, in this study, antenatal ultrasonography was not very helpful in detecting the presence of a morbidly adherent placenta. The authors cited the report written by Baughman et al,[1] who recommended that MRI be used when ultrasonographic findings are ambiguous or in the presence of a posterior placenta previa that is more difficult to assess ultrasonographically.

D. H. Chestnut, MD

Reference

1. Baughman WC, Corteville JE, Shah RR. Placenta accreta: spectrum of US and MR imaging findings. *Radiographics*. 2008;28:1905-1916.

Impact of multiple cesarean deliveries on maternal morbidity: a systematic review
Marshall NE, Fu R, Guise J-M (Oregon Health and Science Univ, Portland)
Am J Obstet Gynecol 205:262.e1-262.e8, 2011

Objective.—The purpose of this study was to determine the impact of increasing numbers of cesarean deliveries on maternal morbidity. This study was performed for the 2010 National Institutes of Health Consensus Development Conference on Vaginal Birth After Cesarean: New Insights.

Study Design.—We conducted a systematic review and meta analysis of observational studies.

Results.—Twenty-one studies (2,282,922 deliveries) were included. The rate of hysterectomy, blood transfusions, adhesions, and surgical injury all increased with increasing number of cesarean deliveries. The incidence of placenta previa increased from 10/1000 deliveries with 1 previous cesarean delivery to 28/1000 with ≥3 cesarean deliveries. Compared with women with previa and no previous cesarean delivery, women with previa and ≥3 cesarean deliveries had a statistically significant increased risk of accreta (3.3–4% vs 50–67%), hysterectomy (0.7–4% vs 50–67%), and composite maternal morbidity (15% vs 83%; odds ratio, 33.6; 95% confidence interval, 14.6–77.4).

Conclusion.—Serious maternal morbidity progressively increased as the number of previous cesarean deliveries increased.

▶ The authors called attention to the decline in the number of eligible women who attempt vaginal birth after cesarean (VBAC) and stated that one-third of hospitals in the United States now ban attempted VBAC. When obstetricians counsel patients with a history of cesarean delivery regarding the delivery options for a subsequent pregnancy, the counseling tends to focus on the risks of a trial of labor and uterine rupture with a scarred uterus rather than the risks of repeat cesarean deliveries in future pregnancies. In this systematic review and meta-analysis, the authors observed that "maternal morbidity increases in a dose-response fashion with each additional cesarean delivery," especially for women with a history of 3 or more previous cesarean deliveries. The authors noted that women with a history of cesarean delivery and a placenta previa in the current pregnancy are at highest risk for morbidity, but they also observed increased maternal morbidity with an increasing number of previous cesarean deliveries, regardless of the placental implantation site. The authors concluded that "women who desire large families should be counseled about the risks of increasing morbidity with multiple cesarean deliveries." Furthermore, "as the rate of cesarean delivery continues to rise, hospitals and physicians must be prepared to optimize the treatment of women with multiple cesarean deliveries and minimize [the risk of] morbidity and death."

D. H. Chestnut, MD

Influence of Patient Comorbidities on the Risk of Near-miss Maternal Morbidity or Mortality

Mhyre JM, Bateman BT, Leffert LR (Univ of Michigan Health System, Ann Arbor; Massachusetts General Hosp, Boston)
Anesthesiology 115:963-972, 2011

Background.—Maternal morbidity and mortality are increased in the United States compared with that of other developed countries. The objective of this investigation is to determine the extent to which it is possible to predict which patients will experience near-miss morbidity or mortality.

Methods.—The authors defined near-miss morbidity as end-organ injury associated with length of stay greater than the 99th percentile or discharge to a second medical facility, and identified all cases of near-miss morbidity or death from admissions for delivery in the 2003—2006 Nationwide Inpatient Sample. Logistic regression was used to examine the effect of maternal characteristics on rates of near-miss morbidity/mortality.

Results.—Approximately 1.3 per 1,000 hospitalizations for delivery was complicated by near-miss morbidity/mortality as defined in this study (95% CI 1.3—1.4). Most of these events (58.3%) occurred in 11.8% of the delivering population—in those women with important medical comorbidities or obstetric complications identified before admission for delivery. The highest rates were noted among women with pulmonary hypertension (98.0 cases per 1,000 deliveries), malignancy (23.4 per 1,000), and systemic lupus erythematosus (21.1 per 1,000).

Conclusions.—Risk for near-miss morbidity or mortality is substantially increased among an identifiable subset of pregnant women. To the extent that antepartum multidisciplinary coordination and high-quality intrapartum care improve delivery outcomes for women with significant antepartum medical and obstetric disease, then public health investments to reduce the national burden of delivery-related near-miss morbidity and mortality will have the greatest effect by focusing resources on identifying and serving these high-risk groups.

▶ The authors noted that "the maternal mortality ratio in the United States has been estimated to be as high as 17 deaths per 100 000 live births, and the rate of annual increase between 1998 and 2008 exceeded that of any other developed country." In the authors' analysis, almost 60% of near-miss morbidity or mortality events occurred in "approximately 10% of women with medical or obstetric conditions known at the time of admission to the labor and delivery unit." The authors observed that the risk of near-miss maternal morbidity/mortality is increased among nonwhite women, and particularly among non-Hispanic black women. The authors also observed that advanced maternal age is "strongly associated with near-miss morbidity/mortality." The authors suggested that "targeted regionalization, specifically, triaging high-risk patients to regional centers with increased capacity to deliver intensive antepartum and peripartum care, may be a viable public health strategy to improve maternal delivery outcomes in the United States."

D. H. Chestnut, MD

Labor Epidural Analgesia and Maternal Fever
Segal S (Brigham and Women's Hosp, Boston, MA)
Anesth Analg 111:1467-1475, 2010

Women in labor who receive epidural analgesia are more likely to experience hyperthermia and overt clinical fever. The gradual development of modest hyperthermia observed in laboring women with epidural analgesia is not seen in those electing other forms of analgesia or unmedicated labor. Clinical fever is also far more likely in women laboring with epidural analgesia. It is possible that the observed slow increase in mean temperature is an artifact of averaging the temperature curves of a small group of women who eventually develop fever with a larger group who remain afebrile throughout labor. Selection bias confounds the association between epidural analgesia and fever, because women at risk for fever—due to longer duration of ruptured membranes, longer labor, more frequent cervical examinations, and other interventions—are also more likely to select epidural analgesia. However, even randomized trials have confirmed a higher incidence of fever in epidural-exposed women, suggesting a causal relationship. The mechanisms of epidural-associated fever remain incompletely understood. Altered thermoregulation and an antipyretic effect of opioids given to women without epidural analgesia may explain part of the phenomenon, but the most likely etiology is inflammation, most commonly in the placenta and membranes (chorioamnionitis). The consequences of maternal fever are diverse. Obstetricians are more likely to intervene surgically in laboring women with fever, and neonatologists are more likely to evaluate neonates of febrile women for sepsis. More ominously, maternal inflammatory fever is associated with neonatal brain injury, manifest as cerebral palsy, encephalopathy, and learning deficits in later childhood. At present, there are no safe and effective means to inhibit epidural-associated fever. Future research should define the etiology of this fever and search for safe and effective interventions to prevent it and to inhibit its potential adverse effects on the neonatal brain.

▶ Laboring women who receive epidural analgesia experience a larger increase in temperature and are more likely to experience overt clinical fever than women who receive other forms of analgesia. The most likely etiology is inflammation. The mechanism by which epidural analgesia enhances noninfectious inflammation and fever remains unclear. In a recent study, Riley et al[1] observed that women with higher interleukin-6 levels on admission to the labor and delivery unit were at increased risk for fever. The authors suggested that intrapartum epidural analgesia plays a role in cytokine activation and that epidural analgesia may increase the risk of noninfectious inflammatory fever in women with evidence of an activated immune system in early labor. Evidence suggests that maternal fever "may harm the fetus, particularly the developing nervous system, and inflammatory causes are likely responsible when the fever occurs in the intrapartum period." It is unclear whether epidural analgesia—associated maternal fever results in neonatal brain injury in the absence of clinical infection. Additional research should focus on the etiology, pathophysiology, consequences, prevention, and treatment of epidural analgesia—associated maternal fever.

D. H. Chestnut, MD

Reference

1. Riley LE, Celi AC, Onderdonk AB, et al. Association of epidural-related fever and noninfectious inflammation in term labor. *Obstet Gynecol.* 2011;117:588-595.

Maternal Obesity and Risk of Postpartum Hemorrhage

Blomberg M (Linköping Univ, Sweden)
Obstet Gynecol 118:561-568, 2011

Objective.—To estimate whether maternal obesity was associated with an increased risk for postpartum hemorrhage more than 1,000 mL and whether there was an association between maternal obesity and causes of postpartum hemorrhage and mode of delivery.

Methods.—A population-based cohort study including 1,114,071 women with singleton pregnancies who gave birth in Sweden from January 1, 1997 through December 31, 2008, who were divided into six body mass index (BMI) classes. Obese women (class I–III) were compared with normal-weight women concerning the risk for postpartum hemorrhage after suitable adjustments. The use of heparin-like drugs over the BMI strata was analyzed in a subgroup.

Results.—There was an increased prevalence of postpartum hemorrhage over the study period associated primarily with changes in maternal characteristics. The risk of atonic uterine hemorrhage increased rapidly with increasing BMI. There was a twofold increased risk in obesity class III (1.8%). No association was found between postpartum hemorrhage with retained placenta and maternal obesity. There was an increased risk for postpartum hemorrhage for women with a BMI of 40 or higher (5.2%) after normal delivery (odds ratio [OR] 1.23, 95% confidence interval [CI] 1.04–1.45]) compared with normal-weight women (4.4%) and even more pronounced (13.6%) after instrumental delivery (OR 1.69, 95% CI 1.22–2.34) compared with normal-weight women (8.8%). Maternal obesity was a risk factor for the use of heparin-like drugs (OR 2.86, 95% CI 2.22–3.68).

Conclusion.—The increased risk for atonic postpartum hemorrhage in the obese group has important clinical implications, such as considering administration of prophylactic postpartum uterotonic drugs to this group.

▶ Abundant evidence indicates that maternal obesity increases the risk of postpartum maternal morbidity and mortality. The author observed a more than twofold increase in the incidence of postpartum hemorrhage secondary to uterine atony in parturients with a body mass index of 40 or more. The author stated that this knowledge "emphasizes the need for active management after delivery of the placenta" in obese parturients.

D. H. Chestnut, MD

Postpartum hemorrhage – update on problems of definitions and diagnosis
Rath WH (Univ Hosp RWTH Aachen, Germany)
Acta Obstet Gynecol Scand 90:421-428, 2011

Maternal mortality due to postpartum hemorrhage (PPH) continues to be one of the most important causes of maternal death worldwide. PPH is a significantly underestimated obstetric problem, primarily because of a lack of definition and diagnosis. The 'traditional' definition of primary PPH based on quantification of blood loss has several limitations. Notoriously, blood loss is not measured or is significantly underestimated by visual estimation and there are no generally accepted cut-offs limits for estimated blood loss. A definition based on hematocrit change is not clinically useful in an emergency such as PPH, as a fall in hematocrit postpartum shows poor correlation with acute blood loss. The need for erythrocyte transfusion alone to define PPH is also of limited value, as the practice of blood transfusion varies widely. Definitions based on symptoms of hemodynamic instability are problematic, as they are late signs of depleted blood volume and commencing failure of compensatory mechanisms threatening the mother's life. There is thus currently no single, satisfactory definition of primary PPH. Proper and timely diagnosis of PPH should above all include accurate estimation of blood loss before vital signs change. Estimation of blood loss by calibrated bags has been shown to be significantly more accurate than visual estimation at vaginal delivery. Careful monitoring of the mother's vital signs, laboratory tests, in particular coagulation testing, and immediate diagnosis of the cause of PPH are important key factors to reduce maternal morbidity and mortality.

▶ Obstetric hemorrhage is the single most important cause of maternal mortality and morbidity worldwide. The author cited evidence that obstetric hemorrhage causes 25% of all maternal deaths and that nearly half of postpartum maternal deaths result from immediate postpartum hemorrhage (PPH). The author suggested that many cases of PPH are not recognized, and therefore, they concluded that the true incidence of maternal death from PPH is likely much higher. The author outlined several principles for the timely diagnosis and treatment of PPH. First, they encouraged the antepartum identification of women at increased risk for PPH. Second, the author affirmed the importance of proper estimation of blood loss before a change in maternal vital signs. They acknowledged the limited value of visual estimation of blood loss, but they called attention to evidence that calibrated collection bags provide a more accurate measurement of postpartum blood loss at vaginal delivery. Third, they emphasized the importance of close monitoring of the mother's vital signs, and they suggested use of an early warning score, such as the Modified Early Obstetric Warning Score (MEOWS).[1] Good care includes continual assessment of the mother's mental response, heart rate, blood pressure, and respiratory rate. The author stated that "smaller changes in all the parameters combined will be noticed earlier than a large change in one parameter alone," and that "a marked drop in blood pressure is usually a late sign of hypovolemia, whereas respiratory rate is one of the most sensitive markers of well being." Fourth, the author affirmed the importance of coagulation testing to facilitate an early diagnosis of impending coagulopathy. Finally, they emphasized the importance of immediate diagnosis of the etiology of PPH to allow timely initiation of appropriate pharmacologic and/or surgical treatment.

D. H. Chestnut, MD

Reference

1. Lewis G, ed. The Confidential Enquiry into Maternal and Child Health (CEMACH): Saving Mothers' Lives: Reviewing Maternal Deaths to Make Motherhood Safe — 2003-2005. The Seventh Report of the Confidential Enquiries into Maternal Deaths in the United Kingdom. London, UK: CEMACH; 2007.

Postpartum Hemorrhage Resulting From Uterine Atony After Vaginal Delivery: Factors Associated With Severity

Driessen M, for the Pithagore6 Group (UPMC Paris, France; et al)
Obstet Gynecol 117:21-31, 2011

Objective.—To identify factors associated with severity of postpartum hemorrhage among characteristics of women and their delivery, the components of initial postpartum hemorrhage management, and the organizational characteristics of maternity units.

Methods.—This population-based cohort study included women with postpartum hemorrhage due to uterine atony after vaginal delivery in 106 French hospitals between December 2004 and November 2006 (N=4,550). Severe postpartum hemorrhage was defined by a peripartum change in hemoglobin of 4 g/dL or more. A multivariable logistic model was used to identify factors independently associated with postpartum hemorrhage severity.

Results.—Severe postpartum hemorrhage occurred in 952 women (20.9%). In women with postpartum hemorrhage, factors independently associated with severity were: primiparity; previous postpartum hemorrhage; previous cesarean delivery; cervical ripening; prolonged labor; and episiotomy; and delay in initial care for postpartum hemorrhage. Also associated with severity was 1) administration of oxytocin more than 10 minutes after postpartum hemorrhage diagnosis (10—20 minutes after, proportion with severe postpartum hemorrhage 24.6% compared with 20.5%, adjusted OR 1.38, 95% CI 1.03—1.85; more than 20 minutes after, 31.8% compared with 20.5%, adjusted OR 1.86, CI 1.45—2.38); 2) manual examination of the uterine cavity more than 20 minutes after (proportion with severe postpartum hemorrhage 28.2% versus 20.7%, adjusted OR 1.83, 95% CI 1.42—2.35); 3) call for additional assistance more than 10 minutes after (proportion with severe postpartum hemorrhage 29.8% versus 24.8%, adjusted OR 1.61, 95% CI 1.23—2.12 for an obstetrician, and 35.1% compared with 29.9%, adjusted OR 1.51, 95% CI 1.14—2.00 for an anesthesiologist); 4) and delivery in a public non-university hospital. Epidural analgesia was found to be a protective factor against severe blood loss in women with postpartum hemorrhage.

Conclusion.—Aspects of labor, delivery, and their management; delay in initial care; and place of delivery are independent risk factors for severe blood loss in women with postpartum hemorrhage caused by atony.

▶ This population-based cohort study assessed outcome for 4550 women with postpartum hemorrhage as a result of uterine atony after vaginal delivery. The author unexpectedly noted that epidural analgesia appeared to be a protective factor against severe blood loss in women with postpartum hemorrhage caused by uterine atony. All of the patients in this study had postpartum hemorrhage caused by uterine atony. Thus, the author did not suggest that epidural analgesia decreases the incidence of uterine atony. Further, they did not suggest that the apparent protective benefit noted in this study resulted from a physiologic effect of epidural analgesia. Rather, they speculated that the presence of epidural analgesia "likely facilitates immediate management of postpartum hemorrhage because some procedures such as examination of the uterine cavity, manual removal of the placenta, or instrumental examination of the vagina and cervix are usually done under anesthesia." Further, the author noted that the need for administration of anesthesia may delay initial management of postpartum hemorrhage and, thus, increase the risk of severe postpartum hemorrhage in women with uterine atony who delivered without epidural analgesia. In this study, the group who delivered without epidural analgesia had a significantly higher proportion of women with no or a delayed examination of the uterine cavity than did the group who delivered with epidural analgesia.

D. H. Chestnut, MD

Predictors of massive blood loss in women with placenta accreta
Wright JD, Pri-Paz S, Herzog TJ, et al (Columbia Univ, NY)
Am J Obstet Gynecol 205:38.e1-38.e6, 2011

Objective.—We examined predictors of massive blood loss for women with placenta accreta who had undergone hysterectomy.

Study Design.—A retrospective review of women who underwent peripartum hysterectomy for pathologically confirmed placenta accreta was performed. Characteristics that are associated with massive blood loss (≥ 5000 mL) and large-volume transfusion (≥ 10 units packed red cells) were examined.

Results.—A total of 77 patients were identified. The median blood loss was 3000 mL, with a median of 5 units of red cells transfused. There was no association among maternal age, gravidity, number of previous deliveries, number of previous cesarean deliveries, degree of placental invasion, or antenatal bleeding and massive blood loss or large-volume transfusion ($P > .05$). Among women with a known diagnosis of placenta accreta, 41.7% had an estimated blood loss of ≥ 5000 mL, compared with 12.0% of those who did not receive the diagnosis antenatally with ultrasound scanning ($P = .01$).

Conclusion.—There are few reliable predictors of massive blood loss in women with placenta accreta.

▶ The authors correctly noted that preoperative diagnosis of placenta accreta facilitates advanced planning and preparation for difficult surgery and massive blood loss. Furthermore, a scheduled cesarean delivery facilitates the immediate availability of additional skilled personnel and the preparation and availability of sufficient blood products. The authors noted that accurate antenatal diagnosis and scheduled delivery have been associated with decreased maternal morbidity in women with placenta accreta. In this study, the authors observed that "there are few reliable predictors of massive blood loss in women with placenta accreta." It is important that women with an antenatal diagnosis of placenta accreta undergo delivery in a facility that is capable of rapid transfusion of large amounts of blood products. This group of investigators previously observed that women who underwent peripartum hysterectomy in a high-volume center are at decreased risk for maternal mortality.[1] The authors recommended referral of all women with a suspected placenta accreta to a tertiary center with expertise in the management of placenta accreta. The authors also called attention to the value of organized simulations of postpartum hemorrhage and the implementation of obstetric hemorrhage protocols.

D. H. Chestnut, MD

Reference

1. Wright JD, Herzog TJ, Shah M, et al. Regionalization of care for obstetric hemorrhage and its effect on maternal mortality. *Obstet Gynecol.* 2010;115:1194-1200.

Pre-eclampsia
Steegers EAP, von Dadelszen P, Duvekot JJ, et al (Univ Med Centre Rotterdam, Netherlands; Univ of British Columbia, Vancouver, Canada; et al)
Lancet 376:631-644, 2010

Pre-eclampsia remains a leading cause of maternal and perinatal mortality and morbidity. It is a pregnancy-specific disease characterised by de-novo development of concurrent hypertension and proteinuria, sometimes progressing into a multiorgan cluster of varying clinical features. Poor early placentation is especially associated with early onset disease. Predisposing cardiovascular or metabolic risks for endothelial dysfunction, as part of an exaggerated systemic inflammatory response, might dominate in the origins of late onset pre-eclampsia. Because the multifactorial pathogenesis of different pre-eclampsia phenotypes has not been fully elucidated, prevention and prediction are still not possible, and symptomatic clinical management should be mainly directed to prevent maternal morbidity (eg, eclampsia) and mortality. Expectant management of women with early onset disease to improve perinatal outcome should not preclude timely delivery—the only definitive cure. Pre-eclampsia foretells raised rates of cardiovascular and metabolic disease in later life, which could be reason for subsequent lifestyle education and intervention.

▶ This concise but thorough review calls attention to the increasing incidence of preeclampsia in the United States. The authors suggest that this finding might be a result of the increased prevalence of predisposing disorders, such as maternal obesity, diabetes, and chronic hypertension. The authors also emphasize that severe preeclampsia is a major cause of severe maternal morbidity and adverse perinatal outcomes, such as intrauterine growth restriction and preterm delivery. The authors call attention to evidence of a 20-fold increase in maternal mortality in women with preeclampsia arising before 32 weeks' gestation when compared with women in whom preeclampsia arises at or beyond 37 weeks' gestation. Therefore, some preeclampsia classification systems now include early onset as a criterion for identifying women with severe preeclampsia. I have long told my residents and students that the earlier the onset of preeclampsia, the sicker the patient. The authors note that magnesium sulphate remains the cornerstone for prevention and treatment of eclampsia seizures. The authors also state that "despite a reduced intravascular volume in preeclampsia, plasma volume expansion has not been proven to provide any benefit." The authors give appropriate emphasis to the importance of the preanesthetic evaluation, including an assessment of the maternal airway and the platelet count. They acknowledge the value of neuraxial anesthesia in avoiding the administration of general anesthesia for emergency cesarean delivery in women at high risk for difficult intubation or severe hypertension. During induction of general anesthesia for emergency cesarean delivery, the authors caution that "measures should be taken to avoid a speed that compromises maternal safety, even in the presence of acute fetal compromise." Of interest, the authors note that preeclampsia, especially early-onset disease, can be followed by maternal symptoms of posttraumatic stress, and they also call attention to the fact that preeclamptic women are at increased risk for future cardiovascular disease.

D. H. Chestnut, MD

Risk of Venous Thromboembolism During the Postpartum Period: A Systematic Review

Jackson E, Curtis KM, Gaffield ME (World Health Organization, Geneva, Switzerland; Ctrs for Disease Control and Prevention, Atlanta, GA)
Obstet Gynecol 117:691-703, 2011

Objective.—To determine, from the literature, the risk of venous thromboembolism during the postpartum period.

Data Sources.—We searched PubMed and Cochrane Library databases for all articles (in all languages) published in peer-reviewed journals from database inception through May 2010 for evidence related to incidence of venous thromboembolism in postpartum women.

Methods of Study Selection.—We included studies reporting relative risk, incidence rate, or cumulative incidence of venous thromboembolism in postpartum women.

Tabulation, Integration, and Results.—We included 15 articles reporting findings from 13 studies. Two studies directly comparing venous thromboembolism during the first 6 weeks postpartum to nonpregnant, nonpostpartum women reported relative effect measures of 21.5 (rate ratio; 95% confidence interval [CI] unable to be calculated) and 84 (odds ratio; 95% CI 31.7−222.6), respectively. A third study reported relative effect measures for deep venous thrombosis (15.2, 95% CI 13.2−17.6; standardized incidence ratio) and pulmonary embolism (9.2, 95% CI 6.5−12.7) separately. Three studies reported incidence rates of venous thromboembolism during the postpartum period (range 25−99 per 10,000 woman-years). We compared these incidence rates to baseline rates among nonpregnant, nonpostpartum women reported in the literature to generate rate ratios; these rate ratios ranged from 2.5 to 21.5. Nine studies reported cumulative incidence proportions of postpartum venous thromboembolism, ranging from 0.14 to 3.24 per 1,000 deliveries at 6 weeks postpartum. Incidence of venous thromboembolism was highest immediately after delivery (standardized incidence ratio for deep venous thrombosis 115.1 [95% CI 96.4−137.0], and for pulmonary embolism 80.7 [95% CI 53.9−117.9]); between 4 and 6 weeks postpartum, risk declined but was still approximately five-times to seven-times that of nonpregnant, nonpostpartum women.

Conclusion.—During the first 6 weeks postpartum, women's risk of venous thromboembolism increased 21.5-fold to 84-fold from baseline in nonpregnant, nonpostpartum women in studies that included an internal reference group. Although incidence of venous thromboembolism declined quickly after delivery, when this risk returns to baseline is not clear from current data.

▶ Half of the cases of thromboembolism in women of childbearing age occur during pregnancy or the puerperium. The higher frequency of thromboembolic disease during and after pregnancy is a result of at least 3 factors: (1) an increase in venous stasis, (2) the hypercoagulable state of pregnancy, and (3) the vascular injury associated with vaginal or cesarean delivery. Pulmonary thromboembolism was the leading cause of maternal death in the United Kingdom between 2003 and 2005.[1] Accordingly, many obstetricians now recommend more aggressive thromboprophylaxis in patients undergoing cesarean delivery. Clark et al[2] called attention to the implementation of a policy of universal pneumatic compression device use for all women undergoing cesarean delivery in their health care system. They concluded that "with appropriate universal thromboembolism prophylaxis ... the excess risk of death because of cesarean delivery may be virtually eliminated."[2]

D. H. Chestnut, MD

References

1. Mhyre JM. Maternal mortality. In: Chestnut's Obstetric Anesthesia: Principles and Practice. 4th ed. Philadelphia, PA: Mosby-Elsevier; 2009:853-865.

2. Clark SL, Belfort MA, Dildy GA, Herbst MA, Meyers JA, Hankins GD. Maternal death in the 21st century: causes, prevention, and relationship to cesarean delivery. *Am J Obstet Gynecol.* 2008;199:36.e1-36.e5.

The Volume of Blood for Epidural Blood Patch in Obstetrics: A Randomized, Blinded Clinical Trial

Paech MJ, Epidural Blood Patch Trial Group (Univ of Western Australia, Crawley, Australia; et al)
Anesth Analg 113:126-133, 2011

Background.—Our aim in this multinational, multicenter, randomized, blinded trial was to determine the optimum of 3 volumes of autologous blood for an epidural blood patch.

Methods.—Obstetric patients requiring epidural blood patch after unintentional dural puncture during epidural catheter insertion were allocated to receive 15, 20, or 30 mL of blood, stratified for the timing of epidural blood patch and center. Participants were followed for 5 days. The primary study end point was a composite of permanent or partial relief of headache, and secondary end points included permanent relief, partial relief, persisting headache severity, and low back pain during or after the procedure.

Results.—One hundred twenty-one women completed the study. The median (interquartile range) volume administered was 15 (15−15), 20 (20−20), and 30 (22−30) mL, with 98%, 81%, and 54% of groups 15, 20, and 30 receiving the allocated volume. Among groups 15, 20, and 30, respectively, the incidence of permanent or partial relief of headache was 61%, 73%, and 67% and that of complete relief of headache was 10%, 32%, and 26%. The 0- to 48-hour area under the curve of headache score versus time was highest in group 15. The incidence of low back pain during or after the epidural blood patch was similar among groups and was of low intensity, although group 15 had the highest postprocedural back pain scores. Serious morbidity was not reported.

Conclusions.—Although the optimum volume of blood remains to be determined, we believe these findings support an attempt to administer 20 mL of autologous blood when treating postdural puncture headache in obstetric patients after unintentional dural puncture.

▶ The authors called attention to the maternal morbidity associated with unintentional dural puncture with an epidural needle in obstetric patients. The risk of postdural puncture headache (PDPH) is high, and persistent PDPH may be accompanied by serious maternal morbidity, such as cranial nerve palsy or subdural hematoma. Although as many as 95% of obstetric patients may experience complete or partial short-term relief of symptoms after a single epidural blood patch, the authors noted that "only 35% to 70% remain headache free after several days." The authors called attention to observational studies that suggest that early performance of epidural blood patch is associated with a higher epidural blood patch failure rate. The authors correctly noted that "it is unclear whether the timing of the procedure actually influences the success rate," or whether patients who receive an early blood patch are different (eg, have a more severe headache) from those patients who receive a later blood patch.

D. H. Chestnut, MD

Use of Recombinant Factor VIIa in Patients with Amniotic Fluid Embolism: A Systematic Review of Case Reports

Leighton BL, Wall MH, Lockhart EM, et al (Washington Univ in Saint Louis School of Medicine, MO; et al)
Anesthesiology 115:1201-1208, 2011

Background.—Patients with amniotic fluid embolism (AFE) (major cardiac and pulmonary symptoms plus consumptive coagulopathy) have high circulating tissue factor concentrations. Recombinant factor VIIa (rVIIa) has been used to treat hemorrhage in AFE patients even though rVIIa can combine with circulating tissue factor and form intravascular clots. A systematic review was done of case reports from 2003 to 2009 of AFE patients with massive hemorrhage who were and were not treated with rVIIa to assess the thrombotic complication risk.

Methods.—MEDLINE was searched for case reports of AFE patients receiving rVIIa (rVIIa cases) and of AFE patients who received surgery to control bleeding but no rVIIa (cohorts who did not receive rVIIa). Additional AFE case reports were obtained from the Food and Drug Administration, the Australian and New Zealand Haemostasis Registry, and scientific meeting abstracts. The risk of a negative outcome (permanent disability or death) in rVIIa cases *versus* cohorts who did not receive rVIIa was calculated using risk ratio and 95% confidence interval.

Results.—Sixteen rVIIa cases and 28 cohorts were identified who did not receive rVIIa. All patients had surgery to control bleeding. Death, permanent disability, and full recovery occurred in 8, 6, and 2 rVIIa cases and 7, 4, and 17 cohorts who did not receive rVIIa (risk ratio 2.2, 95% CI 1.4–3.7 for death or permanent disability *vs.* full recovery).

Conclusion.—Recombinant factor VIIa cases had significantly worse outcomes than cohorts who did not receive rVIIa. It is recommended that rVIIa be used in AFE patients only when the hemorrhage cannot be stopped by massive blood component replacement.

▶ A recent report indicated that amniotic fluid embolism (AFE) is now the second leading cause of direct maternal death in the United States.[1] The maternal mortality rates observed in this systematic review (ie, 50% in the rVIIa cases and 25% in the cohorts who did not receive rVIIa) are consistent with other contemporary reports of maternal mortality from AFE. Given the fact that this was a retrospective study, the authors acknowledged that they could not determine "whether rVIIa caused or was merely associated with poor patient outcome." Further, they acknowledged that "sicker patients, including patients in whom

DIC could not be controlled with blood component therapy, may have been selected to receive rVIIa." Nonetheless, the authors recommended that "the initial therapy of AFE-associated consumptive coagulopathy should consist of blood component replacement, including PRBC, FFP, platelets, cryoprecipitate, and possibly fibrinogen concentrate." Further, they recommended that "rVIIa be used in AFE patients only when the hemorrhage cannot be stopped by massive blood component replacement."

D. H. Chestnut, MD

Reference

1. Clark SL, Belfort MA, Dildy GA, Herbst MA, Meyers JA, Hankins GD. Maternal death in the 21st century: causes, prevention, and relationship to cesarean delivery. *Am J Obstet Gynecol.* 2008;199:36e1-36e5.

Fetal and Neonatal Considerations

Electronic fetal heart rate monitoring and its relationship to neonatal and infant mortality in the United States

Chen H-Y, Chauhan SP, Ananth CV, et al (Univ of Wisconsin—Madison; Eastern Virginia Med School, Norfolk; Columbia Univ, NY; et al)
Am J Obstet Gynecol 204:491.e1-491.e10, 2011

Objective.—To examine the association between electronic fetal heart rate monitoring and neonatal and infant mortality, as well as neonatal morbidity.

Study Design.—We used the United States 2004 linked birth and infant death data. Multivariable log-binomial regression models were fitted to estimate risk ratio for association between electronic fetal heart rate monitoring and mortality, while adjusting for potential confounders.

Results.—In 2004, 89% of singleton pregnancies had electronic fetal heart rate monitoring. Electronic fetal heart rate monitoring was associated with significantly lower infant mortality (adjusted relative risk, 0.75); this was mainly driven by the lower risk of early neonatal mortality (adjusted relative risk, 0.50). In low-risk pregnancies, electronic fetal heart rate monitoring was associated with decreased risk for Apgar scores <4 at 5 minutes (relative risk, 0.54); in high-risk pregnancies, with decreased risk of neonatal seizures (relative risk, 0.65).

Conclusion.—In the United States, the use of electronic fetal heart rate monitoring was associated with a substantial decrease in early neonatal mortality and morbidity that lowered infant mortality.

▶ A 2006 Cochrane review concluded that the use of continuous electronic fetal heart rate (FHR) monitoring increases the operative delivery rate without a concomitant decrease in long-term neonatal outcomes.[1] The investigators for this study suggested that one reason the Cochrane review did not demonstrate a benefit of electronic FHR monitoring was the small sample size of the published reports. The authors concluded that this study demonstrated that in real-life practice in the United States, the use of continuous electronic FHR monitoring was associated with a higher operative delivery rate; however, it was also associated with a substantial decrease in early neonatal mortality and morbidity and, therefore, a decrease in infant mortality. The authors also observed that the benefits of electronic FHR monitoring are gestational-age dependent, with the highest impact demonstrated in preterm infants. The authors noted that preterm fetuses are at greater risk for intrapartum hypoxia and acidosis. The authors also suggested that the better neonatal outcomes associated with the use of electronic FHR monitoring may be a result of appropriate timing of obstetric interventions and delivery because of more accurate and earlier detection of fetal acidemia by electronic FHR monitoring.

D. H. Chestnut, MD

Reference

1. Alfirevic Z, Devane D, Gyte GM. Continuous cardiotocography (CTG) as a form of electronic fetal monitoring (EFM) for fetal assessment during labour. *Cochrane Database Syst Rev.* 2006;(3). CD006066.

Management of Intrapartum Fetal Heart Rate Tracings

American College of Obstetricians and Gynecologists
Obstet Gynecol 116:1232-1240, 2010

Intrapartum electronic fetal monitoring (EFM) is used for most women who give birth in the United States. As such, clinicians are faced daily with the management of fetal heart rate (FHR) tracings. The purpose of this document is to provide obstetric care providers with a framework for evaluation and management of intrapartum EFM patterns based on the new three-tiered categorization.

▶ This American College of Obstetricians and Gynecologists practice bulletin was published following a 2008 workshop that updated electronic fetal monitoring (EFM) nomenclature and recommended the use of a 3-tiered system for evaluation and management of intrapartum EFM patterns.[1] The new terminology includes the use of the term *tachysystole* in patients with more than 5 contractions in 10 minutes, averaged over 30 minutes. Fetal heart rate (FHR) tracings with tachysystole should be categorized by the presence or absence of FHR decelerations. The terms *hyperstimulation* and *hypercontractility* were abandoned.[1] The 3 categories of FHR tracings may be defined as follows: Category I FHR tracings are normal and are not associated with fetal acidemia (Box 1 in the original article). Category II FHR tracings include all FHR patterns that are not classified as category I or category III (Box 1). Category II tracings "require evaluation, continued surveillance, initiation of appropriate corrective measures when indicated, and reevaluation." Category III tracings are abnormal and signal "an increased risk for fetal acidemia at the time of observation"; these tracings have been associated with an increased risk for neonatal encephalopathy, cerebral palsy, and neonatal acidosis. Category III tracings are defined in Box 1. Persistent category III tracings "most often require prompt delivery."

D. H. Chestnut, MD

Reference

1. American College of Obstetricians and Gynecologists. ACOG Practice Bulletin No. 106: Intrapartum fetal heart rate monitoring: nomenclature, interpretation, and general management principles. *Obstet Gynecol.* 2009;114:192-202.

Rats Exposed to Isoflurane *In Utero* during Early Gestation Are Behaviorally Abnormal as Adults

Palanisamy A, Baxter MG, Keel PK, et al (Brigham and Women's Hosp, Boston, MA; Mount Sinai School of Medicine, NY; Florida State Univ, Tallahassee; et al)
Anesthesiology 114:521-528, 2011

Background.—Preclinical evidence suggests that commonly used anesthetic agents induce long-lasting neurobehavioral changes when administered early in life, but there has been virtually no attention to the neurodevelopmental consequences for the fetus of maternal anesthesia. This study tested the hypothesis that fetal rats exposed to isoflurane during maternal anesthesia on gestational day 14, which corresponds to the second trimester in humans, would be behaviorally abnormal as adults.

Methods.—Timed, pregnant rats were randomly assigned on gestational day 14 to receive 1.4% isoflurane in 100% oxygen (n = 3) or 100% oxygen (n = 2) for 4 h. Beginning at 8 weeks of age, male offspring (N = 12−14 in control and anesthesia groups, respectively) were evaluated for spontaneous locomotor activity, hippocampal-dependent learning and memory (*i.e.*, spontaneous alternations, novel object recognition, and radial arm maze), and anxiety (elevated plus maze).

Results.—Isoflurane anesthesia was physiologically well tolerated by the dams. Adult rats exposed prenatally to isoflurane were not different than controls on spontaneous locomotor activity, spontaneous alternations, or object recognition memory, but made more open arm entries on the elevated plus maze and took longer and made more errors of omission on the radial arm maze.

Conclusions.—Rats exposed to isoflurane *in utero* at a time that corresponds to the second trimester in humans have impaired spatial memory acquisition and reduced anxiety, compared with controls. This suggests the fetal brain may be adversely affected by maternal anesthesia, and raises the possibility that vulnerability to deleterious neurodevelopmental effects of isoflurane begins much earlier in life than previously recognized.

▶ Animal studies have demonstrated that exposure to sedative and anesthetic drugs during the critical periods of rapid neural development may cause accelerated neuroapoptosis that is associated with impaired learning and memory. In this study, male rats exposed in utero to a clinically relevant concentration of isoflurane subsequently demonstrated evidence of impaired spatial memory acquisition in young adulthood. The authors noted that the observed behavioral changes were unlikely to be a result of "an indirect adverse effect of isoflurane on maternal well-being because maternal systemic physiology was normal, and there were no differences in noncognitve variables, such as litter size, viability, and weight between the isoflurane-exposed and control animals." In an accompanying editorial, Flood[1] noted that epidemiologic studies have not clearly confirmed whether toxicity observed after administration of anesthesia to young mammals is relevant to human development. Further, other investigators have questioned whether the relatively long duration of intrauterine exposure to anesthesia in animal studies is relevant to the clinical exposure that occurs during surgery in pregnant women. Flood[1] specifically noted that "four hours of isoflurane anesthesia accounts for a much larger portion of the [rat] gestation than a 4-h anesthetic administered to a human mother-fetus pair." The authors of this study acknowledged that their findings seem to differ from a retrospective epidemiologic study that did not find evidence for a linkage between administration of general anesthesia for cesarean delivery and subsequent learning disabilities in childhood.[2] However, the authors correctly noted that the duration of intrauterine fetal exposure to general anesthesia at cesarean delivery was short and occurred at or near term gestation. Flood[1] concluded that the findings of this study should cause "concern but not alarm." She correctly noted that purely elective surgery is not performed during pregnancy, and that "most women who undergo general anesthesia during pregnancy do so to address a medical issue critical to their well-being or that of their fetus." She recommended that "nonurgent surgery should continue to be postponed until after pregnancy" and that "consideration should be made to using regional anesthesia when possible."

D. H. Chestnut, MD

References

1. Flood P. Fetal anesthesia and brain development. *Anesthesiology.* 2011;114: 479-480 [editorial].
2. Sprung J, Flick RP, Wilder RT, et al. Anesthesia for cesarean delivery and learning disabilities in a population-based birth cohort. *Anesthesiology.* 2009;111:302-310.

Special Situations in Obstetric Anesthesia

Anaesthetic considerations for non-obstetric surgery during pregnancy

Reitman E, Flood P (Columbia Univ, NY; Univ of California, San Francisco)
Br J Anaesth 107:i72-i78, 2011

Surgery during pregnancy is complicated by the need to balance the requirements of two patients. Under usual circumstances, surgery is only conducted during pregnancy when it is absolutely necessary for the well-being of the mother, fetus, or both. Even so, the outcome is generally favourable for both the mother and the fetus. All general anaesthetic drugs cross the placenta and there is no optimal general anaesthetic technique. Neither is there convincing evidence that any particular anaesthetic drug is toxic in humans. There is weak evidence that nitrous oxide should be avoided in early pregnancy due to a potential association with pregnancy loss with high exposure. There is evidence in animal models that many general anaesthetic techniques cause inappropriate neuronal apoptosis and behavioural deficits in later life. It is not known whether these considerations affect the human fetus but studies are underway. Given the general considerations of avoiding fetal exposure to unnecessary medication and potential protection of the maternal airway, regional anaesthesia is usually preferred in pregnancy when it is practical for the medical and surgical condition. When surgery is indicated during pregnancy maintenance of maternal oxygenation, perfusion and homeostasis with the least extensive anaesthetic that is practical will assure the best outcome for the fetus.

▶ This excellent review includes a helpful discussion of recent studies that demonstrated accelerated neuronal apoptosis in immature rodent brains that had intrauterine exposure to anesthetic agents. These studies also noted behavioral abnormalities in the rodent offspring after intrauterine exposure to these anesthetic agents. The authors stated that "although evidence for anaesthetic-induced neuronal apoptosis in rodents is convincing, it is less clear that these data can be extrapolated to humans." Further, the authors noted that "the extended period of synaptogenesis in humans could confer protection against persistent behavioural effects of perinatal anaesthetic exposure because the duration of anaesthetic exposure is only for a brief fraction of the vulnerable period." They then stated that "from a developmental perspective, exposing an infant rat to isoflurane for 6 h is roughly the equivalent of producing general anaesthesia for several weeks in a human neonate." Undoubtedly, future studies will address this issue and determine whether the results of these animal studies are relevant to clinical practice.

D. H. Chestnut, MD

Continuous Spinal Anesthesia and Analgesia in Obstetrics
Palmer CM (Univ of Arizona College of Medicine, Tuscon)
Anesth Analg 111:1476-1479, 2010

The development of the technique of continuous spinal anesthesia as it relates to the obstetric population is recounted. The advantages and disadvantages of continuous spinal anesthesia are examined, currently available catheters and kits are reviewed, and strategies for the management of continuous spinal techniques for labor analgesia and surgical anesthesia are discussed. Continuous spinal anesthesia may have particular value over other regional techniques in several specific clinical circumstances.

▶ The author states that currently there are no plans to market a 28-gauge microcatheter for continuous spinal anesthesia in the United States. The only catheters available for continuous spinal anesthesia are the larger catheters included in the commercially available epidural anesthesia kits. Most commercially available epidural anesthesia kits include a 17-gauge or 18-gauge Tuohy-type needle. Unfortunately, dural puncture with needles of this size results in a high risk of postdural puncture headache (PDPH). The author suggests that pediatric epidural catheters (ie, 24-gauge catheters placed through a 20-gauge needle) may also be well suited for continuous spinal anesthesia in obstetric patients, and he speculates that use of these pediatric epidural needles and catheters would be associated with a decreased incidence of PDPH than occurs with the larger, adult epidural needles and catheters. The author identifies 5 situations and/or comorbidities in which continuous spinal anesthesia may be an attractive option in obstetric anesthesia practice: (1) previous spinal surgery (eg, correction or stabilization of scoliosis), (2) significant cardiac disease, (3) morbid obesity, (4) unintentional dural puncture in a patient in whom it has been difficult to identify the epidural space, and (5) anticipated difficult airway. The author acknowledges that the use of continuous spinal anesthesia in this last situation (ie, patients with an anticipated difficult airway) is controversial. Finally, the author correctly cautions that "care must always be taken to clearly identify the spinal catheter as such, to avoid the possibility that it may be mistaken for an epidural catheter." He recommends that "when possible, different infusion pumps and tubing should be used for management of the spinal catheter, ideally pumps and tubing reserved for this purpose."

D. H. Chestnut, MD

Nonobstetric Surgery During Pregnancy
ACOG Committee on Obstetric Practice
Obstet Gynecol 117:420-421, 2011

The American College of Obstetricians and Gynecologists' Committee on Obstetric Practice acknowledges that the issue of nonobstetric surgery during pregnancy is an important concern for physicians who care for women. It is important for a physician to obtain an obstetric consultation before performing nonobstetric surgery and some invasive procedures (eg, cardiac catheterization or colonoscopy) because obstetricians are uniquely qualified to discuss aspects of maternal physiology and anatomy that may affect intraoperative maternal–fetal well-being. Ultimately, each case warrants a team approach (anesthesia and obstetric care providers, surgeons, pediatricians, and nurses) for optimal safety of the woman and the fetus.

▶ I encourage all anesthesiologists who provide care for pregnant women to read this brief American College of Obstetricians and Gynecologists (ACOG) committee opinion in its entirety. This committee opinion provides specific recommendations regarding the use of fetal heart rate (FHR) monitoring before, during, and after nonobstetric surgery during pregnancy. The ACOG stated that "if the fetus is considered previable, it is generally sufficient to ascertain the fetal heart rate by Doppler before and after the procedure." The ACOG also stated that "at a minimum, if the fetus is considered to be viable, simultaneous electronic fetal heart rate and contraction monitoring should be performed before and after the procedure to assess fetal well-being and the absence of contractions." Further, the ACOG opined that intraoperative electronic FHR monitoring "may be appropriate when all of the following apply: 1) the fetus is viable; 2) it is physically possible to perform intraoperative electronic fetal monitoring; 3) a health care provider with obstetric surgery privileges is available and willing to intervene during the surgical procedure for fetal indications; 4) when possible, the woman has given informed consent to emergency cesarean delivery; and 5) the nature of the planned surgery will allow the safe interruption or alteration of the procedure to provide access to perform emergency delivery." The ACOG acknowledged that "in select circumstances, intraoperative fetal monitoring may be considered for previable fetuses to facilitate positioning or oxygenation interventions." I wish that the ACOG had acknowledged that the same considerations may be applicable for surgery for mothers with a viable fetus. The greatest value of intraoperative FHR monitoring is that it allows for the optimization of the maternal condition if the fetus shows signs of compromise. An unexplained change in FHR mandates the evaluation of maternal position, blood pressure, oxygenation, and acid-base status, as well as the inspection of the surgical site to ensure that neither surgeons nor retractors are impairing uterine perfusion.

D. H. Chestnut, MD

Obesity and pregnancy: clinical management of the obese gravida
Gunatilake RP, Perlow JH (Phoenix Perinatal Associates, AZ; Duke Univ Health System, Durham, NC)
Am J Obstet Gynecol 204:106-119, 2011

In recent years, the prevalence of obesity in the United States has risen dramatically, especially among women of reproductive age. Research that has specifically evaluated pregnancy outcomes among obese parturients has allowed for a better understanding of the myriad adverse perinatal complications that are observed with significantly greater frequency in the obese pregnant population. The antepartum, intrapartum, intraoperative, postoperative, and postpartum periods are all times in which the obese pregnant woman is at greater risk for adverse maternal-fetal outcomes, compared with her ideal bodyweight counterpart. Comorbid medical conditions that commonly are associated with obesity further accentuate perinatal risks. All obese pregnant women should be counseled regarding these risks, and strategies should be used to improve perinatal outcome whenever possible. Obese women of reproductive age ideally should be counseled before conception and advised to achieve ideal bodyweight before pregnancy (Table 4).

▶ The authors noted that obesity is associated with an increased risk of instrumental vaginal delivery, shoulder dystocia, and birth trauma (Table 4). Obesity

TABLE 4.—Obesity-Related Peripartum Complications

Problem/Risk	Potential Intervention
Increased respiratory work and myocardial oxygen requirement	Epidural anesthesia, supplemental oxygen, left-lateral laboring position
Difficult peripheral intravenous access	Central intravenous catheter
Inaccurate blood pressure monitoring	Appropriate-sized cuff, arterial line
Increased risk of general anesthesia	Anesthesia consultation, early epidural
Anticipated difficulty with intubation	Capability for awake/fiber-optic intubation
Difficulty with patient transfers	Bariatric lifts and inflatable mattresses, additional personnel
Prolonged cesarean operative time	Combined spinal-epidural anesthesia
Poor operative exposure	Evaluation of maternal anthropometry, panniculus retraction, periumbilical skin incision, atraumatic self-retaining retractor
Enhanced risk of hemorrhage	Blood typed and crossed for transfusion, ligate large subcutaneous vessels, meticulous surgical technique
Enhanced aspiration risk	Prophylactic epidural, H_2 antagonist, sodium citrate with citric acid, metoclopramide, nothing by mouth in labor
Enhanced thromboembolic risk	Early postoperative ambulation, sequential pneumatic compression, heparin until fully ambulatory
Enhanced risk of infectious morbidity	Thorough skin preparation, adequate antimicrobial prophylaxis, avoidance of subpannicular incision, meticulous surgical technique, consideration of subcutaneous drain
Enhanced risk of cesarean delivery	Informed consent, monitoring of labor curve, and intervention for labor dystocia
Enhanced risk of shoulder dystocia	Near-term sonographic fetal weight, caution with operative delivery

is also associated with an increased risk of failed induction of labor. The authors noted that even when labor occurs spontaneously, the labor is less likely to progress according to standard labor curves in an obese parturient. Published studies have consistently demonstrated that obesity is associated with an increased risk of emergency cesarean delivery. The authors outlined the rationale for individualized consideration of elective primary cesarean delivery in women with extreme obesity. They called attention to the fact that the cesarean delivery rate for extremely obese parturients is almost 50%, and extreme obesity may preclude a timely delivery in cases of severe intrapartum fetal compromise. For laboring obese parturients, the authors recommended consideration of the early placement of a prophylactic epidural catheter, even if epidural analgesia is not yet requested or necessary, thereby precluding the need for general anesthesia for emergency cesarean delivery. The authors also called attention to the increased risk of venous thromboembolism in obese parturients, and they outlined a suggested regimen for thromboprophylaxis.

D. H. Chestnut, MD

11 Pain Management

Acute Pain Management

A meta-analysis of the efficacy of wound catheters for post-operative pain management

Gupta A, Favaios S, Perniola A, et al (Örebro Univ Hosp, Sweden; Dept of Anesthesiology of CHTS, EPE, Penafiel, Portugal; et al)
Acta Anaesthesiol Scand 55:785-796, 2011

Local anesthetics (LA) are injected via catheters placed in surgical wounds for post-operative analgesia. The primary aim of this systematic review was to assess whether LA reduce pain intensity when injected via wound catheters. A literature search was performed from Medline via PubMed, EMBASE and the Cochrane database from 1966 until November 2009. The search strategy included the following key words: pain, postoperative, catheters and local anesthetics. Two co-authors independently read every article that was initially included and extracted data into a pre-defined study record form. A total of 753 studies primarily fit the search criteria and 163 were initially extracted. Of these, 32 studies were included in the meta-analysis. Wound catheters provided no significant analgesia at rest or on activity, except in patients undergoing gynecological and obstetric surgery at 48 h ($P = 0.03$). The overall morphine consumption was lower (≈ 13 mg) during 0–24 h ($P < 0.001$) in these patients. No significant differences in side effects were found, except for a lower risk of wound breakdown ($P = 0.048$) and a shorter length of hospital stay ($P = 0.04$) in patients receiving LA. A statistically significant heterogeneity was seen between the studies in most end-points. LA injected via wound catheters did not reduce pain intensity, except at 48 h in a subgroup of patients undergoing obstetric and gynecological surgery. Rescue analgesic consumption was also lower in this group at 0–24 h. The magnitude of these effects was small and compounded by pronounced heterogeneity.

▶ Postoperative local anesthetic wound infiltration is a safe, simple, and, hopefully, low-cost technique for providing improved postoperative analgesia. The results of this extensive review and meta-analysis suggest that the technique may not be worth the time and expense involved. A previous meta-analysis showed more robust benefits[1] but used different methodologies, averaging pain level over 48 hours, which the authors of the current study questioned.

One question that arises is whether local anesthetic wound infusions impede healing. There was no evidence for this among the studies evaluated.

S. E. Abram, MD

Reference

1. Liu SS, Richman JM, Thirlby RC, Wu CL. Efficacy of continuous wound catheters delivering local anesthetic for postoperative analgesia: a quantitative and qualitative systematic review of randomized controlled trials. *J Am Coll Surg*. 2006;203: 914-932.

A systematic review of intravenous ketamine for postoperative analgesia
Laskowski K, Stirling A, McKay WP, et al (Univ of Saskatchewan, Saskatoon, Canada)
Can J Anaesth 58:911-923, 2011

Purpose.—Perioperative intravenous ketamine may be a useful addition in pain management regimens. Previous systematic reviews have included all methods of ketamine administration, and heterogeneity between studies has been substantial. This study addresses this issue by narrowing the inclusion criteria, using a random effects model, and performing subgroup analysis to determine the specific types of patients, surgery, and clinical indications which may benefit from perioperative ketamine administration.

Source.—We included published studies from 1966 to 2010 which were randomized, double-blinded, and placebo controlled using intravenous ketamine (bolus or infusion) to decrease postoperative pain. Studies using any form of regional anesthesia were excluded. No limitation was placed on the ketamine dose, patient age, or language of publication.

Principal Findings.—Ninety-one comparisons in seventy studies involving 4,701 patients met the inclusion criteria (2,652 in ketamine groups and 2,049 in placebo groups). Forty-seven of these studies were appropriate for evaluation in the core meta-analysis, and the remaining 23 studies were used to corroborate the results. A reduction in total opioid consumption and an increase in the time to first analgesic were observed across all studies ($P < 0.001$). The greatest efficacy was found for thoracic, upper abdominal, and major orthopedic surgical subgroups. Despite using less opioid, 25 out of 32 treatment groups (78%) experienced less pain than the placebo groups at some point postoperatively when ketamine was efficacious. This finding implies an improved quality of pain control in addition to decreased opioid consumption. Hallucinations and nightmares were more common with ketamine but sedation was not. When ketamine was efficacious for pain, postoperative nausea and vomiting was less frequent in the ketamine group. The dose-dependent role of ketamine analgesia could not be determined.

Conclusion.—Intravenous ketamine is an effective adjunct for postoperative analgesia. Particular benefit was observed in painful procedures, including upper abdominal, thoracic, and major orthopedic surgeries. The analgesic effect of ketamine was independent of the type of intraoperative opioid administered, timing of ketamine administration, and ketamine dose.

▶ This useful study helps define situations in which ketamine is most useful, that is, surgical interventions that are associated with severe postoperative pain. Other useful information teased out of existing studies includes the lack of effect of timing (no apparent preemptive effect and efficacy at low doses). As the authors point out, regional analgesia is highly effective at reducing postoperative pain and opioid consumption, and ketamine appears to be a good option when severe pain is anticipated and regional analgesia cannot be performed. One situation in which ketamine should be useful is in patients on chronic preoperative opioids. Such a cohort was not among the studies in this analysis.

S. E. Abram, MD

Chronic Opioid Use Prior to Total Knee Arthroplasty

Zywiel MG, Stroh DA, Lee SY, et al (Univ of Toronto, Ontario, Canada; Sinai Hosp of Baltimore, MD; Hallym Univ Med Ctr, Kangdonggu, Seoul, South Korea; et al)
J Bone Joint Surg Am 93:1988-1993, 2011

Background.—Chronic use of opioid medications may lead to dependence or hyperalgesia, both of which might adversely affect perioperative and postoperative pain management, rehabilitation, and clinical outcomes after total knee arthroplasty. The purpose of this study was to evaluate patients who underwent total knee arthroplasty following six or more weeks of chronic opioid use for pain control and to compare them with a matched group who did not use opioids preoperatively.

Methods.—Forty-nine knees in patients who had a mean age of fifty-six years (range, thirty-seven to seventy-eight years) and who had regularly used opioid medications for pain control prior to total knee arthroplasty were compared with a group of patients who had not used them. Length of hospitalization, aseptic complications requiring reoperation, requirement for specialized pain management, and clinical outcomes were assessed for both groups.

Results.—Knee Society scores were significantly lower in the patients who regularly used opioid medications at the time of final follow-up (mean, three years; range, two to seven years); the opioid group had a mean of 79 points (range, 45 to 100 points) as compared with a mean of 92 points (range, 59 to 100 points) in the non-opioid group. A significantly higher prevalence of complications was seen in the opioid group, with five arthroscopic evaluations and eight revisions for persistent stiffness and/or pain, compared with none in the matched group. Ten patients in the opioid group were referred for outpatient pain management, compared with one patient in the non-opioid group.

TABLE 2.—Comparison of Perioperative Pain Management*

	Opioid Group	Non-Opioid Group	P Value
Number of patients who underwent operation under general anesthesia only	24	29	0.265
Number of patients who received regional blocks (epidural and/or nerve blocks) with postoperative infusion	12	10	0.806
Number of patients receiving different postoperative pain regimens			
IV patient-controlled analgesia	31	30	0.476
Continuous catheter infusion analgesia	12	10	
Intermittent IV analgesia	2	5	
Mean morphine-equivalent dose of oral narcotics prescribed at discharge in mg (range [95% CI])	85 (0 to 248 [65 to 106])	91 (36 to 360 [67 to 115])	0.946

*IV = intravenous, and CI = confidence interval.

Conclusions.—Patients who chronically use opioid medications prior to total knee arthroplasty may be at a substantially greater risk for complications and painful prolonged recoveries. Alternative non-opioid pain medications and/or earlier referral to an orthopaedic surgeon prior to habitual opioid use should be considered for patients with painful degenerative disease of the knee.

Level of Evidence.—Therapeutic Level III. See Instructions for Authors for a complete description of levels of evidence (Table 2).

▶ While it is widely accepted that postoperative pain is much more difficult to control for patients using opioids preoperatively, there have been little data to suggest that surgical outcomes may be compromised by chronic presurgical opioid use. The differences in the outcomes tested, most of which were related to continued unresolved joint pain, are striking. The opioid group had longer hospital stays, higher rates of repeated arthroscopic and revision surgery, and more frequent need for pain management services, all of which are costly (Table 2). While opioid use appears to be the culprit, one cannot rule out more extensive presurgical pathology as the reason for more postoperative pain. The authors suggested that preoperative withdrawal of opioids might reduce the likelihood of serious postoperative pain problems. A study randomly assigning opioid users to withdrawal or continued opioid use would help answer this question.

S. E. Abram, MD

Continuous Intercostal Nerve Blockade for Rib Fractures: Ready for Primetime?
Truitt MS, Murry J, Amos J, et al (Methodist Dallas Med Ctr, TX; Denver Health Med Ctr, CO)
J Trauma 71:1548-1552, 2011

Background.—Providing analgesia for patients with rib fractures continues to be a management challenge. The objective of this study was to examine our experience with the use of a continuous intercostal nerve block (CINB). Although this technique is being used, little data have been published documenting its use and efficacy. We hypothesized that a CINB would provide excellent analgesia, improve pulmonary function, and decrease length of stay (LOS).

Methods.—Consecutive adult blunt trauma patients with three or more unilateral rib fractures were prospectively studied over 24 months. The catheters were placed at the bedside in the extrathoracic, paravertebral location, and 0.2% ropivacaine was infused. Respiratory rate, preplacement (PRE) numeric pain scale (NPS) scores, and sustained maximal inspiration (SMI) lung volumes were determined at rest and after coughing. Parameters were repeated 60 minutes after catheter placement (POST). Hospital LOS comparison was made with historical controls using epidural analgesia.

Results.—Over the study period, 102 patients met inclusion criteria. Mean age was 69 (21–96) years, mean injury severity score was 14 (9–16), and the mean number of rib fractures was 5.8 (3–10). Mean NPS improved significantly (PRE NPS at rest = 7.5 vs. POST NPS at rest = 2.6, $p < 0.05$, PRE NPS after cough = 9.4, POST after cough = 3.6, $p < 0.05$) which was associated with an increase in the SMI (PRE SMI = 0.4 L and POST SMI = 1.3 L, $p < 0.05$). Respiratory rate decreased significantly ($p < 0.05$) and only 2 of 102 required mechanical ventilation. Average LOS for the study population was 2.9 days compared with 5.9 days in the historical control. No procedural or drug-related complications occurred.

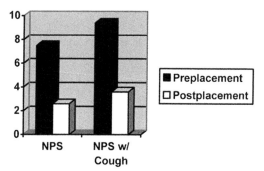

FIGURE 1.—PRE/POST placement pain scores in patients at rest ($p < 0.05$) and after coughing ($p < 0.05$). (Reprinted from Truitt MS, Murry J, Amos J, et al. Continuous intercostal nerve blockade for rib fractures: ready for primetime? *J Trauma.* 2011;71:1548-1552, with permission from Lippincott Williams & Wilkins.)

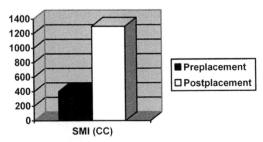

FIGURE 2.—Sustained maximal inspiration before and after placement of continuous intercostal nerve block. (Reprinted from Truitt MS, Murry J, Amos J, et al. Continuous intercostal nerve blockade for rib fractures: ready for primetime? *J Trauma.* 2011;71:1548-1552, with permission from Lippincott Williams & Wilkins.)

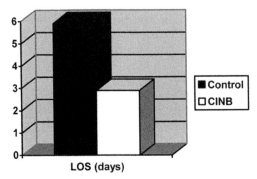

FIGURE 3.—Length of stay in our study population compared to historic control. (Reprinted from Truitt MS, Murry J, Amos J, et al. Continuous intercostal nerve blockade for rib fractures: ready for primetime? *J Trauma.* 2011;71:1548-1552, with permission from Lippincott Williams & Wilkins.)

Conclusion.—Utilization of CINB significantly improved pulmonary function, pain control, and shortens LOS in patients with rib fractures (Figs 1-3).

▶ The placement technique for the intercostal infusions involved a somewhat complicated minor surgical procedure utilizing a tunneling device. Two catheters were placed at the same intercostal level, and each catheter was infused at a rate of 7 mL/h with 0.2% bupivacaine. This is close to the safe upper limit for this drug. It is not clear why 2 catheters were required. It is possible that similar results could be achieved with a simpler technique, such as a single catheter placed through a Tuohy needle.

While this was not a controlled study, the improvement in pain levels and sustained inspiration following implementation of the block was impressive (Figs 1 and 2), and length of stay was reduced compared with historical controls (Fig 3). While this study does not provide evidence for superiority of the technique over epidural analgesia, there are some theoretic advantages, such as avoidance of the risk of epidural hematoma if coagulopathy develops and less likelihood of hypotension.

S. E. Abram, MD

Does Continuous Sciatic Nerve Block Improve Postoperative Analgesia and Early Rehabilitation After Total Knee Arthroplasty? A Prospective, Randomized, Double-Blinded Study
Cappelleri G, Ghisi D, Fanelli A, et al (Azienda Ospedaliera Istituto Ortopedico Gaetano Pini, Milan, Italy; Azienda Ospedaliera di Cremona, Italy; et al)
Reg Anesth Pain Med 36:489-492, 2011

Introduction.—The aim of this prospective, randomized, double-blind study was to evaluate whether continuous sciatic nerve block can improve postoperative pain relief and early rehabilitation compared with single-injection sciatic nerve block in patients undergoing total knee arthroplasty (TKA) and lumbar plexus block.

Methods.—After ethical committee approval and written informed consent, 38 patients with ASA physical status I to II were enrolled. The first group received continuous sciatic and continuous lumbar plexus blocks (group regional or R, n = 19), whereas the second group received a single sciatic nerve block followed by saline infusion through the sciatic catheter and continuous lumbar plexus block (group control or C, n = 19). We assessed morphine consumption, scores for visual analog scale for pain at rest (VASr), and during continuous passive motion (VASi during CPM) for 48 hours postoperatively. Effectiveness of early ambulation was also evaluated.

Results.—Scores for VASr and VASi during CPM, as well as morphine consumption, were significantly higher in group C than in group R (*P* < 0.01). Moreover, patients in group R showed earlier rehabilitation with more effective ambulation (*P* < 0.05).

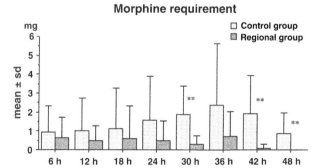

FIGURE 1.—Morphine consumption in the 2 studied groups. Values are shown as mean (SD). **$P < 0.01$. (Reprinted from Cappelleri G, Ghisi D, Fanelli A, et al. Does continuous sciatic nerve block improve postoperative analgesia and early rehabilitation after total knee arthroplasty? A prospective, randomized, double-blinded study. *Reg Anesth Pain Med.* 2011;36:489-492, Copyright 2011, with permission from American Society of Regional Anesthesia and Pain Medicine.)

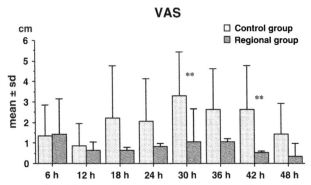

FIGURE 2.—Scores for VASr (0 cm = no pain, 100 mm = worst imaginable pain). Values are shown as mean (SD). **$P < 0.01$. (Reprinted from Cappelleri G, Ghisi D, Fanelli A, et al. Does continuous sciatic nerve block improve postoperative analgesia and early rehabilitation after total knee arthroplasty? A prospective, randomized, double-blinded study. *Reg Anesth Pain Med.* 2011;36:489-492, Copyright 2011, with permission from American Society of Regional Anesthesia and Pain Medicine.)

TABLE 2.—Postoperative Data: VASi Scores (mm) During CPM, Maximum Distance Walked With Walker 48 Hours After Surgery

	Control Group	Regional Group	P
VASi 30 degrees (H8), mean (SD)	10 (12)	10 (12)	NS
VASi 40 degrees (H26), mean (SD)	29 (26)	10 (11)	<0.05
VASi 50 degrees (H32), mean (SD)	38 (30)	7 (14)	<0.01
Maximum knee flexion after 48 h, mean (SD), degrees	60 (12)	102 (10)	<0.01
Ambulation, mean (SD), m	21 (12)	31 (9)	<0.05
Nausea, n (%)	12 (63)	3 (15)	<0.01
Vomiting, n (%)	7 (36)	1 (5)	<0.05

Conclusions.—Continuous sciatic nerve block improves analgesia, decreases morphine request, and improves early rehabilitation compared with single-injection sciatic nerve block in patients undergoing TKA and lumbar plexus block (Figs 1 and 2, Table 2).

▶ This study demonstrates that the addition of a 48-hour continuous sciatic nerve block to a protocol involving continuous lumbar plexus block improves postoperative pain control (Fig 2), reduces morphine consumption (Fig 1), and allows for improved early function (Table 2). The incidence of nausea and vomiting was lower in the sciatic block group as well, presumably because of reduced morphine use. These data confirm that a significant proportion of the nociceptive fibers to the knee joint and surrounding tissues are contained in the sciatic nerve.

S. E. Abram, MD

Effects of pulsed electromagnetic fields on interleukin-1 beta and postoperative pain: a double-blind, placebo-controlled, pilot study in breast reduction patients
Rohde C, Chiang A, Adipoju O, et al (Columbia Univ Med Ctr, NY)
Plast Reconstr Surg 125:1620-1629, 2010

Background.—Surgeons seek new methods of pain control to reduce side effects and speed postoperative recovery. Pulsed electromagnetic fields are effective for bone and wound repair and pain and edema reduction. This study examined whether the effect of pulsed electromagnetic fields on postoperative pain was associated with differences in levels of cytokines and angiogenic factors in the wound bed.

Methods.—In this double-blind, placebo-controlled, randomized study, 24 patients, undergoing breast reduction for symptomatic macromastia received pulsed electromagnetic field therapy configured to modulate the calmodulin-dependent nitric oxide signaling pathway. Pain levels were measured by a visual analogue scale, and narcotic use was recorded. Wound exudates were analyzed for interleukin (IL)-1 beta, tumor necrosis factor-alpha, vascular endothelial growth factor, and fibroblast growth factor-2.

Results.—Pulsed electromagnetic fields produced a 57 percent decrease in mean pain scores at 1 hour ($p < 0.01$) and a 300 percent decrease at 5 hours ($p < 0.001$), persisting to 48 hours postoperatively in the active versus the control group, along with a concomitant 2.2-fold reduction in narcotic use in active patients ($p = 0.002$). Mean IL-1 beta concentration in the wound exudates of treated patients was 275 percent lower ($p < 0.001$). There were no significant differences found for tumor necrosis factor-alpha, vascular endothelial growth factor, or fibroblast growth factor-2 concentrations.

Conclusions.—Pulsed electromagnetic field therapy significantly reduced postoperative pain and narcotic use in the immediate postoperative period. The reduction of IL-1 beta in the wound exudate supports a mechanism that may involve manipulation of the dynamics of endogenous IL-1 beta in the wound bed by means of a pulsed electromagnetic field effect on nitric oxide signaling, which could impact the speed and quality of wound repair.

▶ Pulsed electromagnetic field therapy, which is small changes in electric current, seemed to increased nitric oxide production, decreasing pain, narcotic usage, and edema and speeding healing. Why are we not using this in all patients? It is not clear to me, but this study implies we should be using pulsed electromagnetic field postoperatively and for postoperative pain much more commonly than we are now.

M. F. Roizen, MD

Efficacy and safety of perioperative pregabalin for post-operative pain: a meta-analysis of randomized-controlled trials

Engelman E, Cateloy F (CUB Hopital Erasme, Brussels, Belgium)
Acta Anaesthesiol Scand 55:927-943, 2011

We calculated in a meta-analysis the effect size for the reduction of post-operative pain and post-operative analgesic drugs, which can be obtained by the perioperative administration of pregabalin. Three end-points of efficacy were analysed: early (6 h–7 days) post-operative pain at rest (17 studies) and during movement (seven studies), and the amount of analgesic drugs in the studies that obtained identical results for pain at rest (12 studies). Reported adverse effects were also analysed. The daily dose of pregabalin ranged from 50 to 750 mg/day. The duration of treatment in patients assessed for pain ranged from a single administration to 2 weeks. Pregabalin administration reduced the amount of post-operative analgesic drugs (30.8% of non-overlapping values − odds ratio = 0.43). There was no effect with 150, and 300 or 600 mg/day provided identical results. Pregabalin increased the risk of dizziness or light-headedness and of visual disturbances, and decreased the occurrence of post-operative nausea and vomiting (PONV) in patients who did not receive anti-PONV prophylaxis. The administration of pregabalin during a short perioperative period provides additional analgesia in the short term, but at the cost of additional adverse effects. The lowest effective dose was 225–300 mg/day.

▶ Perioperative administration of pregabalin was associated with modest reduction in postoperative pain scores and with reduction in postoperative analgesic use in studies that failed to show reductions in pain. Although there was some decrease in the incidence of postoperative nausea and vomiting, presumably related to reduced opioid consumption, the overall incidence of side effects was increased. These results do not seem to favor the use of pregabalin over gabapentin, a less expensive drug with more extensive postoperative experience.

S. E. Abram, MD

Efficacy of tramadol versus fentanyl for postoperative analgesia in neonates

de Alencar AJC, Sanudo A, Sampaio VMR, et al (Federal Univ of Ceará, Brazil; Federal Univ of São Paulo, Brazil; Albert Sabin Hosp, Fortaleza, Ceará, Brazil)
Arch Dis Child Fetal Neonatal Ed 97:F24-F29, 2012

Objective.—To assess, in newborn infants submitted to surgical procedures, the efficacy of two opioids—fentanyl and tramadol—regarding time to extubate, time to achieve 100 ml/kg of enteral feeding and pain in the first 72 h after surgery.

Design.—Controlled, blind, randomised clinical trial.

Setting.—Neonatal intensive care unit.

Patients.—160 newborn infants up to 28 days of life requiring major or minor surgeries.

Interventions.—Patients were randomised to receive analgesia with fentanyl (1–2 μg/kg/h intravenously) or tramadol (0.1–0.2 mg/kg/h intravenously) in the first 72 h of the postoperative period, stratified by surgical size and by patient's gender.

Main Outcome Measures.—Pain assessed by validated neonatal scales (Crying, Requires oxygen, Increased vital signs, Expression and Sleepless Scale and the Neonatal Facial Coding System), time until extubation and time to reach 100 ml/kg enteral feeding. Statistical analysis included repeated measures analysis of variance adjusted for confounding variables and Kaplan–Meier curve adjusted by a Cox model of proportional risks.

Results.—Neonatal characteristics were (mean ± SD) birth weight of 2924 ± 702 g, gestational age of 37.6 ± 2.2 weeks and age at surgery of 199 ± 63 h. The main indication of surgery was gastrointestinal malformation (85 newborns; 53%). Neonates who received fentanyl or tramadol were similar regarding time until extubation, time to reach 100 ml/kg of enteral feeding and pain scores in the first 72 h after surgery.

Conclusion.—Tramadol was as effective as fentanyl for postoperative pain relief in neonates but does not appear to offer advantages over fentanyl regarding the duration of mechanical ventilation and time to reach full enteral feeding.

Trial Registration.—NCT00713726.

▶ The efficacy of tramadol for postoperative pain is surprising. Those of us who use oral preparations for treating acute and chronic pain generally observe a much lower initial benefit from tramadol compared with conventional mu opioid agonists. It may be that tramadol is relatively more efficacious in neonates than in adults, or perhaps the intravenous (IV) route of administration offers significant advantage over the oral route. Previous studies of IV tramadol for postoperative pain in adults have shown it to be as effective as conventional opioids. A 2006 study comparing IV patient-controlled analgesia tramadol and morphine for postoperative pain following major surgery showed no difference between the drugs in either pain scores or side effects.[1] Injectable tramadol is not available in the United States. Although there is limited evidence that intravenous tramadol offers substantial benefit over straight mu agonists, there may be individual situations in which it may be a good choice, such as in patients intolerant to conventional opioids or in patients on chronic opioid therapy.

S. E. Abram, MD

Reference

1. Hadi MA, Kamaruljan HS, Saedah A, Abdullah NM. A comparative study of intravenous patient-controlled analgesia morphine and tramadol in patients undergoing major operation. *Med J Malaysia.* 2006;61:570-576.

Is Sciatic Nerve Block Advantageous When Combined With Femoral Nerve Block for Postoperative Analgesia Following Total Knee Arthroplasty?: A Systematic Review

Abdallah FW, Brull R (Univ of Toronto, Ontario, Canada)
Reg Anesth Pain Med 36:493-498, 2011

Sciatic nerve block (SNB) is commonly performed in combination with femoral nerve block (FNB) for postoperative analgesia following total knee arthroplasty (TKA). This systematic review examines the effects of adding SNB to FNB for TKA compared with FNB alone on acute pain and related outcomes. Four intermediate-quality randomized and 3 observational trials, including a total of 391 patients, were identified. Three of 4 trials investigating the addition of single-shot SNB and 2 of 3 trials investigating continuous SNB reported improved early analgesia at rest and reduced early opioid consumption. Only 2 trials specifically assessed posterior knee pain. We were unable to uncover any clinically important analgesic advantages for SNB beyond 24 hours postoperatively. At present, there is inconclusive evidence in the literature to define the effect of adding SNB to FNB on acute pain and related outcomes compared with FNB alone for TKA.

▶ The conclusions of this systematic review are at odds with the findings of a recent, well-designed randomized controlled study that was not considered in the review (it is, however, abstracted in this volume). Meta-analyses and systematic reviews are only as good as the studies they analyze, and the varied quality and methodology of those studies often confound our ability to draw firm conclusions. It is always a good idea to read the well-conducted studies, such as the one cited above, to analyze one's own personal experience and to consider individual patient characteristics when making decisions regarding the choice of regional anesthetic technique.

S. E. Abram, MD

Is Ultrasound Guidance Advantageous for Interventional Pain Management? A Review of Acute Pain Outcomes

Choi S, Brull R (Univ of Toronto, Ontario, Canada)
Anesth Analg 113:596-604, 2011

Background.—Ultrasound (US) guidance for peripheral nerve blockade has gained popularity worldwide. The reported benefits of real-time sonographic visualization compared with traditional nerve localization techniques generally apply to procedural and technical block-related outcomes whereas acute pain—related outcomes are featured less prominently. In this review, we evaluated the effect of US guidance compared with traditional nerve localization techniques for interventional management of acute pain and acute pain—related outcomes.

Methods.—We performed a systematic search of MEDLINE, EMBASE, and the Cochrane Central Register of Controlled Clinical Trials (from January 1990 to January 2011) to identify randomized controlled trials evaluating the effects of US guidance on acute pain and related outcomes compared with traditional nerve localization techniques. Studies were excluded if they did not report at least one of the following acute pain outcomes: pain severity, opioid consumption, sensory block duration, and time to first analgesic request. Related outcomes were classified as follows: patient related (opioid-related adverse effects, patient satisfaction, postoperative cognitive deficit); anesthesia related (unwanted motor block, perineural catheter failure, morbidity, development of chronic pain); surgery related (hospital readmission, ability to ambulate); and hospital related (length of stay, cost). Promising novel applications of US guidance for acute pain management were also sought for discussion purposes.

Results.—We identified 23 randomized controlled trials, including 1674 patients, that compared US guidance with and without peripheral nerve stimulation with peripheral nerve stimulation alone or anatomical landmark techniques. Of the 16 studies that evaluated pain severity, 8 reported improvement with US guidance; however, only 1 study reported a difference between US guidance and the comparator of >1 interval on the numeric rating pain scale. Eight studies evaluated sensory block duration and 3 of these reported prolonged block duration with US guidance. Seven studies evaluated opioid consumption, of which 3 reported a reduction with US guidance. Three studies evaluated time to first analgesic request, of which 2 favored US guidance. We uncovered no significant differences between US guidance and traditional nerve localization techniques for any other related outcome. US guidance was not found to be inferior compared with traditional nerve localization techniques for any outcome. Non-randomized data suggest that US-guided transversus abdominis plane blocks may offer analgesic benefit over standard analgesic therapy, but have not been compared with an anatomical landmark technique.

Conclusions.—At present, there is insufficient evidence in the contemporary literature to define the effect of US guidance on acute pain and related outcomes compared with traditional nerve localization techniques for interventional acute pain management.

▶ For certain nerve blocks and certain clinical conditions, ultrasound guidance offers a clear advantage over other nerve-finding techniques. On the other hand, there are a number of nerve blocks, particularly those targeting superficial nerves or nerves that have a consistent relationship to an easily identified landmark, that can be done quickly and easily without any technological help. The use of ultrasound for such procedures adds unnecessary time and expense. Collection of information regarding the benefit of ultrasound use for specific procedures is a worthwhile endeavor.

S. E. Abram, MD

Thoracic Epidural or Paravertebral Catheter for Analgesia After Lung Resection: Is the Outcome Different?

Elsayed H, McKevith J, McShane J, et al (Liverpool Heart and Chest Hosp, UK)
J Cardiothorac Vasc Anesth 26:78-82, 2012

Objective.—The aim of this study was to determine whether thoracic epidural analgesia (TEA) or a paravertebral catheter block (PVB) with morphine patient-controlled analgesia influenced outcome in patients undergoing thoracotomy for lung resection.

Design.—A retrospective analysis.

Setting.—A tertiary referral center.

Participants.—The study population consisted of 1,592 patients who had undergone thoracotomy for lung resection between May 2000 and April 2008.

Interventions.—Not applicable.

Measurements and Main Results.—Patients who received PVBs were younger, had a higher forced expiratory volume in 1 second, had a higher body mass index, a higher incidence of cardiac comorbidity, fewer pneumonectomies, and more wedge resections. A multivariable logistic regression model was used to develop a propensity-matched score for the probability of patients receiving an epidural or a paravertebral catheter. Four patients with an epidural to one with a paravertebral catheter were matched, with 488 patients and 122 patients, respectively. Postmatching analysis now showed no difference between the groups for preoperative characteristics or operative extent. Postmatching analysis showed no significant difference in outcome between the two groups for the incidence of postoperative respiratory complication ($p = 0.67$), intensive therapy unit (ITU) stay ($p = 0.51$), ITU readmission ($p = 0.66$), or in-hospital mortality ($p = 0.67$). There was a significant reduction in the hospital length of stay in favor of the paravertebral group (6 v 7 days, $p = 0.008$).

Conclusions.—Paravertebral catheter analgesia with morphine patient-controlled analgesia seems as effective as thoracic epidural for reducing the risk of postoperative complications. The authors additionally found that paravertebral catheter use is associated with a shorter hospital stay and may be a better form of analgesia for fast-track thoracic surgery.

▶ Following years of comparisons of these 2 techniques for managing post-thoracotomy pain, it appears that neither technique shows a real advantage. The choice between them should therefore be made on the basis of individual patient characteristics, considering the risks of epidural bleeding and hypotension for epidurals.

S. E. Abram, MD

Transcutaneous spinal direct current stimulation inhibits nociceptive spinal pathway conduction and increases pain tolerance in humans

Truini A, Vergari M, Biasiotta A, et al (Univ "La Sapienza", Rome, Italy; Università di Milano, Italy)

Eur J Pain 15:1023-1027, 2011

Despite concerted efforts from pharmacologic research into neuropathic pain, many patients fail to achieve sufficient pain relief with medication alone. For this reason, increasing interest centres on neurostimulation techniques. We assessed whether transcutaneous spinal direct current stimulation (tsDCS) modulates conduction in ascending nociceptive spinal pathways. We measured changes induced by anodal and cathodal tsDCS over the thoracic spinal cord on face- and foot-laser evoked potentials (LEPs) and foot-cold pressor test responses in 20 healthy subjects. Whereas anodal tsDCS reduced the amplitude of the N1 and N2 components of foot-LEPs ($P < 0.05$) neither anodal nor cathodal tsDCS changed LEPs evoked by face stimulation. Pain tolerance to the cold pressor test was significantly higher after anodal than after cathodal tsDCS ($P < 0.05$). Conversely, no difference was found in the pain threshold or pain ratings to the cold pressor test between the two polarity conditions.

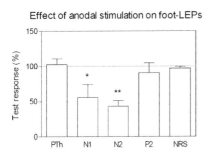

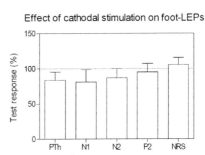

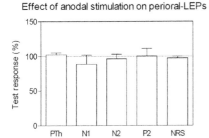

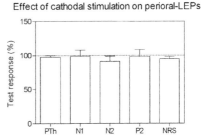

FIGURE 2.—Effects of transcutaneous spinal direct current simulation (tsDCS) on laser-evoked potential (LEP), laser perceptive threshold (PTh) and subjective laser perceptive ratings as assessed by a 11 points numerical rating scale (NRS). Histograms represent the mean ± SE of the conditioned LEP components (amplitude of LEP components after tsDCS expressed as a percentage of those recorded before DC stimulation). $*P = 0.04$; $**P < 0.001$. (Reprinted from Truini A, Vergari M, Biasiotta A, et al. Transcutaneous spinal direct current stimulation inhibits nociceptive spinal pathway conduction and increases pain tolerance in humans. *Eur J Pain.* 2011;15:1023-1027, Copyright 2011, with permission from the European Federation of Chapters of the International Association for the Study of Pain.)

TABLE 2.—Cold Pressor Test Data in the Two Different Polarity Conditions

Cold Pressor Test Data	Anodal Stimulation	Cathodal Stimulation	P
Pain threshold (s)	13.7 ± 3.2	11.6 ± 2.6	0.20
Pain tolerance (s)	83,27 ± 15	54.1 ± 11.5	0.02
Pain ratings (NRS 0–10)	8.3 ± 0.4	9.3 ± 0.8	0.06
Water temperature (°C)	0.4 ± 0.16	0.34 ± 0.14	0.63

Our data suggest that anodal tsDCS over the thoracic spinal cord might impair conduction in the ascending nociceptive spinal pathways, thus modulating LEPs and increasing pain tolerance in healthy subjects (Fig 2, Table 2).

▶ The use of a simple, inexpensive, noninvasive technique to modulate pain perceptions is always intriguing. The study found that anodal stimulation (with the electron source close to the spinal cord) produced reductions in laser-evoked potentials (Fig 2) and increased tolerance to cold-evoked pain (Table 2). In the mid-70s, Sanford Larson[1] found that electrical stimulation across the spinal cord, using anterior and posterior electrodes, produced substantial decreases in somatosensory-evoked potentials, a zone of sensory loss below the level of stimulation, and relief of lower extremity pain caused by malignancy. Such conduction block was much less evident with paired posterior electrodes. The notion that direct current transcutaneous stimulation across the thoracic spinal cord can impair transmission of nociceptive stimulation deserves further study. The use of such a technique to control postoperative pain or cancer pain in opioid-tolerant patients may be a good area of clinical research.

S. E. Abram, MD

Reference

1. Larson SJ, Sances A, Cusick JF, Meyer GA, Swiontek T. A comparison between anterior and posterior spinal implant systems. *Surg Neurol.* 1975;4:180-186.

Uncomplicated Removal of Epidural Catheters in 4365 Patients with International Normalized Ratio Greater Than 1.4 During Initiation of Warfarin Therapy

Liu SS, Buvanendran A, Viscusi ER, et al (Hosp for Special Surgery and the Weill College of Medicine at Cornell Univ, NY; Rush Univ Med Ctr, Chicago, IL; Thomas Jefferson Univ, Philadelphia, PA)
Reg Anesth Pain Med 36:231-235, 2011

Background and Objectives.—Current guidelines from the American Society of Regional Anesthesia state that an international normalized ratio (INR) of 1.4 is the upper limit of warfarin anticoagulation for safe removal of an epidural catheter. However, these guidelines are based

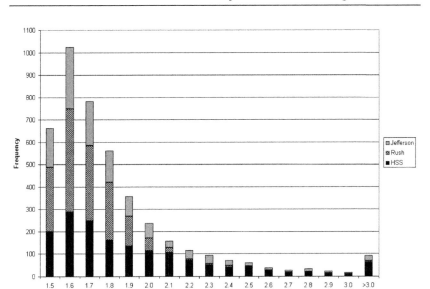

FIGURE 1.—Histogram displaying distribution of international normalized ratio (INR) between institutions at the time of epidural catheter removal. HSS indicates Hospital for Special Surgery; Jefferson, Thomas Jefferson University; Rush, Rush University Medical Center. (Reprinted from Liu SS, Buvanendran A, Viscusi ER, et al. Uncomplicated removal of epidural catheters in 4365 patients with international normalized ratio greater than 1.4 during initiation of warfarin therapy. *Reg Anesth Pain Med.* 2011;36:231-235, Copyright 2011, with permission from American Society of Regional Anesthesia and Pain Medicine.)

primarily on expert consensus, and there is controversy regarding this recommendation as being "too conservative."

Methods.—Prospective (3211) and retrospective (1154) patients undergoing total joint replacement followed by daily warfarin thromboprophylaxis were enrolled in this observational study. All nonsteroidal anti-inflammatory drugs and anticoagulants were held before surgery, and all patients had normal coagulation test results before surgery. Patients were followed twice a day by the acute pain service, no other anticoagulants except nonsteroidal anti-inflammatory drugs were administered, and epidural analgesia was discontinued per institutional protocol. Only patients with INR greater than 1.4 at the time of removal of epidural catheter were included. Neurologic checks were performed for 24 hrs after removal.

Results.—A total of 4365 patients were included, and 79% underwent knee replacement and 18% hip replacement. Mean age was 68 yrs, and mean weight was 81 kg. Mean (SD) duration of epidural analgesia was 2.1 (0.6) days. Mean (SD) INR at the time of epidural removal was 1.9 (0.4), ranging from 1.5 to 7.1. No spinal hematomas were observed (0% incidence with 95% confidence interval, 0%−0.069%).

Conclusions.—Our series of 4365 patients had uncomplicated removal of epidural catheters despite INRs ranging from 1.5 to 5.9. Removal was only during initiation of warfarin therapy (up to approximately 50 hrs after warfarin intake) when several vitamin K factors are likely to still be adequate for hemostasis (Fig 1).

▶ This article helps to fine-tune our understanding of the potential hazards of epidural catheter manipulation during the initiation of warfarin anticoagulation. Catheters were removed in patients with international normalized ratio values ranging from 1.5 to 7.1 with no cases of neurologic injury (see Fig 1). It suggests that there is a wider window of safety that allows a longer period of postoperative epidural analgesia in patients who are being anticoagulated. However, as the authors point out, a high level vigilance is appropriate for patients with these higher values. It should also be emphasized that in all of these patients, catheters were removed during initiation of warfarin therapy. Patients with values in this range during recovery from anticoagulation may be at much higher risk.

S. E. Abram, MD

Cancer Pain Management

A prospective, randomized study of EUS-guided celiac plexus neurolysis for pancreatic cancer: one injection or two?

LeBlanc JK, Al-Haddad M, McHenry L, et al (Indiana Univ Med Ctr/IU Health, Indianapolis; et al)
Gastrointest Endosc 74:1300-1307, 2011

Background.—The technique of alcohol injection during EUS-guided celiac plexus neurolysis (CPN) in patients with pancreatic cancer–related pain has not been standardized.

Objective.—To compare pain relief and safety of alcohol given as 1 versus 2 injections during EUS-guided CPN (EUS-CPN). Secondary outcomes examined were characteristics that predict response and survival.

Design.—Single-blinded, prospective, randomized, parallel-group study.

Setting.—Tertiary-care center.

Patients.—This study involved patients with pancreatic cancer–related pain.

Intervention.—EUS-CPN done by injecting 20 mL of 0.75% bupiva-caine and 10 mL 98% alcohol into 1 or 2 sites at the celiac trunk. Partic-ipants were interviewed by telephone at 24 hours and weekly thereafter.

Main Outcome Measurements.—Time until onset of pain relief, dura-tion of pain relief, complications.

Results.—Fifty patients (mean age 63 years; 24 men) were enrolled and randomized (29 in 1-injection, 21 in 2-injections groups). Pain relief was observed in 37 (74%) patients: 20 (69%) in the 1-injection group and 17 (81%) in the 2-injection group (chi-square $P = .340$). Median onset of pain relief was 1 day for both 1-injection (range 1-28 days) and 2-injection (range 1-21 days) groups (Mann-Whitney $P = .943$). Median duration of pain relief in the 1-injection and 2-injection groups was 11 weeks and 14 weeks, respec-tively (log-rank $P = .612$). Complete pain relief was observed in 4 (8%) patients total, 2 in each group. There were no long-term complications.

Limitations.—Single-blinded study.

Conclusion.—There were no differences in onset or duration of pain relief when either 1 or 2 injections were used. There was no difference in safety or survival between the 2 groups. (Clinical trial registration number: NCT00583479.)

▶ There are many ways to perform neurolytic denervation of the upper abdominal viscera. No matter which technique is used, the overall success rate in most series is around 70%. The reason for some failures may be related to tumor involvement of somatic structures. Denervation of the celiac plexus anterior to the diaphragmatic crura may be unsuccessful if there is substantial tumor or inflammatory tissue encasing the neural structures in the vicinity of the celiac axis. In those cases, splanchnic blocks that denervate visceral afferent fibers adjacent to the anterolateral aspect of the low thoracic vertebral bodies may be more successful. As was the case in this study, opioid dose reduction is not achieved in the majority of cases, and complete pain relief is uncommon.

S. E. Abram, MD

A Strategy for Conversion From Subcutaneous to Oral Ketamine in Cancer Pain Patients: Effect of a 1:1 Ratio

Benítez-Rosario MA, Salinas-Martín A, González-Guillermo T, et al (Univ Hosp La Candelaria, Tenerife, Spain; et al)
J Pain Symptom Manage 41:1098-1105, 2011

Context.—No consensus exists about the most appropriate dose ratio for conversion from parenteral to oral ketamine.

Objectives.—To confirm that a 1:1 dose ratio is suitable for converting subcutaneous (s.c.) to oral ketamine in cancer patients.

Methods.—Patients with opioid poorly responsive cancer pain, who responded to 0.4, 0.6, or 0.8 mg s.c. ketamine bolus, were treated with 0.1, 0.15, or 0.2 mg/kg/h ketamine infusion, respectively. Switching to the oral route, by applying a 1:1 dose ratio, was carried out in patients who experienced adequate pain relief and continued to need ketamine as a coanalgesic. Pain, somnolence, feelings of insobriety, confusion, and cardiovascular parameters were assessed throughout the process.

Results.—Twenty-nine patients were enrolled in the study. Ketamine infusion decreased pain intensity from severe to no pain or slight pain in 23 of 29 and six of 29 patients, respectively. The median of s.c. ketamine doses was 0.2 mg/kg/h (range 0.1–0.5). After oral switching, 27 of 29 patients remained as successfully controlled as when receiving s.c. ketamine. The other two patients needed a slight dose ratio readjustment, to 1:1.3 and 1:1.5, to maintain pain control. The median of oral ketamine doses was 300 mg/day (interquartile range 240–382.5). Seven of 29 patients receiving s.c. ketamine developed moderate and transitory side effects, such as feelings of insobriety and somnolence. No side effects

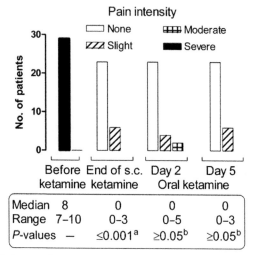

FIGURE 1.—Pain intensity during the conversion from parenteral to oral ketamine. Slight: 1–3/10; moderate: 4–6/10; severe: ≥7/10. The medians and ranges of pain intensity (expressed on a numerical rating scale) and significance levels are in the bottom box. Statistical difference vs. a) "before starting ketamine" and b) "the end of s.c. ketamine" (Friedman-Dunn multiple comparisons test) ($n = 29$ patients). (Reprinted from Benítez-Rosario MA, Salinas-Martín A, González-Guillermo T, et al. A strategy for conversion from subcutaneous to oral ketamine in cancer pain patients: effect of a 1:1 ratio. *J Pain Symptom Manage.* 2011;41:1098-1105, Copyright 2011, with permission from U.S. Cancer Pain Relief Committee.)

TABLE 2.—Subcutaneous Ketamine Dosage Before Switching to the Oral Route

Dose (mg/kg/h)	No. of Patients
0.1	2
0.15	5
0.2	13
0.25	4
0.3	2
0.35	1
0.4	1
0.5	1

were present while receiving oral ketamine. No significant changes were observed in cardiovascular parameters.

Conclusion.—A 1:1 dose ratio for conversion from s.c. to oral ketamine is safe and effective in cancer pain patients (Fig 1, Tables 2 and 4).

▶ There are several appealing aspects to this study. One is the simplicity and lack of technical sophistication involved. All parenteral administrations were subcutaneous. The initial trial involved single subcutaneous injections of 0.4 to 0.8 mg/kg (not milligrams as noted incorrectly in the abstract). Subcutaneous titration determined that a rate of 0.15 to 0.25 mg/kg/h was effective (Table 2) and well tolerated (Table 4) by the majority of the study patients. Likewise,

TABLE 4.—Number of Patients Developing Ketamine Side Effects During Subcutaneous Titration and After the Switch to the Oral Route

Side Effects	Subcutaneous Ketamine	Oral Ketamine
Insobriety level		
None	0	29
Slight	24	0
Moderate	5	0
Severe	0	0
Somnolence		
None	0	29
Slight	25	0
Moderate	4	0
Severe	0	0
Confusion	0	0
Hallucinations	1	0

See description of symptom score evaluation under *Data Collection*.

most patients continued to obtain relief from oral doses of around 300 mg/d given in 3 equally divided doses (Fig 1). Other studies have indicated tremendous variability in the parenteral to oral equivalency ratios (1:0.3–1:8.5).[1]

When ketamine is given orally, there is probably more rapid conversion to norketamine, an active metablolite through first-pass metabolism. The authors point out that norketamine has less affinity for the N-methyl-d-aspartate (NMDA) receptor, so it is likely that much of ketamine's pain-relieving effect in patients with cancer pain is through mechanisms other than NMDA receptor antagonism.

Opioid doses were maintained at preketamine levels during this study.

S. E. Abram, MD

Reference

1. Blonk MI, Koder BG, Van den Bemt PMLA, Huygen FJPM. Use of oral ketamine in chronic pain management: a review. *Eur J Pain*. 2010;14:466-472.

How to switch from morphine or oxycodone to methadone in cancer patients? A randomised clinical phase II trial

Moksnes K, Dale O, Rosland JH, et al (Norwegian Univ of Science and Technology (NTNU), Trondheim, Norway; Haraldsplass Deaconess Hosp, Bergen, Norway)
Eur J Cancer 47:2463-2470, 2011

Aim.—Opioid switching is a treatment strategy in cancer patients with unacceptable pain and/or adverse effects (AEs). We investigated whether patients switched to methadone by the stop and go (SAG) strategy have lower pain intensity (PI) than the patients switched over three days (3DS), and whether the SAG strategy is as safe as the 3DS strategy.

TABLE 1.—Dose Dependent Switching Table and Distribution of Patients in Each Dose Group, $n = 35$

Baseline Morphine Dose (mg)	Protocol Ratio Mo:Me[a]	Final Ratio[b] Mo:Me Mean (Min—Max)	N Stop and go/3-Days Switch
30–90	4:1		0/0
91–300	6:1	4:1 (3.3–4.7)	1/1
301–600	8:1	7.5:1 (4.4–10)	4/4
601–1000	10:1	11.7:1 (7.1–17.3)	5/3
>1000	12:1	14.2:1 (8.6–26.7)	6/11

[a]Mo = morphine, Me = methadone.
[b]Baseline Mo:Me day 14.

Methods.—In this prospective, open, parallel-group, multicentre study, 42 cancer patients on morphine or oxycodone were randomised to the SAG or 3DS switching-strategy to methadone. The methadone dose was calculated using a dose-dependent ratio. PI, AEs and serious adverse events (SAEs) were recorded daily for 14 days. Primary outcome was average PI day 3. Secondary outcomes were PI now and AEs day 3 and 14 and number of SAEs.

Results.—Twenty-one patients were randomised to each group, 16 (SAG) and 19 (3DS) patients received methadone. The mean preswitch morphine doses were 900 mg/day in SAG and 1330 mg/day in 3DS. No differences between groups were found in mean average PI day 3 (mean difference 0.5 (CI −1.2–2.2); SAG 4.1 (CI 2.3–5.9) and 3DS 3.6 (CI 2.9–4.3) or in PI now. The SAG group had more dropouts and three SAEs (two deaths and one severe sedation). No SAEs were observed in the 3DS group.

Conclusion.—The SAG patients reported a trend of more pain, had significantly more dropouts and three SAEs, which indicate that the SAG strategy should not replace the 3DS when switching from high doses of morphine or oxycodone to methadone (Table 1).

▶ A standard strategy for changing to methadone from other oral opioids is the "3-days switch" (3DS) method, which involves reducing the original opioid dose by one-third and substituting one-third the equianalgesic dose of methadone each day over a 3-day period. For the "stop and go" strategy, the current opioid is immediately replaced by methadone. For both strategies, a dose-dependent dose equivalency, in which higher morphine/methadone ratios are used for higher doses, was utilized (Table 1). The actual ratios achieved after titration are also shown in Table 1.

As the authors point out, methadone is commonly selected as a secondary opioid choice. It has high oral bioavailability and no active or toxic metabolites, and its elimination is fairly independent of renal function. Low cost compared with sustained release and transdermal opioids, the other choices for long-acting drugs, is another advantage. A major disadvantage of methadone is the dose-related potential for ventricular arrhythmias, with the risk increasing at doses exceeding 200 mg/d. Q-T intervals should be followed on electrocardiogram at higher doses.

S. E. Abram, MD

Intrathecal combination of ziconotide and morphine for refractory cancer pain: A rapidly acting and effective choice

Alicino I, Giglio M, Manca F, et al (Univ of Bari, Italy)
Pain 153:245-249, 2012

Ziconotide is a nonopioid intrathecal analgesic drug used to manage moderate to severe chronic pain. The aim of this work is to assess the safety and efficacy of intrathecal (IT) combination of ziconotide and morphine in malignant pain refractory to high doses of oral opioids. Patients with malignant pain refractory to high oral opioids doses with a mean visual analogue scale of pain intensity (VASPI) score of ≥70 mm were enrolled. An IT combination therapy was administered: Ziconotide was started at a dose of 2.4 µg/day, followed by increases of 1.2 µg/day at intervals of at least 7 days, and an initial IT daily dose of morphine was calculated based on its oral daily dose. Percentage change in VASPI scores from baseline was calculated at 2 days, at 7 days, and weekly until the first 28 days. The mean percentage change of VASPI score from baseline was used for efficacy assessment. Safety was monitored based on adverse events and routine laboratory values. Twenty patients were enrolled, with a mean daily VASPI score at rest of 90 ± 7. All had a disseminated cancer with bone metastases involving the spine. The percentage changes in VASPI mean scores from baseline to 2 days, 7 days, and 28 days were 39 ± 13% (95% confidence interval [CI] = 13.61−64.49, $P < .001$), 51 ± 12% (95% CI = 27.56−74.56, $P < .001$), and 62 ± 13% (95% CI = 36.03−87.89%, $P < .001$), respectively. Four patients experienced mild adverse events related to the study drugs. In conclusion, an IT combination of low doses of ziconotide and morphine allows safe and rapid control of oral opioid−refractory malignant pain (Fig 1).

▶ The ability to rapidly control severe pain in patients with terminal cancer is essential, given the short remaining life span of these patients, and the results

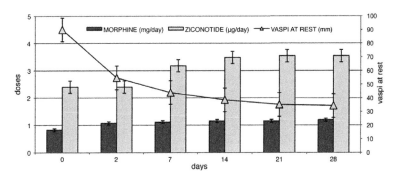

FIGURE 1.—Mean visual analogue scale of pain intensity (VASPI) score and mean doses of morphine (mg/day, filled bars) and ziconotide (µg/day, open bars) among patients at baseline, after 2 days, and weekly during treatment. (Reprinted from Alicino I, Giglio M, Manca F, et al. Intrathecal combination of ziconotide and morphine for refractory cancer pain: a rapidly acting and effective choice. *Pain.* 2012;153:245-249, with permission from International Association for the Study of Pain.)

demonstrated in this study are impressive (Fig 1). The extremely high cost of ziconotide was offset in some of the patients by the use of percutaneous rather than implanted systems in patients with shorter life spans. However, infusion drugs need to be changed frequently because of the degradation of ziconotide when combined with opioids. External intrathecal infusion systems, while more cumbersome than implanted systems, are safe for use over several months and can markedly improve quality of life for patients totally immobilized by pain.

It is not known whether these patients could have experienced expeditious pain control with rapid titration of opioids alone or with opioids combined with other drugs, such as bupivacaine, clonidine, or baclofen. The study does, however, provide a rationale for the initiation of an opioid-ziconotide combination for patients with cancer who fail to respond promptly to intrathecal opioids alone.

S. E. Abram, MD

Preventive or late administration of anti-NGF therapy attenuates tumor-induced nerve sprouting, neuroma formation, and cancer pain

Jimenez-Andrade JM, Ghilardi JR, Castañeda-Corral G, et al (Univ of Arizona, Tucson; VA Med Ctr, Minneapolis, MN)
Pain 152:2564-2574, 2011

Early, preemptive blockade of nerve growth factor (NGF)/tropomyosin receptor kinase A (TrkA) attenuates tumor-induced nerve sprouting and bone cancer pain. A critical unanswered question is whether late blockade of NGF/TrkA can attenuate cancer pain once NGF-induced nerve sprouting and neuroma formation has occurred. By means of a mouse model of

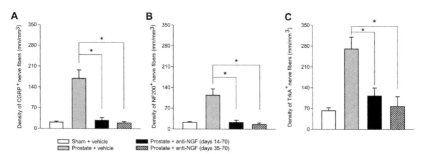

FIGURE 7.—Histograms showing that sustained administration of NGF sequestering therapy, provided either early or late in disease progression, reduces prostate-induced nerve sprouting of CGRP+, NF200+, and TrkA+ nerve fibers. At day 70 after cell injection, the density of CGRP+ (A), NF200+ (B), and TrkA+ (C) nerve fibers is significantly greater in prostate + vehicle-treated mice compared to sham-treated + vehicle-treated mice. At day 70 after tumor injection, tumor-induced nerve sprouting is significantly attenuated by preemptive/sustained administration or anti-NGF (10 mg/kg; i.p.; provided from day 14 to day 70 after cell injection) or by late/sustained administration of anti-NGF (10 mg/kg; i.p., provided from day 35 to day 70 after cell injection). Nerve fiber density was determined by measuring the total length of nerve fibers in areas where viable cancer cells were present. Brackets indicate the groups being compared. *$P < .05$. Bars represent the mean ± SEM for at minimum 6 mice. (Reprinted from Jimenez-Andrade JM, Ghilardi JR, Castañeda-Corral G, et al. Preventive or late administration of anti-NGF therapy attenuates tumor-induced nerve sprouting, neuroma formation, and cancer pain. *Pain.* 2011;152:2564-2574, with permission from International Association for the Study of Pain.)

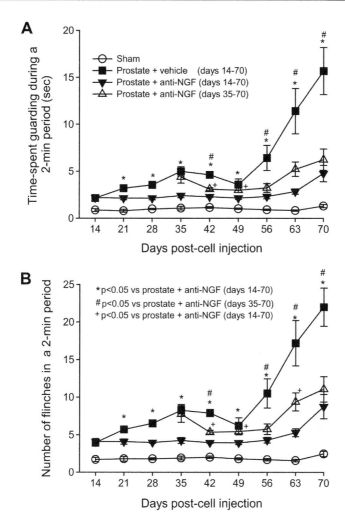

FIGURE 8.—Anti-NGF treatment, when provided early or late in disease progression, attenuates prostate cancer-induced nociceptive behaviors. Nociceptive behaviors including spontaneous guarding (A) and flinching (B) recorded in sham-treated mice (needle placement + injection of culture medium), prostate cancer-bearing mice treated with vehicle, prostate cancer-bearing mice treated preemptively with anti-NGF (from days 14 to 70 after cell injection), and prostate cancer-bearing mice treated late with anti-NGF (from days 35 to 70 after cell injection). Note that nociceptive behaviors in tumor-bearing mice are evident by day 14 after cell injection and are significantly greater than sham-treated mice at all time points shown. Preemptive sustained treatment with anti-NGF commenced at day 14 after tumor cell injection significantly decreased nociceptive behaviors. Importantly, late sustained treatment with anti-NGF commenced at day 35 after tumor injection (when robust sprouting in the parent cell colonies has already occurred) also decreased the nociceptive behaviors. Anti-NGF was provided every 5 days (10 mg/kg, i.p.); each point represents mean ± SEM. (Reprinted from Jimenez-Andrade JM, Ghilardi JR, Castañeda-Corral G, et al. Preventive or late administration of anti-NGF therapy attenuates tumor-induced nerve sprouting, neuroma formation, and cancer pain. *Pain.* 2011;152:2564-2574, with permission from International Association for the Study of Pain.)

prostate cancer-induced bone pain, anti-NGF was either administered preemptively at day 14 after tumor injection when nerve sprouting had yet to occur, or late at day 35, when extensive nerve sprouting had occurred. Animals were humanely killed at day 70 when, in vehicle-treated animals, significant nerve sprouting and neuroma formation was present in the tumor-bearing bone. Although preemptive and sustained administration (days 14–70) of anti-NGF more rapidly attenuated bone cancer nociceptive behaviors than late and sustained administration (days 35–70), by day 70 after tumor injection, both preemptive and late administration of anti-NGF significantly reduced nociceptive behaviors, sensory and sympathetic nerve sprouting, and neuroma formation. In this model, as in most cancers, the individual cancer cell colonies have a limited half-life because they are constantly proliferating, metastasizing, and undergoing necrosis as the parent cancer cell colony outgrows its blood supply. Similarly, the sensory and sympathetic nerve fibers that innervate the tumor undergo sprouting at the viable/leading edge of the parent tumor, degenerate as the parent cancer cell colony becomes necrotic, and resprout in the viable, newly formed daughter cell colonies. These results suggest that preemptive or late-stage blockade of NGF/TrkA can attenuate nerve sprouting and cancer pain (Figs 7 and 8).

▶ Tumor-induced remodeling of nerve fibers occurs rapidly (within days) following the onset of bone cancer in experimental animals. Nerve sprouting and neuroma formation and cancer pain are in part driven by nerve growth factor (NGF) activation of $TrkA^+$ nerve fibers. The authors were concerned that blockade of NGF might only be effective if begun early in the course of the cancer, in which case clinical benefits of such therapy in humans would be limited. What they discovered in this study was that the process of nerve sprouting and sensitization continues as the cancer progresses. Their finding was that late treatment with blockade of NGF/TrkA attenuated the nerve sprouting process (Fig 7) and, importantly, reduced nociceptive pain behaviors (Fig 8). These findings could have important implications for treating cancer pain associated with a wide variety of cancer types. Hopefully, such therapies will provide effective cancer pain control without the side effects and complications associated with opioids, anticonvulsants, neurolytic blocks, and radiation.

S. E. Abram, MD

Prospective Evaluation of Laparoscopic Celiac Plexus Block in Patients with Unresectable Pancreatic Adenocarcinoma
Allen PJ, Chou J, Janakos M, et al (Memorial Sloan-Kettering Cancer Ctr, NY)
Ann Surg Oncol 18:636-641, 2011

Introduction.—The efficacy of laparoscopic celiac plexus block (CPB) in patients with unresectable pancreatic cancer has not been reported.

Methods.—Patients with elevated pain scores scheduled for laparoscopy for diagnosis/staging of unresectable pancreatic adenocarcinoma were eligible. The study was designed to evaluate 20 consecutive patients with validated quality of life (EORTC QLQ-C30, QLQ-PAN26) and validated pain assessment tools [Brief Pain Inventory (BPI)]. Questionnaires were obtained preoperatively, and postoperatively at 1, 4, and 8 weeks. Laparoscopic CPB was performed by bilateral injection of 20 cc 50% alcohol utilizing a recently described laparoscopic technique. Functional and symptom scoring was performed by EORTC scoring manual.

Results.—Median age was 61 years (range 42—80 years), and mean preoperative pain score [worst in 24 h on 0—10 visual analogue scale (VAS)] was 7.8 [standard deviation (SD) 1.6]. Median total operative time (laparoscopy + biopsy + CBP) was 57 min (range 29—92 min), and all patients except one were discharged on day of surgery. No major complications occurred. EORTC functional scales did not change significantly during the postoperative period. EORTC symptomatic pain scores decreased significantly. These findings were also observed in the BPI, with significant decreases in visual analogue score for reported mean (preoperative versus week 4, mean: 5.7 versus 2.7; $p < 0.01$) and worst (preoperative versus week 4, mean: 7.8 versus 5.1; $p < 0.01$) pain during a 24-h period.

Conclusions.—This study documents the efficacy of laparoscopic CPB. The procedure was associated with minimal morbidity, brief operative times, outpatient management, and reduction in pain scores similar to that reported with other approaches to celiac neurolysis (Figs 2 and 3, Table 3).

▶ At first glance, this study suggests that early treatment with neurolytic celiac plexus block is associated with reduced pain levels during the following 2 months (Table 3, Figs 2 and 3). While pain levels decreased, opioid use remained unchanged.

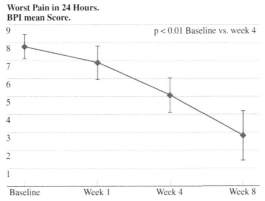

FIGURE 2.—Mean visual analogue scores (±SD) for Brief Pain Inventory question evaluating "worst pain in 24 h." (Reprinted from Allen PJ, Chou J, Janakos M, et al. Prospective evaluation of laparoscopic celiac plexus block in patients with unresectable pancreatic adenocarcinoma. *Ann Surg Oncol.* 2011;18: 636-641, with kind permission from Springer Science+Business Media: Annals of Surgical Oncology.)

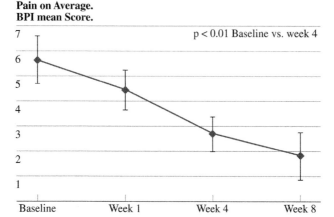

Pain on Average.
BPI mean Score.

p < 0.01 Baseline vs. week 4

FIGURE 3.—Mean visual analogue scores (±SD) for Brief Pain Inventory question evaluating "pain on average." (Reprinted from Allen PJ, Chou J, Janakos M, et al. Prospective evaluation of laparoscopic celiac plexus block in patients with unresectable pancreatic adenocarcinoma. *Ann Surg Oncol.* 2011;18: 636-641, with kind permission from Springer Science+Business Media: Annals of Surgical Oncology.)

TABLE 3.—Pain Severity Scores (BPI) for the 20 Patients Who Underwent Laparoscopic CPB

BPI	Preoperative (n = 20) Mean	SD	Week 1 (n = 20) Mean	SD	Week 4 (n = 20) Mean	SD	Baseline−Week 4 p
Worst (24 h)	7.8	1.6	6.9	2.1	5.1	2.2	<0.01
Least (24 h)	3.7	2.8	2.1	2.1	1.4	1.7	<0.01
Average	5.7	2.2	4.5	1.9	2.7	1.6	<0.01
Right now	5.3	2.4	3.3	2.4	1.9	1.9	<0.01

Comparison of means made between preoperative and postoperative week 4 time points.

There are several problems with this study that make it difficult to conclude that the block produced ongoing pain relief, not the least of which is the lack of blinding and controls. Pain levels in these continued to decline over the 8-week study period, which would not be expected following a single neurolytic block. Much of the pain reduction might be attributed to chemotherapy (received by 100% of patients) or radiation (received by 20%).

My own experience has been that splanchnic, or retrocrural, neurolytic blockade is a more effective technique than injection around the celiac plexus itself. That conclusion is based in part on the success of splanchnic blocks following failed transcrural injections. Given the high success rates with percutaneous splanchnic or combined splanchnic/celiac plexus blocks (about 70% in our recent unpublished series), it might be more reasonable to perform neurolytic blocks early for those patients with particularly severe pain and watch responses to chemotherapy and radiation therapy initially for patients with pain that is fairly well controlled with opioids.

S. E. Abram, MD

Chronic Pain Management

A Modified Microsurgical DREZotomy Procedure for Refractory Neuropathic Pain

Chun H-J, Kim YS, Yi H-J (Hanyang Univ Med Ctr, Seoul, Korea)
World Neurosurg 75:551-557, 2011

Objective.—Control of neuropathic pain secondary to spinal cord injury is difficult; microsurgical DREZotomy (MDT) is the currently preferred treatment modality. According to previous reports, traditional MDT has poor outcomes when addressing diffuse (infralesional), thermal, and continuous pain. Here, we report improvements in surgical outcomes in these neuropathic pain conditions using a modified MDT technique.

Methods.—Patients with segmental, mechanical, or intermittent pain underwent MDT using the traditional (Sindou's) technique performed at the indicated cord level based on pain distribution. Patients suffering from diffuse, thermal, or continuous pain underwent a modified MDT procedure in the "lump" and "irritative" zones, as well as another procedure, whereby an attempt was made to cut every injured and fused rootlet.

Results.—In 38 patients with paraplegic pain resulting from a spinal cord injury occurring within the preceding 7 years, 11 of 15 patients (73%) with a diffuse pain distribution had a good reduction in pain. Thirteen patients (86%) with continuous pain noted good pain relief. In patients with thermal pain, only one patient (20%) demonstrated a good response to the investigational procedure.

TABLE 4.—Results of Advanced Microsurgical DREZotomy According to Pain Characteristics

| | Surgical Outcome (%) | | | |
	Good	Fair	Poor	Total
Topography				
Segmental	19 (82.6%)	2 (8.7%)	2 (8.7%)	23
Diffuse	11 (73.3%)	2 (13.3%)	2 (13.3%)	15
Total	30 (78.9%)	4 (10.5%)	4 (10.5%)	38
Nature				
Mechanical	19 (82.6%)	2 (8.7%)	2 (8.7%)	23
Thermal	1 (20%)	2 (40%)	2 (40%)	5
Combined	10 (100%)	0	0	10
Total	30	4	4	38
Frequency				
Intermittent	18 (78.2%)	2 (8.6%)	3 (13.0%)	23
Continuous	12 (80.0%)	2 (13.3%)	1 (6.7%)	15
Total	30	4	4	38

DREZ, dorsal root entry zone.

Conclusion.—These procedures, including the modified MDT technique, may be helpful in controlling paraplegic pain in patients suffering from diffuse, thermal, or continuous pain (Table 4).

▶ Pain associated with spinal cord injury is notoriously difficult to treat. "At-level" pain is likely to improve following dorsal root entry zone lesions performed at and immediately above the level of injury. Diffuse, constant, "below-level" pain is generally considered unresponsive to this surgical intervention. The authors present a modified approach to neuroablation for patients with diffuse, constant, and thermal pain that involves more extensive resection of nerve rootlets, even if they feed into uninjured portions of the spinal cord. Their success rate was impressive with the exception of those patients with solely thermal pain (see Table 4).

S. E. Abram, MD

A Peripherally Acting Na$_v$1.7 Sodium Channel Blocker Reverses Hyperalgesia and Allodynia on Rat Models of Inflammatory and Neuropathic Pain
McGowan E, Hoyt SB, Li X, et al (Dept of Pharmacology and Medicinal Chemistry, Rahway, NJ)
Anesth Analg 109:951-958, 2009

Background.—Voltage-gated sodium channels (Na$_v$1) are expressed in primary sensory neurons where they influence excitability via their role in the generation and propagation of action potentials. Recently, human genetic data have shown that one sodium channel subtype, Na$_v$1.7, plays a major role in pain. We performed these studies to characterize the antinociceptive effects of N-[(R)-1-((R)-7-chloro-1-isopropyl-2-oxo-2,3,4,5-tetrahydro-1H-benzo[b]azepin- 3-ylcarbamoyl)-2-(2- fluorophenyl)-ethyl]-4-fluoro-2-trifluoromethyl-benzamide (BZP), a non-central nervous system (CNS) penetrant small molecule with high affinity and preferential selectivity for Na$_v$1.7 over Na$_v$1.8 and Na$_v$1.5.

Methods.—BZP was evaluated in rat preclinical models of inflammatory and neuropathic pain and compared with standard analgesics. Two models were used: the complete Freund's adjuvant model of inflammatory pain and the spinal nerve ligation model of neuropathic pain. BZP was also evaluated in a motor coordination assay to assess its propensity for CNS side effects.

Results.—In preclinical models of chronic pain, BZP displayed efficacy comparable with that of leading analgesics. In the complete Freund's adjuvant model, BZP produced reversal of hyperalgesia comparable with nonsteroidal antiinflammatory drugs, and in the spinal nerve ligation model, BZP produced reversal of allodynia comparable with gabapentin and mexiletine. Unlike the CNS penetrant compounds gabapentin and mexiletine, BZP did not induce any impairment of motor coordination.

Conclusions.—These data suggest that a peripherally acting sodium channel blocker, preferentially acting through Na$_v$1.7, could provide clinical relief of chronic pain without the CNS side effects typical of many existing pain treatments.

▶ Years of research have been carried out in the search for sodium channel blockers that selectively block channels that are specific to pain perception and/or are upregulated in neuropathic pain states. Lidocaine is a fairly nonspecific sodium channel blocker that is effective in a number of painful conditions, but it is relatively ineffective orally (one-pass metabolism to a toxic metabolite, MEGX), and it has a narrow therapeutic index and significant central nervous system (CNS) side effects. Mexiletine, which is available as an oral preparation, is also nonspecific, is rarely effective for neuropathic pain, and has a high incidence of intolerable side effects. Several anticonvulsants have sodium blocking effects (topiramate, carbamazepine, oxcarbazepine, lamotrigine), but their effects are also nonspecific and can produce significant central effects. NAV1.3 is upregulated in certain neuropathic pain states, whereas NAV1.7 produces a painful disorder when genetically overexpressed (erythromelalgia) and insensitivity to pain when underexpressed. This study showed that a peripherally acting NAV1.7 blocker, BZP reversed hyperalgesia associated with inflammatory and neuropathic pain without significant CNS effects in rats. If such a drug provides similar benefits clinically, it could be extremely useful in managing both acute and chronic pain states.

S. E. Abram, MD

A Randomized, Controlled, Double-Blind Trial of Fluoroscopic Caudal Epidural Injections in the Treatment of Lumbar Disc Herniation and Radiculitis

Manchikanti L, Singh V, Cash KA, et al (Pain Management Ctr of Paducah, KY; Pain Diagnostics Associates, Niagara, WI; et al)
Spine 36:1897-1905, 2011

Study Design.—A randomized, controlled, double-blind trial.

Objective.—To assess the effectiveness of fluoroscopically directed caudal epidural injections in managing chronic low back and lower extremity pain in patients with disc herniation and radiculitis with local anesthetic with or without steroids.

Summary of Background Data.—The available literature on the effectiveness of epidural injections in managing chronic low back pain secondary to disc herniation is highly variable.

Methods.—One hundred twenty patients suffering with low back and lower extremity pain with disc herniation and radiculitis were randomized to one of the two groups: group I received caudal epidural injections with an injection of local anesthetic, lidocaine 0.5%, 10 mL; group II patients received caudal epidural injections with 0.5% lidocaine, 9 mL, mixed with 1 mL of steroid.

The Numeric Rating Scale (NRS), the Oswestry Disability Index 2.0 (ODI), employment status, and opioid intake were utilized with assessment at 3, 6, and 12 months posttreatment.

TABLE 1.—Baseline Demographic Characteristics

	Group 1 (60)	Group II (60)	P
Sex			
Men	32% (19)	38% (23)	0.566
Women	68% (41)	62% (37)	
Age, mean ± SD	48.7 ± 14.1	43.0 ± 14.5	0.031
Weight, mean ± SD	208.3 ± 53.9	177.5 ± 46.8	0.001
Height, mean ± SD	66.2 ± 3.5	66.6 ± 4.0	0.580
Duration of pain (mo), mean ± SD	93.4 ± 86.9	81.3 ± 81.7	0.436
Onset of pain			
Gradual	72% (43)	52% (31)	0.034
Injury	28% (17)	48% (29)	
Low back pain distribution			
Bilateral	75% (45)	67% (40)	0.422
Left or right	25% (15)	33% (20)	
Numeric Rating Score Mean ± SD	8.1 ± 0.9	7.8 ± 0.9	0.077
Oswestry Disability Index Mean ± SD	29.2 ± 4.6	27.9 ± 4.8	0.158
Disc herniation (levels)*			
L3/L4	8% (5)	5% (3)	NS
L4/L5	67% (40)	70% (42)	
L5/S1	58% (35)	50% (30)	

*Multiple patients presented with disc herniation at more than one level.

Results.—The percentage of patients with significant pain relief of 50% or greater and/or improvement in functional status with 50% or more reduction in ODI scores was seen in 70% and 67% in group I and 77% and 75% in group II with average procedures per year of 3.8 ± 1.4 in group I and 3.6 + 1.1 in group II. However, the relief with first and second procedures was significantly higher in the steroid group. The number of injections performed was also higher in local anesthetic group even though overall relief was without any significant difference among the groups. There was no difference among the patients receiving steroids.

Conclusion.—Caudal epidural injection with local anesthetic with or without steroids might be effective in patients with disc herniation or radiculitis. The present evidence illustrates potential superiority of steroids compared with local anesthetic at 1-year follow-up (Tables 1-3).

▶ This study differs from most previous trials of epidural injections for low back/leg pain in that it evaluates the benefit of repeated procedures for patients with very chronic pain (mean duration > 7 years, see Table 1). The randomized controlled trial compared protocols that provided multiple injections per year containing either local anesthetic alone or local anesthetic plus steroid. Patients received on average more than 3 procedures per year in each group. The steroid group experienced slightly better pain reduction with the initial 2 procedures; otherwise there was little difference in benefit (see Tables 2 and 3).

There are several obvious deficiencies of this study. First, and perhaps the most concerning, is that the authors did not identify the patients in each group who exhibited radicular versus axial pain. Nearly every previous study has noted a much higher success in patients with true radicular pain. Second, the caudal

TABLE 2.—Pain Relief Characteristics

Numeric Rating Score	Group I (60) (Mean ± SD)	Group II (60) (Mean ± SD)	P (Between Group I and Group II)
Baseline	8.1 ± 0.9	7.8 ± 0.9	0.077
3 mo	4.1* ± 1.8	3.4* ± 1.7	0.022
6 mo	3.9* ± 1.8	3.5* ± 1.7	0.206
12 mo	4.1* ± 1.8	3.5* ± 1.9	0.058

*Significant difference with baseline values within the Group (P < 0.001).

TABLE 3.—Functional Assessment Evaluated by Oswestry Disability Index

Oswestry Disability Index	Group I (60) (Mean ± SD)	Group II (60) (Mean ± SD)	P (Between Group I and Group II)
Baseline	29.2 ± 4.6	27.9 ± 4.8	0.158
3 mo	16.5* ± 7.2	13.6* ± 6.5	0.023
6 mo	15.5* ± 7.3	13.7* ± 7.0	0.167
12 mo	15.5* ± 7.74	13.1* ± 7.0	0.073

*Significant difference with baseline values within the Group (P < 0.001).

route may not provide the best opportunity for steroids to have an effect, because very little of the steroid reaches the affected nerve root(s) given the distance from the injection site and the high dilution. A better assessment of steroid effect might be seen with deposition of the drug in higher concentrations and lower volumes close to the affected root. Again, a higher steroid efficacy might be seen if the patient selection were confined to patients with radicular pain. The last concern is that multiple steroid preparations were used.

Most physicians (and most insurance carriers) are convinced that epidural steroid injections provide at least transient relief for patients with radicular pain. Studies that allow practitioners to target those patients most likely to benefit are still needed.

S. E. Abram, MD

Absence of long-term analgesic effect from a short-term S-ketamine infusion on fibromyalgia pain: A randomized, prospective, double blind, active placebo-controlled trial

Noppers I, Niesters M, Swartjes M, et al (Leiden Univ Med Ctr, The Netherlands)
Eur J Pain 15:942-949, 2011

To assess the analgesic efficacy of the N-methyl-D-aspartate receptor antagonist S(+)-ketamine on fibromyalgia pain, the authors performed a randomized double blind, active placebo-controlled trial. Twenty-four fibromyalgia patients were randomized to receive a 30-min intravenous infusion with

S(+)-ketamine (total dose 0.5 mg/kg, $n = 12$) or the active placebo, midazolam (5 mg, $n = 12$). Visual Analogue Pain Scores (VAS) and ketamine plasma samples were obtained for 2.5-h following termination of treatment; pain scores derived from the fibromyalgia impact questionnaire (FIQ) were collected weekly during an 8-week follow-up. Fifteen min after termination of infusion the number of patients showing a reduction in pain scores >50% was 8 vs. 3 ($P < 0.05$), at $t = 180$ min 6 vs. 2 (ns), at the end of week-1 2 vs. 0 (ns) and at end of week-8 2 vs. 2 in the ketamine and midazolam groups, respectively. Ketamine effect on VAS closely followed ketamine plasma concentrations. For VAS and FIQ scores no significant differences in treatment effects were observed in the 2.5-h following infusion or during the 8-week follow-up. Side effects as measured by the Bowdle questionnaire (which scores for 13 separate psychedelic symptoms) were mild to moderate in both study groups and declined rapidly, indicating adequate blinding of treatments. Efficacy of ketamine was limited and restricted in duration to its pharmacokinetics. The authors argue that a short-term infusion of ketamine is insufficient to induce long-term analgesic effects in fibromyalgia patients (Figs 2-4).

▶ The administration of ketamine at subdissociative doses provides reliable analgesia for a variety of painful conditions while maintaining plasma levels within a target range. There is much less evidence that the drug provides pain reduction for prolonged periods following its administration, as was originally hoped. This study demonstrates acute reduction of clinical pain in fibromyalgia patients as well as reduction in experimental heat pain that correspond to ketamine plasma levels (see Figs 2 and 4). However, as seen in Fig 3, the reduction in clinical pain does not continue beyond the day of treatment.

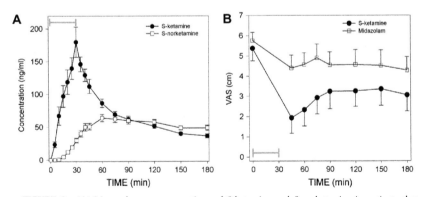

FIGURE 2.—(A) Mean plasma concentrations of S-ketamine and S-norketamine in patients that received a 30-min S-ketamine infusion (gray bar). (B) Effect of a 30-min treatment with S-ketamine (0.5 mg/kg, closed circles, $n = 12$) and midazolam (5 mg, open squares, $n = 12$) on pain scores in fibromyalgia patients. No significant differences in pain relief between the two treatment was observed during the treatment recovery phase ($t = 45$ to $t = 180$ min). The gray bar indicates the treatment period. Data are mean ± SEM. (Reprinted from Noppers I, Niesters M, Swartjes M, et al. Absence of long-term analgesic effect from a short-term S-ketamine infusion on fibromyalgia pain: a randomized, prospective, double blind, active placebo-controlled trial. *Eur J Pain.* 2011;15:942-949, Copyright 2011, with permission from European Federation of International Association for the Study of Pain Chapters.)

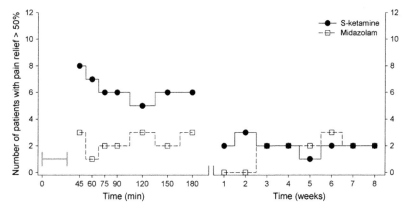

FIGURE 3.—Number of fibromyalgia patients with pain relief >50%. Left graph: Data derived from the assessment of spontaneous fibromyalgia pain following treatment ($t = 45–180$ min following the 30-min treatment period). Right graph: Data derived from the weekly fibromyalgia impact questionnaires, which assess the mean pain score over the previous week. A difference in number of patients that had a pain score >50% was significant at time $t = 45$ and $t = 60$ min only. The gray bar indicates the treatment period. (Reprinted from Noppers I, Niesters M, Swartjes M, et al. Absence of long-term analgesic effect from a short-term S-ketamine infusion on fibromyalgia pain: a randomized, prospective, double blind, active placebo-controlled trial. *Eur J Pain.* 2011;15:942-949, Copyright 2011, with permission from European Federation of International Association for the Study of Pain Chapters.)

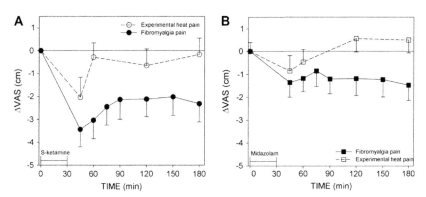

FIGURE 4.—Effect of S-ketamine and midazolam treatment on experimental heat pain intensity scores. (A) Scores following S-ketamine treatment. (B) Scores following midazolam treatment. No differences between treatments on experimental pain scores were observed. For comparison, the effects of treatment of the fibromyalgia pain scores are included. The gray bar indicates the treatment period. Data are mean ± SEM. (Reprinted from Noppers I, Niesters M, Swartjes M, et al. Absence of long-term analgesic effect from a short-term S-ketamine infusion on fibromyalgia pain: a randomized, prospective, double blind, active placebo-controlled trial. *Eur J Pain.* 2011;15:942-949, Copyright 2011, with permission from European Federation of International Association for the Study of Pain Chapters.)

Ketamine has significant and profound analgesic effects that are unrelated to its *N*-methyl-D-aspartate (NMDA) antagonist effects. In animal studies, NMDA antagonists that are devoid of other receptor affinities have minimal effect on acute pain but can block or reverse central sensitization resulting from nociceptive or neuropathic pain. To date, such benefits for patients with either nociceptive or neuropathic pain have been elusive. Ketamine can provide analgesia for opioid-resistant or opioid-tolerant patients. It has modest efficacy in reducing early postoperative pain when given intraoperatively but does not seem to be effective at reversing established central sensitization.

S. E. Abram, MD

Are Sympathetic Blocks Useful for Diagnostic Purposes?

Krumova EK, Gussone C, Regeniter S, et al (Ruhr-Univ of Bochum, Germany)
Reg Anesth Pain Med 36:560-567, 2011

Background.—Sympathetically maintained pain (SMP) can occur in patients with neuropathic pain. Sympathetically maintained pain is frequently diagnosed clinically by assessing the analgesic effect of an appropriate sympathetic block (SB). The diagnostic value of such blocks depends on both the degree of sympathetic activity disruption achieved and its duration without unintentional concomitant sensory block.

Methods.—This pilot study evaluated the rate of diagnostically valuable SBs performed by experienced anesthesiologists in 19 patients (stellate/thoracic blocks: n = 11, lumbar blocks: n = 12). Monitoring included pain rating before SB; 10 and 30 minutes; and at 1, 3, and 6 hours after SB; bilateral skin temperature 30 minutes before SB through 120 minutes after SB; and detection of bilateral thresholds for cold, warmth, tactile, and vibration stimuli before and after.

Results.—Ten (43%) of 23 SBs were not eligible for SMP diagnosis (4 had insufficient skin temperature increase; and 6 had cold or tactile detection threshold increases in the painful area). In 11 of the SBs, no significant sensory threshold change was detected; however, 2 individuals demonstrated marked reductions in the cold or tactile sensory thresholds. Sympathetically maintained pain was diagnosed in 3 (25%) of the 12 patients who had at least 1 SB with the required skin temperature increase without concomitant somatosensory block.

Conclusions.—Sympathetic blocks are useful in the diagnosis of SMP. However, their value is limited by the potential for false positives (unintentional sensory block) or false negatives (insufficient SB). Adequate monitoring of the sympathetic and somatosensory function for a minimum of 90 minutes after the intervention is essential to ensure that a valid diagnosis of SMP is made.

▶ This study again details the problems involved in determining whether there is sympathetically maintained pain in patients with symptoms consistent with complex regional pain syndrome. False-positive responses are associated with sensory changes from spread of local anesthetic somatic nerves, particularly with upper extremity blocks. False-negative responses are encountered when sympathetic blockade is incomplete. The development of a Horner response without appreciable increase in skin temperature of the hand is fairly common. In addition, bilateral increases in skin temperature are frequently seen following stellate block, making interpretation of the response questionable. Even when there is pain relief following a block after which sympathetic denervation is documented and somatic block is absent, placebo response cannot be ruled out.

Perhaps even more important is the question of how the diagnosis of sympathetically maintained pain will influence treatment. Systemically administered adrenergic blocking agents are often poorly tolerated and rarely provide significant relief. Perhaps pain relief following sympathetic block is predictive only of pain relief following subsequent sympathetic blocks.

S. E. Abram, MD

Associations between recreational exercise and chronic pain in the general population: Evidence from the HUNT 3 study

Landmark T, Romundstad P, Borchgrevink PC, et al (Norwegian Univ of Science and Technology, Trondheim, Norway; St Olavs Univ Hosp, Trondheim, Norway)
Pain 152:2241-2247, 2011

The evidence for an association between leisure-time physical activity and prevalence of pain is insufficient. This study investigated associations between frequency, duration, and intensity of recreational exercise and chronic pain in a cross-sectional survey of the adult population of a Norwegian county (the Nord-Trøndelag Health Study; HUNT 3). Of the 94,194

TABLE 1.—Characteristics of Study Population, and Prevalence of Chronic Pain[a] and Non-Exercise[b]

	Women			Men		
	n (%)	Chronic Pain (%)	Nonexercise (%)	n (%)	Chronic Pain (%)	Nonexercise (%)
Age, years						
20–34	4085 (16)	15	18	2835 (13)	11	29
35–49	7443 (30)	28	17	6030 (28)	22	33
50–64	8249 (33)	41	17	7642 (36)	32	28
65–79	4351 (17)	41	22	4145 (19)	28	24
80+	996 (4)	43	42	757 (4)	30	36
Smoke						
Nonsmoker	11,447 (45)	27	16	9029 (42)	19	24
Previous smoker	6187 (25)	38	16	6468 (30)	30	27
Current smoker	7490 (30)	39	26	5912 (28)	30	39
Education						
Elementary	5214 (21)	45	28	4023 (19)	35	36
Secondary	12,203 (48)	36	19	12,456 (58)	27	31
Higher	7707 (31)	21	13	4930 (23)	15	18
Organ disease*						
No	18,545 (74)	29	17	14,927 (70)	22	29
One	5030 (20)	40	22	4581 (21)	30	29
Two or more	1549 (6)	58	32	1901 (9)	41	31
HADS-D <8	19,094 (91)	32	17	14,929 (90)	24	26
HADS-D ≥8	2817 (9)	53	30	1728 (10)	43	38
Total	25,124 (100)	33	19	21,409 (100)	26	29

HADS-D, Hospital Anxiety and Depression Scale-Depression.
*Based on self report of the following: myocardial infarction (heart attack), angina pectoris (chest pain), other heart disease, stroke/brain haemorrhage, kidney disease, diabetes, cancer, epilepsy, chronic bronchitis, emphysema, asthma or COPD (chronic obstructive pulmonary disease).
[a]Pain lasting more than 6 months and of at least moderate intensity during last month.
[b]Reports of no exercise or less than once a week or < 15 minutes duration.

TABLE 2.—Prevalence Ratios (PR) for Chronic Pain With 95% Confidence Intervals (CI) by Frequency, Duration, and Intensity of Exercise in the HUNT 3 Study

| | 20–64 Years | | | | | | 65 Years or More | | | | | |
| | Women | | | Men | | | Women | | | Men | | |
	n	PR*	95% CI	n	PR*	95% CI	n	PR*	95% CI	n	PR*	95% CI
Frequency												
Nonexercise[a]	3471	1	Ref	4982	1	Ref	1393	1	Ref	1267	1	Ref
1 time/week	4231	0.92	0.86–0.97	3811	0.90	0.84–0.97	817	0.76	0.69–0.84	748	0.90	0.79–0.95
2–3 times/week	8524	0.90	0.85–0.94	5643	0.88	0.83–0.94	1909	0.73	0.67–0.79	1680	0.73	065–0.82
≥4 times/week	3551	1.00	0.94–1.07	2071	1.03	0.95–1.11	1228	0.66	0.60–0.72	1207	0.79	0.70–0.89
Duration												
Nonexercise[a]	3471	1	Ref	4982	1	Ref	1393	1	Ref	1267	1	Ref
15–30minutes	2213	1.00	0.93–1.07	1618	0.98	0.90–1.07	961	0.79	0.72–0.86	713	0.95	0.83–1.08
30–60 minutes	10,959	0.92	0.87–0.97	6584	0.90	0.85–0.96	2413	0.70	0.65–0.76	2017	0.75	0.68–0.84
≥60 minutes	3134	0.87	0.81–0.93	3323	0.91	0.84–0.98	580	0.62	0.55–0.71	905	0.72	0.62–0.83
Intensity												
Nonexercise[a]	3471	1	Ref	4982	1	Ref	1393	1	Ref	1267	1	Ref
Light	5491	0.97	0.92–1.02	3031	0.99	0.92–1.06	2797	0.73	0.68–0.78	1882	0.85	0.77–0.94
Moderate	10,228	0.90	0.86–0.95	7529	0.89	0.84–0.94	1069	0.66	0.59–0.73	1691	0.69	0.61–0.78
Hard	473	0.68	0.55–0.84	904	0.77	0.65–0.91	18	0.54	0.25–1.12	29	0.89	0.50–1.60

*Adjusted for age (15-year categories), smoking (never, past, current), and education (primary, secondary, tertiary).
[a]Exercising less than once a week or for <15 minutes each time.

invited to participate, complete data were obtained from 46,533 participants. Separate analyses were performed for the working-age population (20—64 years) and the older population (65 years or more). When defined as pain lasting longer than 6 months, and of at least moderate intensity during the past month, the overall prevalence of chronic pain was 29%. We found that increased frequency, duration, and intensity of exercise were associated with less chronic pain in analyses adjusted for age, education, and smoking. For those aged 20—64 years, the prevalence of chronic pain was 10—12% lower for those exercising 1—3 times a week for at least 30 minutes duration or of moderate intensity, relative to those not exercising. Dependent on the load of exercise, the prevalence of chronic pain was 21—38% lower among older women who exercised, relative to those not exercising. Similar, but somewhat weaker, associations were seen for older men. This study shows consistent and linear associations between frequency, duration, and intensity of recreational exercise and chronic pain for the older population, and associations without an apparent linear shape for the working-age population (Tables 1 and 2).

▶ In addition to the outcomes regarding the link between exercise and chronic pain, there is a great deal of data in this study relating the prevalence of chronic pain to other variables (Table 1). Smoking, lower educational levels, and organ system dysfunction were all associated with increased prevalence of chronic pain (smokers and individuals with lower educational levels were less likely to exercise). There was some association between age and chronic pain prevalence, but the elderly were no more likely to have pain than middle-aged patients.

Prevalence of chronic pain was based on positive responses to presence of pain for at least 6 months (39% for this question alone) and presence of moderate to severe pain currently (29% for both questions).

The association between amount and intensity of exercise and lower incidence of chronic pain was most robust for older patients (Table 2). For the working-age population, the prevalence of chronic pain was higher for those exercising daily than for those exercising 2 to 3 times a week, suggesting that excessive physical activity may have deleterious effects.

S. E. Abram, MD

Chronic postsurgical pain after nitrous oxide anesthesia

Chan MTV, Wan ACM, Gin T, et al (Chinese Univ of Hong Kong, Shatin, NT; et al)
Pain 152:2514-2520, 2011

Nitrous oxide is an antagonist at the N-methyl-D-aspartate receptor and may prevent the development of chronic postsurgical pain. We conducted a follow-up study in the Evaluation of Nitrous Oxide in the Gas Mixture for Anaesthesia (ENIGMA) trial patients to evaluate the preventive analgesic efficacy of nitrous oxide after major surgery. The ENIGMA trial was a randomized controlled trial of nitrous oxide-based or nitrous oxide-free general anesthesia in patients presenting for noncardiac surgery lasting more than 2 hours.

Using a structured telephone interview, we contacted all ENIGMA trial patients recruited in Hong Kong (n = 640). We recorded the severity of postsurgical pain of at least 3 months' duration that was not due to disease recurrence or a pre-existing pain syndrome, using the modified Brief Pain Inventory. The impact of postsurgical pain on quality of life was also measured. Pain intensity, opioid and other analgesic requirements during the first week of surgery, were retrieved from the trial case report form and medical records. A total of 46 (10.9%) patients reported pain that persisted from the index surgery, and 39 (9.2%) patients had severe pain. In

TABLE 6.—Factors Associated with Mild-to-Moderate Chronic Postsurgical Pain

Factors	Patients (n)	Patients with Severe Chronic Postsurgical Pain	Univariate OR (95% CI)	P Value	Multivariate OR (95% CI)	P Value
Age (y)	423	62.4 ± 12.5 (n = 46)	1.01 (0.99—1.05)	.24		
Gender						
Male	235	23 (9.8%)	Reference			
Female	188	23 (12.2%)	1.29 (0.69—2.37)	.44		
Wound type						
Others	199	17 (7.6%)	Reference			
Supraumbilical wound	224	29 (14.6%)	2.08 (1.10—3.91)	.03		
Wound length (cm)	423	19.3 ± 3.7 (n = 46)	1.17 (1.10—1.25)	.01	1.14 (1.04—1.26)	0.04
Minimally invasive surgery						
No	363	44 (12.1%)	Reference			
Yes	60	2 (3.3%)	0.25 (0.06—1.00)	.05		
Regional block						
No	352	42 (11.9%)	Reference			
Yes	71	4 (5.6%)	0.44 (0.15—1.27)	.08		
Severe acute postoperative pain						
No	378	26 (6.9%)	Reference			
Yes	45	20 (44.4%)	10.8 (5.32—22.0)	<.001	9.10 (2.58—32.1)	0.001
Anxiety[a]	423	11 (2—17) (n = 46)	2.38 (1.92—2.94)	<.001	2.28 (1.76—2.95)	<0.001
Wound infection						
No	365	28 (7.7%)	Reference			
Yes	58	18 (31.0%)	5.42 (2.75—10.7)	.001	4.80 (1.48—15.6)	0.01
Nitrous oxide administration						
No	209	31 (14.8%)	Reference			
Yes	214	15 (7.0%)	0.43 (0.23—0.83)	.01	0.48 (0.33—0.93)	0.04
Pre-existing pain problem elsewhere						
No	403	42 (10.4%)	Reference			
Yes	20	4 (20.0%)	2.15 (0.69—6.73)	.26		
Inspired oxygen concentration[b]						
21%—40%	43	7 (16.3%)	Reference			
41%—60%	60	9 (15.0%)	1.28 (0.48—3.42)	.63		
>61%	106	14 (13.2%)	1.16 (0.47—2.87)	.75		

Values are n (%), mean ± standard deviation, or median (range).
[a]Range of possible scores 0 (lowest level) to 21.
[b]This analysis included only those patients receiving nitrous oxide-free anesthesia.

addition, patients with chronic pain rated poorly in all attributes of the quality-of-life measures compared with those who were pain free. In a multivariate analysis, nitrous oxide decreased the risk of chronic postsurgical pain. In addition, severe pain in the first postoperative week, wound complication, and abdominal incision increased the risk of chronic pain. In conclusion, chronic postsurgical pain was common after major surgery in the ENIGMA trial. Intraoperative nitrous oxide administration was associated with a reduced risk of chronic postsurgical pain (Table 6).

▶ The use of intraoperative nitrous oxide was independently predictive of an incidence of postoperative chronic pain that was half that for patients not receiving it (Table 6). Nitrous oxide is often excluded from general anesthetic techniques in high-altitude locations because partial pressures attained with safe concentrations provide little additional intraoperative analgesia or central nervous system suppression. It would be useful to know the threshold partial pressures that provide this protective effect on the generation of chronic pain.

Other interesting information was generated from this study, such as the contribution of wound length, wound infection, and severity of immediate postoperative pain on the development of chronic pain. If acute postoperative pain intensity is associated with the development of chronic pain, the use of aggressive postoperative regional analgesia would be expected to reduce the incidence. There are studies that support this notion.

S. E. Abram, MD

Correlation between Preoperative Pain Duration and Percutaneous Vertebroplasty Outcome
Ehteshami Rad A, Kallmes DF (Mayo Clinic, Rochester, MN)
AJNR Am J Neuroradiol 32:1842-1845, 2011

Background and Purpose.—The duration of the fracture is considered by many practitioners to be an important predictor of outcome following vertebroplasty. We sought to define the impact of preprocedural pain duration on outcomes, including pain relief, improvement in function, and medication usage among patients treated with single-level vertebroplasty.

Materials and Methods.—Institutional review board approval was obtained before conducting this retrospective analysis of 321 patients undergoing single-level vertebroplasty at our institution. Fractures were categorized as acute (≤6 weeks, $n = 153$), subacute (6—24 weeks, $n = 124$), and chronic (>24 weeks, $n = 44$). Pain NRS (0—10) scores at rest and with activity and RDS were compared among 3 groups at baseline and postprocedure. Also absolute and proportional improvement of pain NRS and RDS were compared among 3 groups by using ANOVA. Linear regression was performed between preoperative pain duration and symptom improvement for each group.

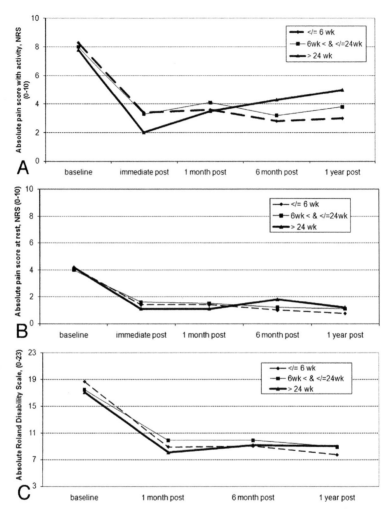

FIGURE 1.—Pain scores at rest (A), with activity (B), and RDS improvement (C). (Reprinted from Ehteshami Rad A, Kallmes DF. Correlation between preoperative pain duration and percutaneous vertebroplasty outcome. *AJNR Am J Neuroradiol.* 2011;32:1842-1845, with permission from American Society of Neuroradiology.)

Results.—Baseline RDS and pain NRS with activity and at rest were not significantly different among groups ($P =.09$, .30, and .91, respectively). Mean improvement in pain NRS with activity at 1 month postvertebroplasty in acute (improvement $= 4.9 \pm 3.5$), subacute (improvement $= 4.2 \pm 3.2$), and chronic fractures (improvement $= 4.5 \pm 3.2$) was similar among groups ($P =.28$). Mean improvement in RDS at 1 month postprocedure was 9.6, 8.3, and 9.9, for acute, subacute, and chronic fractures, respectively ($P =.56$). There was no strong correlation between length of pain and symptom improvement.

Conclusions.—The age of fracture has minimal impact on outcome following single-level vertebroplasty, with good outcomes noted among patients with acute, subacute, and chronic fractures (Fig 1).

▶ If there is no reduction in efficacy of vertebroplasty with increasing duration of fracture, as suggested by this study (Fig 1), then it seems reasonable to manage cases of vertebral compression fractures conservatively for several weeks, as pain resolves spontaneously in many cases, and delay in initiating vertebroplasty does not appear to reduce success. Because there is evidence that vertebroplasty increases the risk of fracture at adjacent levels, there is additional rationale for trying to avoid this treatment.

Because this is an uncontrolled, retrospective study, the evidence for lack of effect with symptom duration is not terribly robust and should be confirmed with prospective controlled studies.

S. E. Abram, MD

Drug-induced liver injury following a repeated course of ketamine treatment for chronic pain in CRPS type 1 patients: A report of 3 cases
Noppers IM, Niesters M, Aarts LPHJ, et al (Leiden Univ Med Ctr, The Netherlands; et al)
Pain 152:2173-2178, 2011

Studies on the efficacy of ketamine in the treatment of chronic pain indicate that prolonged or repetitive infusions are required to ensure prolonged pain relief. Few studies address ketamine-induced toxicity. Here we present data on the occurrence of ketamine-induced liver injury during repeated administrations of S(+)-ketamine for treatment of chronic pain in patients with complex regional pain syndrome type 1 as part of a larger study exploring possible time frames for ketamine re-administration. Six patients were scheduled to receive 2 continuous intravenous 100-hour S(+)-ketamine infusions (infusion rate 10–20 mg/h) separated by 16 days. Three of these patients developed hepatotoxicity. Patient A, a 65-year-old woman, developed an itching rash and fever during her second exposure. Blood tests revealed elevated liver enzymes (alanine transaminase, alkaline phosphatase, aspartate transaminase, and γ-glutamyl transferase, all ≥3 times the upper limit of normal) and modestly increased eosinophilic leukocytes. Patient E, a 48-year-old woman, developed elevated liver enzymes of similar pattern as Patient A during her second ketamine administration and a weakly positive response to antinuclear antibodies. In a third patient, Patient F, a 46-year-old man, elevated liver enzymes (alanine transaminase and γ-glutamyl transferase) were detected on the first day of his second exposure. In all patients, the ketamine infusion was promptly terminated and the liver enzymes slowly returned to reference values within 2 months. Our data suggest an increased risk for development of ketamine-induced liver injury when the infusion is prolonged and/or repeated within a short time frame. Regular measurements of liver function are therefore required during such treatments.

▶ As the use of ketamine for chronic pain management becomes more frequent, uncommon side effects and complications will become increasingly evident. For most patients, persistent reduction in chronic pain cannot be achieved with a single ketamine exposure. These reports indicate that repeated exposure can produce liver injury. The study involved the use of the S(+) enantiomer, which is the form that is active for pain management, rather than the more widely used racemic mixture, so elimination of the S(−) form is not protective. Liver dysfunction has been reported with ketamine administration for surgical anesthesia, and both liver and kidney failure have been reported among recreational ketamine users. Liver failure has so far not been reported among patients using oral ketamine, but it would seem likely that it could occur with prolonged use. There are few data regarding the safety of prolonged oral ketamine use. In one case series, 4 of 20 patients trialed with oral ketamine obtained long-term benefit (> 1 year) using doses of 100 to 500 mg/d.[1] No adverse effects were reported.

S. E. Abram, MD

Reference

1. Enarson MC, Hays H, Woodroffe MA. Clinical experience with oral ketamine. *J Pain Symptom Manage.* 1999;17:384-386.

Effects of Yoga Interventions on Pain and Pain-Associated Disability: A Meta-Analysis
Büssing A, Ostermann T, Lüdtke R, et al (Univ of Witten/Herdecke, Germany; Karl und Veronica Carstens-Stiftung, Essen, Germany; et al)
J Pain 13:1-9, 2012

We searched databases for controlled clinical studies, and performed a meta-analysis on the effectiveness of yoga interventions on pain and associated disability. Five randomized studies reported single-blinding and had a higher methodological quality; 7 studies were randomized but not blinded and had moderate quality; and 4 nonrandomized studies had low quality. In 6 studies, yoga was used to treat patients with back pain; in 2 studies to treat rheumatoid arthritis; in 2 studies to treat patients with headache/migraine; and 6 studies enrolled individuals for other indications. All studies reported positive effects in favor of the yoga interventions. With respect to pain, a random effect meta-analysis estimated the overall treatment effect at SMD = −.74 (CI: −.97; −.52, $P < .0001$), and an overall treatment effect at SMD = −.79 (CI: −1.02; −.56, $P < .0001$) for pain-related disability. Despite some limitations, there is evidence that yoga may be useful for several pain-associated disorders. Moreover, there are hints that even short-term interventions might be effective. Nevertheless,

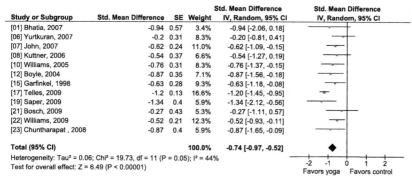

FIGURE 2.—Standardized mean differences on pain. The size of circles represents the weight of the study in meta-regression. (Reprinted from Büssing A, Ostermann T, Lüdtke R, et al. Effects of yoga interventions on pain and pain-associated disability: a meta-analysis. *J Pain*. 2012;13:1-9, with permission from the American Pain Society.)

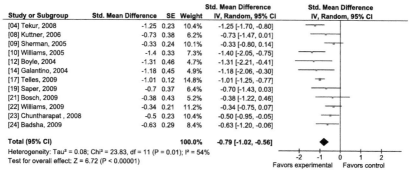

FIGURE 3.—Standardized treatment effects (SMD and confidence intervals) on pain-related disability. The size of circles represents the weight of the study in meta-regression. (Reprinted from Büssing A, Ostermann T, Lüdtke R, et al. Effects of yoga interventions on pain and pain-associated disability: a meta-analysis. *J Pain*. 2012;13:1-9, with permission from the American Pain Society.)

large-scale further studies have to identify which patients may benefit from the respective interventions.

Perspective.—This meta-analysis suggests that yoga is a useful supplementary approach with moderate effect sizes on pain and associated disability (Figs 2 and 3).

▶ Virtually all of the studies that met the methodological criteria showed significant benefit or trends toward benefit with respect to pain levels (Fig 2) and disability (Fig 3). The obvious methodological concern is that it is impossible to provide a blinded control group. Nevertheless, the evidence that patients can achieve improvement in function and quality of life with these programs is robust, and the cost and risks are minimal. Major advantages to yoga are that it shifts the locus of control from the practitioner to the patient and helps to dispel the sense of helplessness.

S. E. Abram, MD

Efficacy and Safety of Lumbar Epidural Dexamethasone Versus Methylprednisolone in the Treatment of Lumbar Radiculopathy: A Comparison of Soluble Versus Particulate Steroids
Kim D, Brown J (Henry Ford Hosp, Detroit, MI)
Clin J Pain 27:518-522, 2011

Introduction.—The literature is limited in the comparative efficacy and safety of dexamethasone phosphate (DP) compared with methylprednisolone acetate (MPA) in the treatment of lumbar radiculopathy by epidural injection. This study attempts to test the hypothesis that 2 corticosteroids are equivalent in efficacy and side effects.

Methods.—Patients with lumbar radicular symptoms for at least 6 months were randomized to equipotent doses of MPA 80 mg or DP 15 mg by lumbar translaminar epidurals administered under fluoroscopy. The epidurals were administered by different nonblinded practitioners other than the authors. Preprocedure Visual Analog Scale (VAS) pain scores by preoperative pain clinic nursing staff not involved in the study. On follow-up for the second epidural at 1 to 2 months, VAS scores and any reports of adverse side effects were obtained by pain clinic nursing staff who were blinded to the type of corticosteroid used. Electronic records were also reviewed for intervening changes in medication, additional therapeutic modalities, emergency room visits, and any other complications missed on nursing follow-up.

Results.—There were no significant demographic differences between the DP group (N = 30) and MPA group (N = 30). The mean days to follow-up was less for the DP group (41.1) versus the MPA group (51.1), although the difference was not statistically significant ($P = 0.4284$). Comparing the DP group and MPA group, there was a smaller mean decrease in VAS for the DP group (−19.7%) versus the MPA group (−27.2%), although the difference was not statistically significant ($P = 0.3672$). Eighty-seven percent of patients in the MPA group and 90% in the DP group had decreases in postprocedure VAS with no statistically significant difference between the 2 groups ($P = 0.999$). Thirteen percent of the MPA group and 10% of the DP group had increases in postprocedure VAS with no significant difference between the 2 groups ($P = 0.999$). The percentage increase in postprocedure VAS for those who had increase in pain was 34.3% and 31.7% for the MPA and DP group, respectively, with no statistically significant difference noted ($P = 0.8657$). Review of electronic medical records showed no change in pain medication prescribed, emergency room visits for pain, or any new treatments for pain in either group. No complications were reported by patients on nursing follow-up or seen in review of medical records including new neurological symptoms or new areas of pain.

Conclusions.—Nonparticulate DP seems to be close to the safety and effectiveness of particulate MPA in the treatment of lumbar radiculopathy. There is, however, a statistically nonsignificant trend toward less pain relief and shorter duration of action that may be clarified in a larger and longer duration study.

▶ Reports of catastrophic neurological complications following cervical, thoracic, and lumbar transforaminal epidural steroid injections have created concerns that injection of particulate material into a radicular artery can lead to embolization and injury to the spinal cord. The use of nonparticulate steroids might eliminate that hazard, but to date there is little evidence that they have equivalent efficacy. This study provides evidence that the nonparticulate steroid preparation dexamethasone phosphate provides equivalent or nearly equivalent efficacy compared with equipotent doses of the particulate steroid preparation methylprednisolone acetate for patients undergoing interlaminar epidural injections. It remains to be determined whether the same results would apply for transforaminal epidurals. There is such great concern about the safety of cervical transforaminal injections of particulate steroids that there would be some ethical concerns raised about a proposed study comparing the 2 drugs for that application. On the other hand, the data from this study would justify doing a prospective noncontrolled study of transforaminal dexamethasone phosphate injections for cervical radiculopathy.

Another consideration regarding this issue is whether transforaminal epidural steroid injections are more efficacious than interlaminar injections, for which the use of particulate steroids are safe. There are few data to indicate that transforaminal epidurals are more effective or which patient subgroups are more likely to benefit from transforaminals. Costs to the health care system are higher for transforaminal injections, particularly when multiple levels are injected.

S. E. Abram, MD

Increased adolescent opioid use and complications reported to a poison control center following the 2000 JCAHO pain initiative
Tormoehlen LM, Mowry JB, Bodle JD, et al (Indiana Univ School of Medicine, Indianapolis; Indiana Poison Ctr, Indianapolis)
Clin Toxicol 49:492-498, 2011

Context.—Adolescents are at risk to abuse opioid analgesics for many reasons, including inaccurate perception of risk and increased drug availability. In 2000, the Joint Commission on Accreditation of Healthcare Organizations (JCAHO) released pain management standards that emphasized pain control as a patient rights issue. This focus on analgesia may have increased both the prescribing and use of opioid analgesics, thereby increasing availability.

Objective.—Using data from a US poison center, this study aims to compare the number of adolescent opioid cases and their outcome severity before and after the 2000 JCAHO pain initiative.

Methods.—Retrospective case series of opioid exposures involving persons 12–18 years of age reported to a US poison center from 1994 to 2007. The main outcome measure was the number of adolescent opioid

TABLE 1.—Adolescent Opioid Cases by Age, Sex, and Opioid

Characteristics	1994–2000 (n = 632) n (%)	2001–2007 (n = 1002) n (%)	p-Value
Age (years)*			
12	32 (5.1)	38 (3.8)	0.533[‡]
13	51 (8.1)	62 (6.2)	
14	76 (12.0)	109 (10.9)	
15	107 (16.9)	159 (15.9)	
16	124 (19.6)	183 (18.3)	
17	124 (19.6)	244 (24.4)	
18	117 (18.5)	196 (19.6)	
Teen[†]	1 (0.2)	11 (1.1)	
Sex*			
Female	423 (66.9)	556 (55.5)	0.001[‡]
Male	209 (33.1)	445 (44.4)	
Unknown	0 (0)	1 (0.1)	
Opioid*			
Hydrocodone	71 (11.2)	480 (47.9)	0.001
Morphine	16 (2.5)	31 (3.1)	0.999
Codeine	242 (38.3)	124 (12.4)	0.001
Methadone	8 (1.3)	72 (7.2)	0.001
Oxycodone	48 (7.6)	100 (10.0)	0.660
Meperidine	6 (1.0)	10 (1.0)	>0.99
Fentanyl	3 (0.5)	14 (1.4)	0.581
Propoxyphene	237 (37.5)	164 (16.4)	0.001
Buprenorphine	0 (0)	2 (0.2)	>0.99
Hydromorphone	1 (0.2)	5 (0.5)	>0.99
Oxymorphone	0 (0)	0 (0)	>0.99

*Number of cases for each.
[†]Cases in which age was listed only as teen.
[‡]p-value for age/sex distribution of entire group.

cases reported for 1994–2000 compared to 2001–2007. Secondary outcomes included outcome severity, number of cases involving specific opioids, and correlation between the number of cases and the amount of opioids distributed to the state.

Results.—There were 1634 adolescent opioid-related cases with 187 cases developing medical complications. Compared with 1994–2000, the rate ratio of cases involving adolescents and opioid analgesics for the years 2001–2007 was 1.69 (95% CI: 1.53, 1.86), and these cases were 2.84 (95% CI: 2.06, 3.91) times more likely to have had medical complications. Medical complications involving methadone ($p = 0.001$) increased after the JCAHO initiative, while complications related to codeine ($p = 0.001$) and propoxyphene ($p = 0.030$) decreased. There were 15 deaths in 2001–2007 and none in 1994–2000 ($p = 0.012$). Lastly, there was a correlation between the rate of adolescent opioid cases and the amount of opioids distributed to the state ($r^2 = 0.90$; $p < 0.001$).

Conclusion.—In the 7 years following the JCAHO pain standards, there was an increase in the number and severity of adolescent opioid-related poison center cases. The increase correlates with statewide availability of opioids. These data may prove useful in drug education and prevention programs targeting adolescents (Table 1).

▶ There is general agreement that there has been a steady increase in the recreational use of prescription opioids among adolescents over the past decade (Table 1). The authors point to adolescents' attitudes toward prescription opioids as a factor. They cited a 2008 survey of more than 20 million teenagers reported by the Partnership for a Drug-Free America, stating that 41% of teenagers believed that prescription drugs were safer than illegal drugs, and 29% believed that prescription analgesics were not addictive.[1] There is no question that the number of opioid doses prescribed by physicians for legitimate medical purposes as well as by unscrupulous physicians working out of "pill mills" has increased dramatically in recent years. However, to suggest that the increase in adolescent overdose is a consequence of the Joint Commission on Accreditation of Healthcare Organizations (JCAHO's) Pain as the Fifth Vital sign initiative may be a bit of a stretch. The JCAHO initiative liberalized inpatient opioid use and may have led to an increase in the amount of opioids prescribed at the time of hospital discharge, but it seems more likely that outpatient clinic prescriptions as well as "rogue internet" sources have played a more significant role in making opioids more accessible. There may, however, be another unintended consequence of the JCAHO initiative, namely, an increase in the number of inpatient opioid overdose cases resulting from policies that require active treatment based on numerical pain ratings.[2]

S. E. Abram, MD

References

1. The Partnership Attitude Tracking Study (PATS): Teens 2008 Report. *The Partnership for a Drug-Free America*, http://www.doj.mt.gov/rxabuse/docs/2008PATSreport.pdf; 2009.
2. Lucas CE, Vlahos AL, Ledgerwood AM. Kindness kills: the negative impact of pain as the fifth vital sign. *J Am Coll Surg.* 2007;205:101-107.

Interventional management of intractable sympathetically mediated pain by computed tomography-guided catheter implantation for block and neuroablation of the thoracic sympathetic chain: technical approach and review of 322 procedures

Agarwal-Kozlowski K, Lorke DE, Habermann CR, et al (Centre for Palliative Care and Pain Management (T.I.P.S.), Stade, Germany; Florida International Univ, Miami; Univ Med Centre Hamburg-Eppendorf, Germany)
Anaesthesia 66:699-708, 2011

We retrospectively evaluated the safety and efficacy of computed tomography-guided placement of percutaneous catheters in close proximity to the thoracic sympathetic chain by rating pain intensity and systematically reviewing charts and computed tomography scans. Interventions were performed 322 times in 293 patients of mean (SD) age 59.4 (17.0) years, and male to female ratio 105:188, with postherpetic neuralgia (n = 103, 35.1%), various neuralgias (n = 88, 30.0%), complex regional pain syndrome (n = 69, 23.6%), facial pain (n = 17, 5.8%), ischaemic limb pain (n = 7, 2.4%), phantom limb pain (n = 4, 1.4%), pain following cerebrovascular accident (n = 2, 0.7%), syringomyelia (n = 2, 0.7%) and palmar hyperhidrosis (n = 1, 0.3%). The interventions were associated with a total of 23 adverse events (7.1% of all procedures): catheter dislocation (n = 9, 2.8%); increase in pain intensity (n = 8, 2.5%); pneumothorax (n = 3, 0.9%); local infection (n = 2, 0.6%); and puncture of the spinal cord (n = 1, 0.3%). Continuous infusion of 10 ml.h^{-1} ropivacaine 0.2% through the catheters decreased median (IQR [range]) pain scores from 8 (6−9 [2−10]) to 2 (1−3 [0−10]) (p < 0.0001). Chemical neuroablation was necessary in 137 patients (46.8%). We conclude that this procedure leads to a significant reduction of pain intensity in otherwise obstinate burning or stabbing pain and is associated with few hazards (Fig 2).

▶ Whereas lumbar sympathetic blocks are commonly performed for a variety of conditions, thoracic sympathetic blocks are performed infrequently, presumably

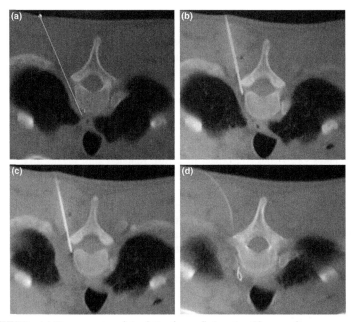

FIGURE 2.—(a) Measurements and simulation for needle insertion. The exact distances are measured from the metal marker to the intended point of puncture. The direction of the needle is simulated on the screen. (b) CT images showing the relationship of lung and vertebra. The needle is inserted as far as possible without damaging the lung. (c) CT images following injection of 40 ml saline 0.9%. Note the distance of the lung from the vertebra that allows the needle to pass without causing harm or pneumothorax. (d) CT images showing the catheter in place after subcutaneous placement to avoid infection. (Reprinted from Agarwal-Kozlowski K, Lorke DE, Habermann CR, et al. Interventional management of intractable sympathetically mediated pain by computed tomography-guided catheter implantation for block and neuroablation of the thoracic sympathetic chain: technical approach and review of 322 procedures. *Anaesthesia.* 2011;66:699-708, with permission from The Authors.)

because of the fairly high risk of pneumothorax. The use of CT guidance reduced the incidence to less than 1% in this series. Images shown in Fig 2 demonstrate the proximity of the needle path to the lung.

S. E. Abram, MD

Multiple Active Myofascial Trigger Points Reproduce the Overall Spontaneous Pain Pattern in Women With Fibromyalgia and Are Related to Widespread Mechanical Hypersensitivity
Alonso-Blanco C, Fernández-de-las-Peñas C, Morales-Cabezas M, et al (Universidad Rey Juan Carlos, Madrid, Spain; et al)
Clin J Pain 27:405-413, 2011

Objectives.—To determine whether the local and referred pain from active myofascial trigger points (MTrPs) reproduce the overall spontaneous fibromyalgia syndrome (FMS) pain pattern and whether widespread pressure hypersensitivity is related to the presence of widespread active MTrPs in FMS.

Methods.—Forty-four women with FMS (mean age: 47 ± 8 y) and 50 comparable healthy women (age: 48 ± 7 y) participated in the study. MTrPs in the temporalis, masseter, upper trapezius, splenius capitis, sternocleidomastoid, suboccipital, levator scapulae, scalene, pectoralis major, extensor carpi radialis brevis, extensor digitorum communis, gluteus maximus, piriformis, vastus medialis, and tibialis anterior muscles were explored. Pressure pain thresholds over 18 tender points specified in the 1990 American College of Rheumatology for FMS were also assessed by an assessor blinded to the condition of the participants.

Results.—The mean ± SD number of MTrPs for each woman with FMS was 11 ± 3, of which 10 ± 2 were active MTrPs and the remaining 1 ± 1 were latent. Healthy controls only had latent MTrPs (mean ± SD: 2 ± 1). The combination of the referred pain patterns from active MTrPs fully reproduced the overall spontaneous clinical pain area in patients with FMS. Patients with FMS had significant lower PPT compared with controls ($P < 0.001$). Within FMS, a significant positive correlation was found between the number of active MTrPs and spontaneous pain intensity ($r_s = 0.455$; $P = 0.002$).

Conclusions.—The local and referred pain elicited from widespread active MTrPs fully reproduced the overall spontaneous clinical pain area in patients with FMS. Widespread mechanical pain hypersensitivity was related to a greater number of active MTrPs. This study suggests that nociceptive inputs from active MTrPs may contribute to central sensitization in FMS (Figs 1 and 2).

▶ Older discussions of myofascial pain and fibromyalgia identify "trigger points" in myofascial pain patients and "tender points" in fibromyalgia patients. Myofascial pain is generally associated with 1 or several trigger points, fibromyalgia with multiple, usually bilateral sites. This study suggests that there is more similarity between these conditions than previously thought. The authors

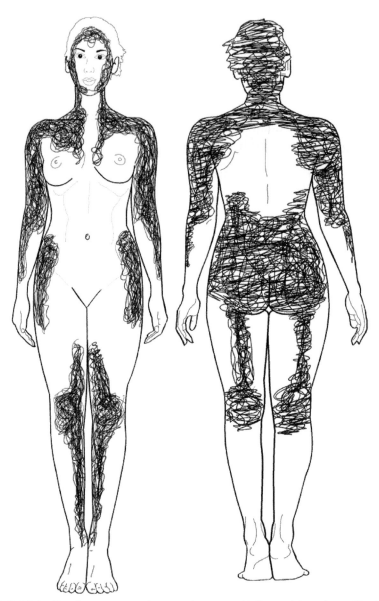

FIGURE 1.—Overall spontaneous pain pattern in women with fibromyalgia syndrome. (Reprinted from Alonso-Blanco C, Fernández-de-las-Peñas C, Morales-Cabezas M, et al. Multiple active myofascial trigger points reproduce the overall spontaneous pain pattern in women with fibromyalgia and are related to widespread mechanical hypersensitivity. *Clin J Pain*. 2011;27:405-413, with permission from Lippincott Williams & Wilkins.)

found a high correlation between the referred pain associated with palpation of selected trigger points and the spontaneous pain described by fibromyalgia patients (Fig 1 and 2). While trigger point injections are generally not

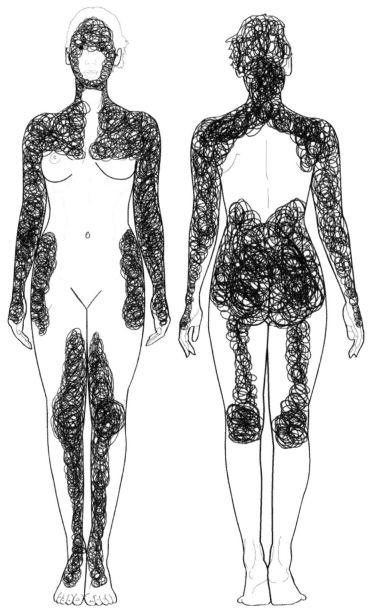

FIGURE 2.—Induced pain pattern from active MTrPs. Note that the combination of the referred pain patterns from active MTrPs fully reproduced the overall spontaneous clinical pain pattern seen in Figure 1. MTrP indicates myofascial trigger point. (Reprinted from Alonso-Blanco C, Fernández-de-las-Peñas C, Morales-Cabezas M, et al. Multiple active myofascial trigger points reproduce the overall spontaneous pain pattern in women with fibromyalgia and are related to widespread mechanical hypersensitivity. *Clin J Pain.* 2011;27:405-413, with permission from Lippincott Williams & Wilkins.)

recommended for fibromyalgia patients, the procedure, though tedious and time consuming given the large number of sites to inject, can provide relief, lasting as long as several weeks, for some patients. A confounding issue is the presence of multiple bony tender points in fibromyalgia patients. This characteristic suggests a mechanism that is not simply a widespread form of myofascial pain.

S. E. Abram, MD

Opioid Use, Misuse, and Abuse in Patients Labeled as Fibromyalgia
Fitzcharles M-A, Ste-Marie PA, Gamsa A, et al (McGill Univ Health Ctr, Montreal, Quebec, Canada; Université de Montréal, Quebec, Canada)
Am J Med 124:955-960, 2011

Background.—As pain is the cardinal symptom of fibromyalgia, it is logical that treatments directed toward pain relief will be commonly used. Analgesic drug therapy remains the traditional treatment intervention for most chronic pain conditions, with a progressive increased use of opioids in the past 20 years. Concerns about efficacy, risk-benefit ratio, and possible long-term effects of chronic opioid therapy have been raised. There is limited information about opioid treatment in fibromyalgia, with all current guidelines discouraging opioid use.

Methods.—A chart review of all patients referred to a tertiary care pain center clinic with a referring diagnosis of fibromyalgia was conducted to evaluate use of opioid medications.

Results.—We have recorded opioid use by 32% of 457 patients referred to a multidisciplinary fibromyalgia clinic, with over two thirds using strong opioids. Opioid use was more commonly associated with lower education, unemployment, disability payments, current unstable psychiatric disorder, a history of substance abuse, and previous suicide attempts.

Conclusion.—We have observed negative health and psychosocial status in patients using opioids and labeled as fibromyalgia. Prolonged use of opioids in fibromyalgia requires evaluation.

▶ There is widespread agreement that opioids are a poor therapeutic choice for patients with fibromyalgia. The authors of this study point out that many of the negative effects of opioids, which include fatigue, sleep disturbance, hyperalgesia, and depressed mood, are common symptoms of fibromyalgia. Nevertheless, one-third of fibromyalgia patients referred to this tertiary pain center were being treated with opioids. As is commonly seen with opioid treatment of other conditions, the use of opioids in this group did not appear to improve pain, mood, or function. Rather, the opioid patients exhibited more evidence of disability, psychiatric disorders, and suicide attempts.

S. E. Abram, MD

Psychoactive Medications and Crash Involvement Requiring Hospitalization for Older Drivers: A Population-Based Study

Meuleners LB, Duke J, Lee AH, et al (Curtin Univ, Perth, Western Australia)
J Am Geriatr Soc 59:1575-1580, 2011

Objectives.—To determine the association between psychoactive medications and crash risk in drivers aged 60 and older.

Design.—Retrospective population-based case-crossover study.

Setting.—A database study that linked the Western Australian Hospital Morbidity Data System and the Pharmaceutical Benefits Scheme.

Participants.—Six hundred sixteen individuals aged 60 and older who were hospitalized as the result of a motor vehicle crash between 2002 and 2008 in Western Australia.

Measurements.—Hospitalization after a motor vehicle crash.

Results.—Greater risk for a hospitalization crash was found for older drivers prescribed benzodiazepines (odds ratio (OR)=5.3, 95% confidence interval (CI)=3.6−7.8, $P < .001$), antidepressants (OR = 1.8, 95% CI = 1.0−3.3, $P = .04$), and opioid analgesics (OR = 1.5, 95% CI = 1.0−2.3, $P = .05$). Crash risk was significantly greater in men prescribed a benzodiazepine (OR = 6.2, 95% CI = 3.2−12.2, $P < .001$) or an antidepressant (OR = 2.7, 95% CI = 1.1−6.9, $P = .03$). Women prescribed benzodiazepines

TABLE 2.—Use of Psychoactive Medications and Risk of a Motor Vehicle Crash Requiring Hospitalization

Medication	Odds Ratio (95% Confidence Interval)	P-Value
Benzodiazepine		
All exposed subjects	5.3 (3.6−7.8)	<.001
Subgroup analyses		
Sex		
Male	6.2 (3.2−12.2)	<.001
Female	4.9 (3.1−7.8)	<.001
Chronic condition		
No	6.0 (3.8−9.5)	<.001
Yes	4.0 (2.9−8.1)	<.001
Antidepressant		
All exposed subjects	1.8 (1.0−3.3)	.04
Subgroup analyses		
Sex		
Male	2.7 (1.1−6.9)	.03
Female	1.4 (0.6−3.0)	.44
Chronic condition		
No	1.2 (0.6−2.7)	.63
Yes	3.4 (1.3−8.5)	.01
Opioid analgesic		
All exposed subjects	1.5 (1.0−2.3)	.05
Subgroup analyses		
Sex		
Male	1.2 (0.6−2.4)	.66
Female	1.8 (1.1−3.0)	.03
Chronic condition		
No	1.4 (0.8−2.3)	.20
Yes	2.1 (0.9−4.7)	.09

(OR = 4.9, 95% CI = 3.1−7.8, P < .001) or opioid analgesics (OR = 1.8, 95% CI = 1.1−3.0, P =.03) also had a significantly greater crash risk. Subgroup analyses further suggested that drivers with (OR = 4.0, 95% CI = 2.9−8.1, P < .001) and without (OR = 6.0, 95% CI = 3.8−9.5, P < .001) a chronic condition who were prescribed benzodiazepines were at greater crash risk. Drivers with a chronic condition taking antidepressants (OR = 3.4, 95% CI = 1.3−8.5, P =.01) also had a greater crash risk.

Conclusion.—Psychoactive medication usage was associated with greater risk of a motor vehicle crash requiring hospitalization in older drivers (Table 2).

▶ Tests of reaction time and driving simulations have demonstrated significant impairment by benzodiazepines. The chronic use of opioids has not been shown to produce substantial adverse effects on such test results. However, during initiation of opioid therapy, interference with driving skills and reduced attention may be evident. This study clearly implicates the use of benzodiazepines as a risk factor for motor vehicle accidents among older patients. While the effects for opioids and antidepressants are not as robust, they are still significant (Table 2). This study indicates that older patients should be apprised of the risks associated with driving wile using any of these medications. When benzodiazepines are used as well, all patients should be strongly advised against driving.

S. E. Abram, MD

Randomized controlled trial of percutaneous vertebroplasty versus optimal medical management for the relief of pain and disability in acute osteoporotic vertebral compression fractures
Farrokhi MR, Alibai E, Maghami Z (Shiraz Univ of Med Sciences, Iran)
J Neurosurg Spine 14:561-569, 2011

Object.—Osteoporotic vertebral compression fractures (VCFs) are a major cause of increased morbidity in older patients. This randomized controlled trial compared the efficacy of percutaneous vertebroplasty (PV) versus optimal medical therapy (OMT) in controlling pain and improving the quality of life (QOL) in patients with VCFs. Efficacy was measured as the incidence of new vertebral fractures after PV, restoration of vertebral body height (VBH), and correction of deformity.

Methods.—Of 105 patients with acute osteoporotic VCFs, 82 were eligible for participation: 40 patients underwent PV and 42 received OMT. Primary outcomes were control of pain and improvement in QOL before treatment, and these were measured at 1 week and at 2, 6, 12, 24, and 36 months after the beginning of the treatment. Radiological evaluation to measure VBH and sagittal index was performed before and after treatment in both groups and after 36 months of follow-up.

Results.—The authors found a statistically significant improvement in pain in the PV group compared with the OMT group at 1 week (difference

−3.1, 95% CI −3.72 to −2.28; p < 0.001). The QOL improved significantly in the PV group (difference −14, 95% CI −15 to −12.82; p < 0.028). One week after PV, the average VBH restoration was 8 mm and the correction of deformity was 8°. The incidence of new fractures in the OMT group (13.3%) was higher than in the PV group (2.2%; p < 0.01).

Conclusions.—The PV group had statistically significant improvements in visual analog scale and QOL scores maintained over 24 months, improved VBH maintained over 36 months, and fewer adjacent-level fractures compared with the OMT group (Tables 2 and 3).

▶ The results of this study are at odds with 2 previous randomized trials that failed to show significant reductions in pain or function in patients undergoing vertebroplasty for osteoporotic fractures.[1,2] This study showed immediate and persistent improvement in pain levels and Oswestry scores (Table 2). The authors of this study point out several potential flaws in the Buchbinder and Kallmes studies, such as less vigorous inclusion criteria, shorter follow-up, non-randomization in 1 study, liberal opioid use, and higher complication rates.

An interesting statistic from this study is a lower incidence of subsequent adjacent fractures in the vertebroplasty group than in the control group, again a different finding than in some previous studies. This study showed better restoration of vertebral body height and deformity angle (see Table 3) than many previous studies. In fact, the authors stated that the degree of restoration was similar to that produced by kyphoplasty. This is puzzling, particularly in light of the relatively low cement volumes used in this study. It is particularly hard to understand why the deformity angle in the treated patients continued to improve over time (Table 3). The authors suggest that the relative

---

TABLE 2.—Primary Outcome According to Group in 82 Patients Treated for VCFs*

Outcome Measure	PV Group	OMT Group	Mean Difference, Treatment Effect (95% CI)	p Value
VAS for pain				
baseline	8.4 ± 1.6	7.2 ± 1.7		
1 wk	3.3 ± 1.5	6.4 ± 2.1	−3.1 (−3.72 to −2.28)	<0.001
2 mos	3.2 ± 2.2	6.1 ± 2.1	−2.9 (−4.9 to −0.82)	<0.011
6 mos	2.2 ± 2.1	4.1 ± 1.5	−1.9 (−3.25 to −0.55)	<0.021
12 mos	2.2 ± 2.1	4.1 ± 1.8	−1.9 (−2.9 to 0.9)	<0.11
24 mos	2.8 ± 2.0	3.7 ± 2.0	−0.5 (−1.39 to 0.5)	<0.37
36 mos	1.8 ± 1.7	3.7 ± 2.5	−1.5 (−9.85 to 6.85)	<0.81
Oswestry LBP score for QOL				
baseline	52.2 ± 2.4	50.4 ± 2.8		
1 wk	30.1 ± 3.0	44.0 ± 2.5	−14.0 (−15.0 to −12.82)	<0.028
2 mos	15.0 ± 2.2	30.0 ± 3.1	−15.0 (−16.76 to −13.24)	<0.019
6 mos	10.0 ± 2.0	21.0 ± 2.5	−11.0 (−12.17 to −7.83)	<0.011
12 mos	8.0 ± 3.2	20.0 ± 1.7	−12.0 (−13.5 to −11.5)	<0.021
24 mos	8.0 ± 2.2	20.0 ± 2.0	−12.0 (−13.32 to −10.68)	<0.041
36 mos	8.0 ± 1.7	22.0 ± 1.2	−14.0 (−14.91 to −13.09)	<0.01

In the OMT group there were 42 patients at baseline, 1 week, and 2 and 6 months; and 39 at 12, 24, and 36 months. See Fig. 1 for details.

*In the PV group there were 40 patients at baseline, 1 week, and 2 and 6 months; 38 at 12 and 24 months; and 37 at 36 months.

TABLE 3.—Radiological Outcome According to Group in 82 Patients Treated for VCFs*

Measure	PV Group	OMT Group	Mean Difference, Treatment Effect (95% CI)	p Value
VBH (cm)				
baseline	2.8 ± 1.5	2.5 ± 1.3		
1 wk	3.2 ± 1.1	2.0 ± 1.0	1.2 (1.73−0.67)	<0.011
6 mos	3.2 ± 1.1	1.9 ± 1.4	1.3 (2.05−0.55)	<0.027
12 mos	3.2 ± 1.5	2.0 ± 1.2	1.2 (2.03−0.37)	<0.001
24 mos	3.0 ± 1.5	2.1 ± 1.2	0.9 (1.75−0.05)	<0.04
36 mos	3.0 ± 1.2	2.0 ± 1.0	2.0 (1.5−0.44)	<0.01
SI (°)				
baseline	20.0 ± 5.5	21.0 ± 4.2		
1 wk	10.0 ± 2.5	22.0 ± 2.2	−12.0 (−12.96 to −11.04)	<0.027
6 mos	10.1 ± 2.6	23.0 ± 2.1	−13.0 (−13.73 to −11.37)	<0.031
12 mos	10.0 ± 1.0	23.0 ± 2.0	−13.0 (−13.47 to −12.53)	<0.001
24 mos	9.0 ± 1.0	23.0 ± 2.3	−14.0 (−14.53 to −13.57)	<0.001
36 mos	8.9 ± 1.0	23.0 ± 2.0	−14.0 (−14.96 to −13.04)	<0.011

*In the PV group there were 40 patients at baseline, 1 week, and 6 months; 38 at 12 and 24 months; and 37 at 36 months. In the OMT group there were 42 patients at baseline, 1 week, and 6 months; and 39 at 12, 24, and 36 months. See Fig. 1 for details.

preservation of vertebral body height and angulation actually reduces the risk of subsequent fractures in adjacent bodies.

S. E. Abram, MD

References

1. Buchbinder R, Osborne RH, Ebeling PR, et al. A randomized trial of vertebro-plasty for painful osteoporotic vertebral fractures. *N Engl J Med.* 2009;361:557-568.
2. Kallmes DF, Comstock BA, Heagerty PJ, et al. A randomized trial of vertebro-plasty for osteoporotic spinal fractures. *N Engl J Med.* 2009;361:569-579.

Safety Assessment and Pharmacokinetics of Intrathecal Methylprednisolone Acetate in Dogs

Rijsdijk M, van Wijck AJM, Kalkman CJ, et al (Univ Med Ctr Utrecht, The Netherlands; et al)
Anesthesiology 116:170-181, 2012

Background.—Intrathecal methylprednisolone acetate (MPA) has been used in patients with chronic pain syndromes. Its safety has been debated after reports of adverse events. No systematic preclinical evaluation of MPA has been reported. In the current study, the acute and long-term effects of intrathecal MPA on dog spinal tissue was studied with the injec-tate reformulated to include minimal adjuvants.

Methods.—Seventeen dogs were implanted with intrathecal catheters and randomized to three groups: vehicle (lidocaine; 4 dogs), MPA 20 mg/ml (human dose; 7 dogs), and MPA 80 mg/ml (maximum deliverable dose; 6 dogs). In parallel with the human protocols, dogs received four injections at 7-day intervals. Clinical observations and plasma methylprednisolone measurements were done before and at intervals after intrathecal delivery. One week (acute) or 6 weeks (long-term) after the last injection, animals were sacrificed and spinal tissues harvested for histopathology.

Results.—Other than a brief motor block, no adverse clinical event occurred in any animal. Group A (vehicle) showed minimal histologic changes (median histology-score; acute: 1.3, long-term: 1.0). Group B (MPA 20 mg/ml) had a diffuse inflammatory reaction (acute: 2.0, long-term: 3.0), group C (MPA 80 mg/ml) a severe inflammatory response, with large inflammatory masses (acute: 4.0, long-term: 7.0) The severity of the inflammatory reaction increased significantly with increasing dose at long-term sacrifice (acute $P = 0.167$, long-term $P = 0.014$). No neuronal injury, demyelination, or gliosis was seen in any animal.

Conclusion.—These results, showing dose-dependent intrathecal inflammatory reactions at MPA doses and injectate concentrations comparable to those used in humans, indicate that the continued use of this modality in humans is not recommended (Table 1).

▶ The debate over the safety of intrathecally administered suspensions of corticosteroids has gone on for years. Clinically, the concern that arachnoiditis could result from intrathecal Depo Medrol was somewhat allayed by a lack of adverse effects among patients with postherpetic neuralgia who were treated with multiple intrathecal (IT) injections of that drug.[1] However, the concern remains that the devastating complication of arachnoiditis might occur sporadically. In the 1970s, I reported several patients treated with IT methylprednisolone acetate or triamcinolone diacetate who experienced transient symptoms compatible with aseptic meningitis (bilateral leg pain, fever, difficulty voiding), suggesting at least transient inflammatory response.[2]

This study by Yaksh's group is one that should have preceded all the IT steroid trials. It was done in a laboratory with a great deal of experience with preclinical safety testing of neuraxially administered drugs. (Their dog model was positive for development of intrathecal granulomas following high-dose IT morphine infusions.) This study demonstrated inflammatory changes in the

TABLE 1.—Overview of Histopathology Results

Treatment	Survival	N	Dura Scores	Arachnoid Scores	Spinal Cord Scores	Total Histology Score
Vehicle	1 wk	2	0/0	0.5/2	0/0	0.5/2
Vehicle	6 wk	2	0.5/1	0/0.5	0/0	0.5/1.5
MPA 20 mg/ml	1 wk	4	1/4/1/1	0.5/3/1/1	0/1/0/0	1.5/8/2/2
MPA 20 mg/ml	6 wk	3	1/1/2	0.5/1/1	0/1/0	1.5/3/3
MPA 80mg/ml	1 wk	3	2/1/3	2/2/4	0/0/1	4/3/8
MPA 80mg/ml	6 wk	3	2/4/2	4/4/2	1/1/1	7/9/5

The histopathology scores are based on the lumbar and sacral sections. Dura, arachnoid, and spinal cord are examined for the presence, location, and type of inflammatory reaction, including inflammatory cell infiltrates, granulation tissue, and fibrosis. Scoring system from 0 to 4: 0 being no inflammatory response and 4 being the maximal response observed in this cohort. Total histology score was the sum of the scores for dura, arachnoid, and spinal cord (possible score of 0–12). MPA = methylprednisolone acetate; N = Number of dogs; wk = weeks after the last intrathecal MPA dose.

dura and arachnoid that were particularly prominent 6 weeks after drug administration (see Table 1). The authors' conclusions regarding the possible adverse effects of this treatment have implications for the intentional IT administration of particulate steroids as well as for epidural steroid injection immediately following accidental dural puncture.

S. E. Abram, MD

References

1. Kotani N, Kushikata T, Hashimoto H, et al. Intrathecal methylprednisolone for intractable postherpetic neuralgia. *N Engl J Med.* 2000;343:1514-1519.
2. Abram SE. Subarachnoid corticosteroid injection following inadequate response to epidural steroids for sciatica. *Anesth Analg.* 1978;57:313-315.

Spinal Cord Stimulation Is Effective in Management of Complex Regional Pain Syndrome I: Fact or Fiction
Kumar K, Rizvi S, Bnurs SB (Univ of Saskatchewan, Regina, Canada)
Neurosurgery 69:566-580, 2011

Background.—Complex regional pain syndrome (CRPS) I is a debilitating neuropathic pain disorder characterized by burning pain and allodynia. Spinal cord stimulation (SCS) is effective in the treatment of CRPS I in the medium term but its long-term efficacy and ability to improve functional status remains controversial.

Objective.—To evaluate the ability of SCS to improve pain, functional status, and quality of life in the long term.

Methods.—We retrospectively analyzed 25 patients over a mean follow-up period of 88 months. The parameters for evaluation were visual analog scale (VAS), Oswestry Disability Index (ODI), Beck Depression Inventory (BDI), EuroQoL-5D (EQ-5D) and Short Form 36 (SF-36), and drug consumption. Evaluations were conducted at point of entry, 3 months, 12 months, and last follow-up at 88 months (mean).

Results.—At baseline, the mean scores were VAS 8.4, ODI 70%, BDI 28, EQ-5D 0.30, and SF-36 24. In general, maximum improvement was recorded at follow-up at 3 months (VAS 4.8, ODI 45%, BDI 15, EQ-5D 0.57, and SF-36 45). At last follow-up, scores were 5.6, 50%, 19, 0.57, and 40, respectively. Despite some regression, at last follow-up benefits were maintained and found to be statistically significant ($P < .001$) compared with baseline. Medication usage declined. SCS did not prevent disease spread to other limbs. Best results were achieved in stage I CRPS I, patients under 40 years of age, and those receiving SCS within 1 year of disease onset.

Conclusion.—SCS improves pain, quality of life, and functional status over the long term and consequently merits early consideration in the treatment continuum.

▶ While this was not a controlled study, it is valuable in that it documents ongoing benefit from spinal cord stimulation (SCS) over long time periods.

The fact that disease progression (spread to other limbs, increased involvement within a limb) occurred during treatment suggests that SCS provides symptomatic relief rather than reversing the underlying pathologic mechanism. While cost-benefit estimates were not included, documented reductions in medication use could offset some of the expenses of stimulation.

The majority of patients were treated using older electrode technology (single quad electrode). Newer techniques (octapolar, multiple leads, retrograde leads) might further improve long-term outcomes.

S. E. Abram, MD

The association between psychological factors and the development of complex regional pain syndrome type 1 (CRPS1) — A prospective multicenter study
Beerthuizen A, Stronks DL, Huygen FJPM, et al (Erasmus MC, Rotterdam, The Netherlands; et al)
Eur J Pain 15:971-975, 2011

The objective of this study was to investigate the association between psychological factors and complex regional pain syndrome type 1 (CRPS1). A prospective multicenter cohort study was performed involving the emergency room of three hospitals, and patients age 18 years or older, with a single fracture, were included in the study. At baseline (T0), participants completed a questionnaire covering demographic, psychological (Symptom Checklist-90), and medical variables. At plaster removal (T1) and at T2, the participants completed a questionnaire addressing symptoms of CRPS1. Psychological factors that were analysed were agoraphobia, depression, somatization, insufficiency, (interpersonal) sensitivity, insomnia, and life events. In total, 596 consecutive patients were included in the study, and 7.0% were diagnosed with CRPS1. None of the psychological factors predicted the development of CRPS1. The scores on the Symptom Checklist-90 subscales fell into the range of the general population and were, in most cases, average or below average when compared with those of pain patients or psychiatric patients. No empirical evidence supports a diagnosis of CRPS1 patients as psychologically different, and the current results indicate that there is no association between psychological factors and CRPS1.

▶ Several previous studies have failed to show that patients with complex regional pain syndrome (CRPS) (or reflex sympathetic dystrophy) exhibited more psychopathology or abnormal personality traits than other individuals with chronic pain. This study goes a step further and indicates that patients who develop CRPS are no more likely to have pre-existing psychopathology than patients who do not develop CRPS following minor hand, wrist, foot, or ankle fractures. This study provides some interesting epidemiologic data, providing a CRPS incidence of 7% among patients with these minor distal extremity fractures.

S. E. Abram, MD

The Red Wine Polyphenol Resveratrol Shows Promising Potential for the Treatment of Nucleus Pulposus–Mediated Pain *In Vitro* and *In Vivo*
Wuertz K, Quero L, Sekiguchi M, et al (Univ of Zurich, Switzerland; Fukushima Med Univ, Japan; et al)
Spine 36:E1372-E1384, 2011

Study Design.—Descriptive and mechanistic investigation of the anti-inflammatory and anticatabolic effect of resveratrol in intervertebral discs (IVDs) *in vitro* and of the analgetic effect *in vivo*.

Objective.—To determine whether resveratrol may be useful in treating nucleus pulposus (NP)—mediated pain.

Summary of Background Data.—Proinflammatory cytokines seem to be key mediators in the development of NP-mediated pain. Patients with discogenic or radiculopathic pain may substantially benefit from anti-inflammatory substances that could be used in a minimal-invasive treatment approach. Resveratrol, a polyphenolic phytoalexin found in red wine exhibits anti-inflammatory effects in various cell types and tissues, but no data exists so far with regards to the IVD in the context of low back and leg pain.

Methods.—In part 1, the anti-inflammatory and anticatabolic effect of resveratrol was investigated in a cell culture model on interleukin 1β (IL-1β) prestimulated human IVD cells on the gene and protein expression level. In part 2, the molecular mechanisms underlying the effects observed upon resveratrol treatment were investigated (toll-like receptors, nuclear factor κB, sirtuin 1 (SIRT1), mitogen-activated protein (MAP) kinases p38/ERK/JNK). In part 3, the analgetic effects of resveratrol were investigated *in vivo* using a rodent model of radiculopathy and von Frey filament testing. All quantitative data were statistically evaluated either by Mann-Whitney U test or by one-way analysis of variance and Bonferroni *post hoc* testing ($P < 0.05$).

Results.—*In vitro*, resveratrol exhibited an anti-inflammatory and anti-catabolic effect on the messenger RNA and protein level for IL-6, IL-8, MMP1, MMP3 and MMP13. This effect does not seem to be mediated via the MAP kinase pathways (p38, ERK, JNK) or via the NF-κB/SIRT1 pathway, although toll-like receptor 2 was regulated to a minor extent. *In vivo*, resveratrol significantly reduced pain behavior triggered by application of NP tissue on the dorsal root ganglion for up to 14 days.

Conclusion.—Resveratrol was able to reduce levels of proinflammatory cytokines *in vitro* and showed analgetic potential *in vivo*. A decrease in proinflammatory cytokines may possibly be the underlying mechanism of pain reduction observed *in vivo*. Resveratrol seems to have considerable

Pain Behavior *in vivo*

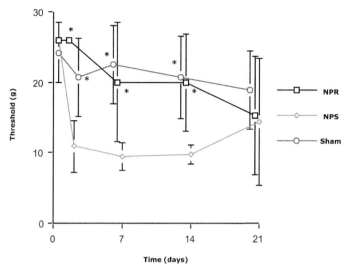

FIGURE 7.—Resveratrol reduces pain behavior *in vivo*. This figure shows results of the *in vivo* testing of resveratrol, using a rodent pain model. Compared with sham animals, application of nucleus pulposus tissue (+ saline) (NPS group) reduced mechanical sensitivity thresholds primarily up to day 14. If coapplication of nucleus pulposus tissue and resveratrol was performed at the DRG (NPR group), thresholds were significantly higher than in the NPS group at days 2 ($P < 0.0001$), 7 ($P = 0.037$), and 14 ($P = 0.0044$) and very similar to the sham group (indicative of pain reduction by resveratrol treatment). Data were obtained by von Frey filament testing and are presented as Mean and SD (n = 6). Asterisks indicate statistical significance ($P < 0.05$). (Reprinted from Wuertz K, Quero L, Sekiguchi M, et al. The red wine polyphenol resveratrol shows promising potential for the treatment of nucleus pulposus—mediated pain *in vitro* and *in vivo*. *Spine*. 2011;36:E1372-E1384, with permission from Lippincott Williams & Wilkins.)

potential for the treatment of NP-mediated pain and may thus be an alternative to other currently discussed (biological) treatment options (Fig 7).

▶ Increased levels of proinflammatory cytokines appear in the spinal cord dorsal horn and in the dorsal root ganglia of animals subjected to inflammatory and neuropathic insults, such as application of nucleus pulposus tissue to the diagnosis-related groups. Drugs that block the development of glial activation in animal pain models, such as pentoxifylline and minocycline, have been shown to reduce pain behavior, but they have been disappointing in human trials. The development of safe and effective drugs that can reverse the development of neuroimmune responses would be a real step forward. While this study suggests potential for a substance found in red wine, the reduction in pain behavior (Fig 7) was produced by direct application of the drug to the DRG at the time of injury. This suggests that an epidural or transforaminal route would be required, and it remains to be seen if the drug is effective in already established radiculopathy.

S. E. Abram, MD

Time-scheduled vs. pain-contingent opioid dosing in chronic opioid therapy

Von Korff M, Merrill JO, Rutter CM, et al (Group Health Res Inst, Seattle, WA; Univ of Washington School of Medicine, Seattle; et al)

Pain 152:1256-1262, 2011

Some expert guidelines recommend time-scheduled opioid dosing over pain-contingent dosing for patients receiving chronic opioid therapy (COT). The premise is that time-scheduled dosing results in more stable opioid blood levels and better pain relief, fewer adverse effects, less reinforcement of pain behaviors, and lower addiction risk. We report results of a survey of 1781 patients receiving COT for chronic noncancer pain, in which 967 reported time-scheduled opioid dosing only and 325 reported pain-contingent opioid dosing only. Opioid-related problems and concerns were assessed with the Prescribed Opioids Difficulties Scale. We hypothesized that respondents using time-scheduled opioid dosing would report significantly fewer problems and concerns than those using pain-contingent dosing. Patients receiving time-scheduled dosing received substantially higher average daily opioid doses than those using pain-contingent dosing (97.2 vs. 37.2 mg average daily dose morphine equivalents, $P < .0001$). Contrary to expectation, time-scheduled opioid dosing was associated with higher levels of patient opioid control concerns than pain-contingent dosing (6.2 vs. 4.8, $P = .008$), after adjusting for patient and drug regimen differences. Opioid-related psychosocial problems were somewhat greater among patients using time-scheduled dosing, but this difference was nonsignificant after controlling for patient and drug regimen differences (5.9 vs. 5.0, $P = .14$). Time-scheduled dosing typically involved higher dosage levels

TABLE 4.—Specific Problems and Concerns Attributed to Opioids by Patients

Problem/Concern	A: Pain-Contingent Dosing Only	B: Time-Scheduled Dosing Only (%)	P Value (A vs. B)	Both A and B (%)	Neither A nor B (%)
Opioid control concerns					
Preoccupied with opioids	4.4	8.7	.03	11.9	5.1
Could not control opioid use	1.6	6.1	.0002	6.5	2.0
Need higher opioid dose for same effect	25.6	28.3	.51	22.5	29.9
Worry about opioid dependence	15.5	35.9	<.0001	33.6	23.2
Wanted to stop or cut down	43.2	43.8	.89	39.8	31.4
Problems with family/friends/coworkers	3.6	5.4	.20	7.8	3.4
Family/friends thought might be dependent	4.6	17.6	<.0001	12.8	9.6
Psychosocial problems attributed by patient to use of opioids					
Loss of interest in usual activities	8.5	6.9	.45	15.9	5.6
Trouble concentrating or remembering	12.3	17.9	.07	14.2	7.4
Slowed down, sluggish, sedated	17.2	18.3	.75	16.2	14.4
Depressed or anxious	6.5	8.9	.27	10.1	5.6
Interference with work-family-social activities	17.8	21.9	.22	17.7	13.5
Hard to think clearly	9.0	19.5	.0004	11.2	9.3
Less alert driving or when needed	19.6	30.2	.004	23.8	19.2
Bothersome adverse effects	27.4	34.1	.10	21.2	23.5

and was associated with higher levels of patient concerns about opioid use. Controlled comparative effectiveness research is needed to assess benefits and risks of time-scheduled opioid dosing relative to pain-contingent opioid dosing among COT patients in ambulatory care (Table 4).

▶ Although this was not a randomized, controlled study, the results are both interesting and iconoclastic. For the past 2 decades, the conventional wisdom has been that we will attain better pain control if we prescribe long-acting opioids and use time-scheduled dosing. In this study, a higher percentage of the time-scheduled patients was using long-acting drugs (43% vs 11%). There did not appear to be any advantage to using time-scheduled dosing, and a number of outcomes favored pain-contingent dosing. Time-scheduled patients used higher doses and had more opioid control concerns and more psychosocial problems (Table 4).

The use of long-acting opioids has not been proven to offer substantial advantages over short-acting drugs. A recent systematic review indicated that the only advantage for long-acting drugs was a tendency toward better sleep and more patient convenience.[1] Those benefits may not be worth the added cost of sustained-release medications.

S. E. Abram, MD

Reference

1. Rauck RL. What is the case for prescribing long-acting opioids over short-acting opioids for patients with chronic pain? A critical review. *Pain Pract.* 2009;9: 468-479.

Topical capsaicin for pain management: therapeutic potential and mechanisms of action of the new high-concentration capsaicin 8% patch
Anand P, Bley K (Hammersmith Hosp, London, UK; NeurogesX, Inc, San Mateo, CA)
Br J Anaesth 107:490-502, 2011

Topical capsaicin formulations are used for pain management. Safety and modest efficacy of low-concentration capsaicin formulations, which require repeated daily self-administration, are supported by meta-analyses of numerous studies. A high-concentration capsaicin 8 patch (Qutenza™) was recently approved in the EU and USA. A single 60-min application in patients with neuropathic pain produced effective pain relief for up to 12 weeks. Advantages of the high-concentration capsaicin patch include longer duration of effect, patient compliance, and low risk for systemic effects or drug-drug interactions. The mechanism of action of topical capsaicin has been ascribed to depletion of substance P. However, experimental and clinical studies show that depletion of substance P from nociceptors is only a correlate of capsaicin treatment and has little, if any, causative role in pain relief. Rather, topical capsaicin acts in the skin to attenuate cutaneous hypersensitivity and reduce pain by a process best described as 'defunctionalization' of nociceptor fibres. Defunctionalization is due to a number of effects that include temporary loss of membrane potential, inability to transport neurotrophic factors leading to altered phenotype, and reversible retraction of epidermal and dermal nerve fibre terminals. Peripheral neuropathic hypersensitivity is mediated by diverse mechanisms, including altered expression of the capsaicin receptor TRPV1 or other key ion channels in affected or intact adjacent peripheral nociceptive nerve fibres, aberrant re-innervation, and collateral sprouting, all of which are defunctionalized by topical capsaicin. Evidence suggests that the utility of topical capsaicin may extend beyond painful peripheral neuropathies.

▶ Depletion of substance P from nociceptive fibers, the putative mechanism of analgesic action of topical capsaicin, fails to explain the antinociceptive action of high-dose capsaicin. Prolonged inactivation by capsaicin of cutaneous nerve fibers that express TRPV1 ion channels has been documented. Although some neuropathic pain disorders are associated with loss of intraepidermal nerve fibers (postherpetic neuralgia, painful diabetic neuropathy, painful human immunodeficiency virus—associated neuropathy, small fiber neuropathy, and others) remaining nociceptive fibers may become hypersensitized by nerve growth factor glial cell line—derived neurotrophic factor (GDNF) and pro-inflammatory cytokines. The defunctionalization of these remaining, highly active axons can produce reduction in spontaneous pain and allodynia for up to 3 months with a single application. The treatment is expensive (approximately $800 for each application), and additional costs may be involved with the production of cutaneous anesthesia required before the patch application.

S. E. Abram, MD

Value of bone SPECT-CT to predict chronic pain relief after percutaneous vertebroplasty in vertebral fractures
Solá M, Pérez R, Cuadras P, et al (Hospital Universitari Germans Trias i Pujol. Badalona, Spain)
Spine J 11:1102-1107, 2011

Background Context.—Longer life span has resulted in increased risk of vertebral osteoporotic fractures. Among minimally invasive procedures, percutaneous vertebroplasty (PV) has shown excellent results in the treatment of chronic vertebral pain. The role of preintervention bone single photon emission computed tomography—computed tomography (SPECT-CT) has not been clearly established for the management of these patients.
Purpose.—To determine the value of bone SPECT-CT in patient selection, treatment planning, and prediction of response to PV. A comparison with magnetic resonance imaging (MRI) was also aimed.
Study Design.—Prospective consecutive series.

Patient Sample.—We studied the performance of bone SPECT-CT on 33 consecutive patients with chronic pain because of vertebral fracture intended for PV.

Outcome Measures.—Improvement of clinical status was based on comparison of preprocedure and postprocedure outcome measurements of pain, mobility, and analgesic use.

Methods.—Bone SPECT was done using a dual-detector variable-angle gamma camera coupled with a two-slice CT scanner (Symbia T2 System; Siemens, Munich, Germany). Magnetic resonance imaging was done using a magnet of 1.5 T (Giroscan System ACS NT Intera; Philips, Amsterdam, The Netherlands).

Results.—Of the 33 patients, 24 finally underwent PV. Positive SPECT-CT images predicted clinical improvement in 91% (21 of 23) of them. Agreement between SPECT-CT and MRI was 80% (20 of 25). Single photon emission computed tomography—computed tomography images showed an alternative cause of pain in some cases, such as new fractures or multiple coexisting fractures, persisting bone remodeling in a previous cemented vertebra, and facet or discal degenerative disease. Single photon emission computed tomography—computed tomography was mandatory in eight patients that could no receive MRI, all of whom improved after PV.

Conclusions.—Positive bone SPECT-CT seems a good predictor of post-procedural response. It also adds valuable information as to the cause of back pain and facilitates complete patient evaluation in patients that can not receive MRI.

▶ Despite recent studies that questioned the benefit of vertebroplasty for osteoporotic compression fractures, there is mounting evidence that the procedure is effective in many cases and can shorten the duration of pain. Several recent studies have focused on predictors of improved outcomes. MRI evidence of edema, which is associated with more recent fractures, provides some help, although there is also evidence that some patients with old fractures can obtain relief. This study represents an additional effort to predict which patients will respond. The authors conclude: "Bone scan may provide additional important functional information, as it shows abnormal tracer uptake as the broken bone increases its metabolic turnover in the attempt to heal…Edema on MRI and increased bone turnover on planar or single photon emission computed tomography (SPECT) bone scans are different physiological features on the same sequence of fracture healing. Therefore, either or both techniques may be able to signal the specific vertebral body to be treated."

The editors' comments, published with the article, are worth reading: "The article provides some good general information regarding the use of this diagnostic test. However, formal conclusions cannot be drawn. The outcome measures are not validated. Prognostic value (PPV) cannot be derived from the data, nor can diagnostic value as there were insufficient SPECT-negative or pain-negative patients included. Thus, further research is needed before routine implementation of bone SPECT-CT as a pre-procedural prognostic tool."

S. E. Abram, MD

12 Geriatric Medicine

Activity Energy Expenditure and Incident Cognitive Impairment in Older Adults

Middleton LE, Manini TM, Simonsick EM, et al (Sunnybrook Health Sciences Centre, Toronto, Ontario, Canada; Univ of Florida, Gainesville; Natl Inst on Aging, Bethesda, MD; et al)
Arch Intern Med 171:1251-1257, 2011

Background.—Studies suggest that physically active people have reduced risk of incident cognitive impairment in late life. However, these studies are limited by reliance on self-reports of physical activity, which only moderately correlate with objective measures and often exclude activity not readily quantifiable by frequency and duration. The objective of this study was to investigate the relationship between activity energy expenditure (AEE), an objective measure of total activity, and incidence of cognitive impairment.

Methods.—We calculated AEE as 90% of total energy expenditure (assessed during 2 weeks using doubly labeled water) minus resting metabolic rate (measured using indirect calorimetry) in 197 men and women (mean age, 74.8 years) who were free of mobility and cognitive impairments at study baseline (1998-1999). Cognitive function was assessed at baseline and 2 or 5 years later using the Modified Mini-Mental State Examination. Cognitive impairment was defined as a decline of at least 1.0 SD (9 points) between baseline and follow-up evaluations.

Results.—After adjustment for baseline Modified Mini-Mental State Examination scores, demographics, fat-free mass, sleep duration, self-reported health, and diabetes mellitus, older adults in the highest sex-specific tertile of AEE had lower odds of incident cognitive impairment than those in the lowest tertile (odds ratio, 0.09; 95% confidence interval, 0.01-0.79). There was also a significant dose response between AEE and incidence of cognitive impairment ($P = .05$ for trend over tertiles).

Conclusions.—These findings indicate that greater AEE may be protective against cognitive impairment in a dose-response manner. The significance of overall activity in contrast to vigorous or light activity should be determined.

▶ The abstract says it all: The more physical activity you do, the smarter you are. I think the best treatment or preventative for brain dysfunction is physical activity. Whether it is causing new neurons to grow through release of brain-derived neurotrophic growth factor as is believed in Parkinson's patients or whether it is clearing out arteries and decreasing inflammation is unclear. But the data are clear—the more physical activity you do, the better your brain will be.

M. F. Roizen, MD

Association Between Serum Cathepsin S and Mortality in Older Adults
Jobs E, Ingelsson E, Risérus U, et al (Uppsala Univ, Sweden)
JAMA 306:1113-1121, 2011

Context.—Experimental data suggest that cathepsin S, a cysteine protease, is involved in the complex pathways leading to cardiovascular disease and cancer. However, prospective data concerning a potential association between circulating cathepsin S levels and mortality are lacking.

Objective.—To investigate associations between circulating cathepsin S levels and mortality in 2 independent cohorts of elderly men and women.

Design, Setting, and Participants.—Prospective study using 2 community-based cohorts, the Uppsala Longitudinal Study of Adult Men (ULSAM; n = 1009; mean age: 71 years; baseline period: 1991-1995; median follow-up: 12.6 years; end of follow-up: 2006) and the Prospective Investigation of the Vasculature in Uppsala Seniors (PIVUS; n = 987; 50% women; mean age: 70 years; baseline period: 2001-2004; median follow-up: 7.9 years; end of follow-up: 2010). Serum samples were used to measure cathepsin S.

Main Outcome Measure.—Total mortality.

Results.—During follow-up, 413 participants died in the ULSAM cohort (incidence rate: 3.59/100 person-years at risk) and 100 participants died in the PIVUS cohort (incidence rate: 1.32/100 person-years at risk). In multivariable Cox regression models adjusted for age, systolic blood pressure, diabetes, smoking status, body mass index, total cholesterol, high-density lipoprotein cholesterol, antihypertensive treatment, lipid-lowering treatment, and history of cardiovascular disease, higher serum cathepsin S was associated with an increased risk for mortality (ULSAM cohort: hazard ratio [HR] for 1-unit increase of cathepsin S, 1.04 [95% CI, 1.01-1.06], $P = .009$; PIVUS cohort: HR for 1-unit increase of cathepsin S, 1.03 [95% CI, 1.00-1.07], $P = .04$). In the ULSAM cohort, serum cathepsin S also was associated with cardiovascular mortality (131 deaths; HR for quintile 5 vs quintiles 1-4, 1.62 [95% CI, 1.11-2.37]; $P = .01$) and cancer mortality (148 deaths; HR for 1-unit increase of cathepsin S, 1.05 [95% CI, 1.01-1.10]; $P = .01$).

Conclusions.—Among elderly individuals in 2 independent cohorts, higher serum cathepsin S levels were associated with increased mortality risk. Additional research is needed to delineate the role of cathepsin S and whether its measurement might have clinical utility.

▶ Okay. Admit it. You didn't know what cathepsin S was. I didn't either before reading this study. This is another marker of inflammation that appears sensitive and independent of many other risk factors for mortality. The risk factor difference in normal treatment is almost 60%. What is your cathepsin S level? I have never had mine measured.

M. F. Roizen, MD

Brains and Aging: Comment on "Physical Activity and Cognition in Women With Vascular Conditions" and "Activity Energy Expenditure and Incident Cognitive Impairment in Older Adults"
Larson EB (Group Health Res Inst, Seattle, WA)
Arch Intern Med 171:1258-1259, 2011

Background.—A growing body of evidence suggests that habitual physical activity and fitness are associated with age-related alterations in cognition and dementia risk. With increasing numbers of very old persons, appreciation of the personal and public health consequences of dementia, and an urgent need to learn how to modify age-related decline, it is important to improve the current understanding of how activity affects brain function in later life, particularly since physical activity is a modifiable quantity.

Current Evidence.—Various studies have linked physical activity and cognitive decline and/or risk of dementia related to age. Using data from the Women's Antioxidant Cardiac Study, researchers found that women with the lowest levels of physical activity had significantly more pronounced cognitive decline than women with higher physical activity levels. It was concluded that older women at high vascular risk are also at high risk for cognitive decline. The relationships between energy expenditure and self-reported physical activity and incident cognitive impairment were explored using data from the Health, Aging, and Body Composition (Health ABC) study. Persons with the highest average energy expenditure (AEE) scores had significantly lower odds of cognitive impairment than persons with the lowest AEE scores. An Australian randomized clinical trial of a community-based walking intervention revealed that increased levels of activity were protective of cognition. Having a regular walking program, which qualifies as moderate exercise, has also been found to reduce mental decline and diminish the need for admission to a nursing home with behavioral problems. Finally, a randomized controlled trial studied the effect of aerobic exercise training on memory and the hippocampus, which shrinks in late adulthood. The reduced hippocampal volume (especially that of the anterior area) is associated with impaired memory and increased risk of dementia. The anterior hippocampus increased in size, the patients had better spatial memory, and other brain areas were unaffected by aerobic exercise training in these older adults.

Implications.—Alzheimer disease research has focused largely on amyloid deposition and the role of tau proteins. More recent research suggests that other so-called mixed pathologic processes contribute to late-life dementias. Vascular degenerative processes evidently play an important role, and vascular risk factors such as limited physical activity, midlife hypertension, and smoking are associated with late-life dementia. It can be difficult to clinically distinguish vascular dementia from Alzheimer disease. Since physical activity and other vascular risk factors can be modified, there may be the potential for reducing late-life cognitive impairment.

Conclusions.—Research should now be directed toward developing effective ways to change behavior and promote engagement in habitual physical activity, ideally throughout one's lifetime. Such exercise is especially needed during middle and late life. Further research is needed to understand how other vascular risk factors might reduce late-life cognitive decline and dementia risk, how newly discovered growth factors may function, and what are the potential long-term effects of widely dispensed anticholinergic drugs.

▶ This article buttresses our belief that habitual physical activity and intensity of physical activity are important for decreasing cognitive dysfunction and improving spatial memory. What this means to me is that I am going to keep exercising as long as I can and justify it by how much it is going to help my brain.

M. F. Roizen, MD

Dietary Supplements and Mortality Rate in Older Women: The Iowa Women's Health Study

Mursu J, Robien K, Harnack LJ, et al (Univ of Eastern Finland, Kuopio, Finland; Univ of Minnesota, Minneapolis; et al)
Arch Intern Med 171:1625-1633, 2011

Background.—Although dietary supplements are commonly taken to prevent chronic disease, the long-term health consequences of many compounds are unknown.

Methods.—We assessed the use of vitamin and mineral supplements in relation to total mortality in 38 772 older women in the Iowa Women's Health Study; mean age was 61.6 years at baseline in 1986. Supplement use was self-reported in 1986, 1997, and 2004. Through December 31, 2008, a total of 15 594 deaths (40.2%) were identified through the State Health Registry of Iowa and the National Death Index.

Results.—In multivariable adjusted proportional hazards regression models, the use of multivitamins (hazard ratio, 1.06; 95% CI, 1.02-1.10; absolute risk increase, 2.4%), vitamin B_6 (1.10; 1.01-1.21; 4.1%), folic acid (1.15; 1.00-1.32; 5.9%), iron (1.10; 1.03-1.17; 3.9%), magnesium (1.08; 1.01-1.15; 3.6%), zinc (1.08; 1.01-1.15; 3.0%), and copper (1.45; 1.20-1.75; 18.0%) were associated with increased risk of total mortality when compared with corresponding nonuse. Use of calcium was inversely related (hazard ratio, 0.91; 95% confidence interval, 0.88-0.94; absolute risk reduction, 3.8%). Findings for iron and calcium were replicated in separate, shorter-term analyses (10-year, 6-year, and 4-year follow-up), each with approximately 15% of the original participants having died, starting in 1986, 1997, and 2004.

Conclusions.—In older women, several commonly used dietary vitamin and mineral supplements may be associated with increased total mortality risk; this association is strongest with supplemental iron. In contrast to the findings of many studies, calcium is associated with decreased risk.

▶ This study brings up important issues, although also highlighted by the fact that the same week, a randomized controlled trial assessing the effect of extra vitamin E or selenium on development of prostate cancer was published. These studies showed an increased risk from these therapies. So let me give you my take on these 2 studies.

A. A multivitamin is an insurance policy against inadequate diet in people aged over 55 (those in the study); multivitamin and docosahexaenoic acid (DHA) use is much more important in women of child-bearing age.

B. These Iowa women consumed an average of 6.3 servings of fruit and veggies a day, more than twice the average in the United States and Canada. So maybe they didn't need this insurance policy.

C. We know that extra iron for 50-year-old or older women and men who do not have iron deficiencies is harmful. Even so, the incremental hazard ratio was under 10% range. We typically look for hazard ratios that decrease risk by 40% or increase risk to 240% of baseline in epidemiologic association studies such as the Iowa study before we put a lot of faith in them or act on them before randomized studies.

D. We know vitamin D is beneficial because most of us do not get enough from our diet, so that is why it is included, yet this study showed that vitamin D was hazardous. Why? That is not clear.

E. We know that extra vitamin E, large amounts seen in this Iowa study and in the prostate study, are harmful from randomized studies, yet a benefit was shown in the Iowa study. Additionally, extra magnesium in elderly individuals has been shown to be beneficial yet is indicated as harmful in this Iowa study. This is the problem with epidemiologic studies. You use them to suggest questions that need answering, but they often don't answer a lot by themselves. We need to do further studies.

F. Quality-of-life measures, such as the decreased memory degradation or decreases in eye-sight loss with the DHA, or decreased bone fractures from vitamin D3, were not examined in this Iowa study. My overall impression is that this study changes nothing and reinforces iron and copper as a hazard. Avoiding these 2 in multivitamins if not of child-bearing age is important. What this leaves me with is more puzzles and questions for future studies to solve. My own take home is this: I'm still taking (because data supports such) a multivitamin without iron and with only a low dose of vitamin A (< 3500 IU a day) and low amounts of vitamin E (as mixed tocopherols of about 30 IU). I split my multivitamin in half and take half in the morning and half at night; I also take 1200 IU of vitamin D3 a day, DHA 900 mg a day, lutein 20 mg a day, a probiotic, 2 baby aspirins with plenty of water, and a little extra calcium and magnesium (600 and 300 a day).

M. F. Roizen, MD

13 Medical Education and Simulation

2007 American College of Cardiology/American Heart Association (ACC/AHA) Guidelines on Perioperative Cardiac Evaluation Are Usually Incorrectly Applied by Anesthesiology Residents Evaluating Simulated Patients

Vigoda MM, Sweitzer B, Miljkovic N, et al (Univ of Miami Miller School of Medicine, FL; Univ of Chicago, IL; Univ of Nebraska Med Ctr, Omaha)
Anesth Analg 112:940-949, 2011

Background.—The 2007 American College of Cardiology/American Heart Association (ACC/AHA) Guidelines on Perioperative Cardiac Evaluation and Care for Noncardiac Surgery is the accepted standard for perioperative cardiac evaluation. Anesthesiology training programs are required to teach these algorithms. We estimated the percentage of residents nationwide who correctly applied suggested testing algorithms from the ACC/AHA guidelines when they evaluated simulated patients in common clinical scenarios.

Methods.—Anesthesiology resident volunteers at 24 training programs were presented with 6 scenarios characterized by surgical procedure, patient's risk factors, and patient's functional capacity. Scenarios and 5 possible recommendations per scenario were both presented in randomized orders. Senior anesthesiologists at 24 different United States training programs along with the first author of the 2007 ACC/AHA guidelines validated the appropriate recommendation to this web-based survey before distribution.

Results.—The 548 resident participants, representing 12% of anesthesiology trainees in the United States, included 48 PGY-1s (preliminary year before anesthesia training), 166 Clinical Anesthesia Year 1 (CA-1) residents, 161 CA-2s, and 173 CA-3s. For patients with an active cardiac condition, the upper 95% confidence bound for the percent of residents who recommended evaluations consistent with the guidelines was 78%. However, for the remaining 5 scenarios, the upper 95% confidence bound for the percent of residents with an appropriate recommendation was 46%.

Conclusions.—The results show that fewer than half of anesthesiology residents nationwide correctly demonstrate the approach considered the standard of care for preoperative cardiac evaluation. Further study is necessary to elucidate the correct intervention(s), such as use of decision support tools, increased clarity of guidelines for routine use, adjustment in educational programs, and/or greater familiarity of responsible faculty with the material.

▶ It is not common that learning in residency programs is assessed as critically as reported in this study. More frequently, instructors administer pre- and post-tests to document that their teaching has improved residents' understanding of a topic. However, the questions in those tests are not as carefully constructed as those in this study, in which correct responses were validated by a panel of experts, including directors of preanesthesia clinics who wrote the questions, residency program directors, additional directors of preanesthesia clinics, chiefs of anesthesia, cardiac anesthesiologists, a neuroanesthesiologist, an intensivist, and a director of quality improvement. Additionally, the lead author of the American College of Cardiology/American Heart Association (ACC/AHA) guidelines reviewed the questions and their answers and agreed that they were consistent with the evidence-based guidelines.

This study found that less than 50% of residents correctly applied the guidelines defining standard of care for preoperative cardiac evaluation. Although it was not part of the scope of this study, it would have been interesting to see how faculty applied these same guidelines. As the authors suggest, in addition to learning from the material they read, residents learn from those who supervise them.

Although all programs required resident rotation through preoperative clinics and most had a yearly teaching session on the guidelines, the manner of teaching the ACC/AHA guidelines likely varied from one program to the next. It would be interesting to learn whether the specific nature of the teaching—whether through suggested reading, simulation, specific individual discussion of the guidelines while evaluating patients in preoperative clinics, or lectures—resulted in a better understanding of the material and a greater tendency to appropriately apply the guidelines. Educational plans need to be constantly revised and updated so that those being taught actually learn the material.

C. Lien, MD

Technology-enhanced simulation for health professions education: a systematic review and meta-analysis
Cook DA, Hatala R, Brydges R, et al (Mayo Med School, Rochester, MN; Univ of British Columbia, Vancouver, Canada; Univ of Toronto, Ontario, Canada; et al)
JAMA 306:978-988, 2011

Context.—Although technology-enhanced simulation has widespread appeal, its effectiveness remains uncertain. A comprehensive synthesis of evidence may inform the use of simulation in health professions education.

Objective.—To summarize the outcomes of technology-enhanced simulation training for health professions learners in comparison with no intervention.

Data Source.—Systematic search of MEDLINE, EMBASE, CINAHL, ERIC, PsychINFO, Scopus, key journals, and previous review bibliographies through May 2011.

Study Selection.—Original research in any language evaluating simulation compared with no intervention for training practicing and student physicians, nurses, dentists, and other health care professionals.

Data Extraction.—Reviewers working in duplicate evaluated quality and abstracted information on learners, instructional design (curricular integration, distributing training over multiple days, feedback, mastery learning, and repetitive practice), and outcomes. We coded skills (performance in a test setting) separately for time, process, and product measures, and similarly classified patient care behaviors.

Data Synthesis.—From a pool of 10,903 articles, we identified 609 eligible studies enrolling 35,226 trainees. Of these, 137 were randomized studies, 67 were nonrandomized studies with 2 or more groups, and 405 used a single-group pretest-posttest design. We pooled effect sizes using random effects. Heterogeneity was large ($I^2 > 50\%$) in all main analyses. In comparison with no intervention, pooled effect sizes were 1.20 (95% CI, 1.04-1.35) for knowledge outcomes (n = 118 studies), 1.14 (95% CI, 1.03-1.25) for time skills (n = 210), 1.09 (95% CI, 1.03-1.16) for process skills (n = 426), 1.18 (95% CI, 0.98-1.37) for product skills (n = 54), 0.79 (95% CI, 0.47-1.10) for time behaviors (n = 20), 0.81 (95% CI, 0.66-0.96) for other behaviors (n = 50), and 0.50 (95% CI, 0.34-0.66) for direct effects on patients (n = 32). Subgroup analyses revealed no consistent statistically significant interactions between simulation training and instructional design features or study quality.

Conclusion.—In comparison with no intervention, technology-enhanced simulation training in health professions education is consistently associated with large effects for outcomes of knowledge, skills, and behaviors and moderate effects for patient-related outcomes.

▶ This study shows that we learn better with simulation, at least in the short term. Whether it results in better postoperative outcomes still may be in doubt, but the number of articles favoring simulation is 27, even if the effect size for this benefit is very small. For all of those who question simulation, this article may be your bible. For all of those who believe in it, this article may be your bible. For the rest of us, it is a fascinating article that indicates may be simulation really is a true benefit.

M. F. Roizen, MD

14 Anesthesia Outside the Operating Room

Neurointerventional procedures for unruptured intracranial aneurysms under procedural sedation and local anesthesia: a large-volume, single-center experience
Ogilvy CS, Yang X, Jamil OA, et al (Massachusetts General Hosp, Boston; et al)
J Neurosurg 114:120-128, 2011

Object.—In this paper, the authors' goal was to report the outcome of patients with unruptured intracranial aneurysms undergoing endovascular treatment under conscious sedation (local anesthesia).

Methods.—Between November 5, 2001, and February 5, 2009, the authors treated 340 patients with 358 unruptured aneurysms by using neuro-interventional procedures at Millard Fillmore Gates Hospital (Buffalo, New York). The data were retrospectively reviewed for periprocedural safety and long-term follow-up.

Results.—A total of 496 procedures were performed under local anesthesia. Of those, 370 procedures (74.6%) were completed successfully. In 82 procedures (16.5%), an associated medical or technical event occurred. Forty-four procedures (8.9%) were aborted. Rates of overall procedure-related morbidity and mortality were 1.2% (6 of 496) and 0.6% (3 of 496), respectively. The average hospital stay was 1.5 ± 2.5 days. Long-term follow-up was available in 261 (82.1%) of 318 patients whose procedures were performed with local anesthesia. Of those, 246 patients (94.3%) had a good outcome (modified Rankin Scale score ≤ 2), 6 patients (2.3%) had an unfavorable outcome, not related to the procedure, and 9 patients (3.4%) had a poor outcome (modified Rankin Scale score > 2) as a result of the intervention.

Conclusions.—Interventional treatment under conscious sedation (local anesthesia) can be effectively performed in most patients with unruptured intracranial aneurysms and is associated with a short hospital stay and low morbidity and mortality.

▶ In this article, the authors describe a series of cases over the course of 8 years in which patients with unruptured intracranial aneurysms received either local anesthesia or sedation for neurointerventional management of their intracranial vascular lesions. The authors describe several reasons to proceed with local anesthesia or sedation rather than general anesthesia. These include decreased time required for turnover of the procedure room, less intensive monitoring of the patient, shorter length of hospital stay, and earlier recognition of mishaps during the procedure. However, in more than 25% of their procedures performed under sedation or local anesthesia, there was an adverse event, and in some of these the patient returned for a subsequent procedure. In others, the anesthetic was converted to a general anesthetic.

It would have been interesting to know what percentage of patients who initially had their procedures performed under a general anesthetic had to return for a second procedure because of inability to complete the procedure on the first attempt. Forty-two of the patients undergoing similar procedures received general anesthesia, yet why these patients were not considered for local anesthesia or sedation is not described, nor is their outcome in terms of either the number of procedures needed to treat their intracranial vascular lesions or their morbidity and mortality.

Emergent intubation and induction of general anesthesia in the interventional neuroradiology suite because of coil migration or rupture of an intracranial aneurysm is not technically easy because of the location of the fluoroscopy arms and the ongoing need to image a patient as initial radiologic treatment, such as balloon placement, is begun. Additionally, in this situation, patients are frequently not appropriately monitored, and, as described by the authors, the anesthesiologists are not necessarily present in the INR suite.

Before the management of anesthesia for treatment of unruptured aneurysms described by these authors can become routine, larger multicenter trials, over a shorter time period, comparing the risks and benefits with those of patients receiving general anesthesia for management of the same lesions need to be conducted. Additionally, in series such as this, the rationale for determining who receives general anesthesia and who receives local anesthesia or sedation must be described so that clinicians can offer the option of local anesthesia or sedation to appropriate patients.

C. Lien, MD

15 Practice Management and Professionalism

Association Between Physician Billing and Cardiac Stress Testing Patterns Following Coronary Revascularization
Shah BR, Cowper PA, O'Brien SM, et al (Duke Univ Med Ctr, Durham, NC; et al)
JAMA 306:1993-2000, 2011

Context.—The degree to which financial factors may influence use of cardiac stress imaging procedures is unknown.

Objective.—To examine the association of physician billing and nuclear stress and stress echocardiography testing following coronary revascularization.

Design, Setting, and Patients.—Using data from a national health insurance carrier, 17 847 patients were identified between November 1, 2004, and June 30, 2007, who had coronary revascularization and an index cardiac outpatient visit more than 90 days following the procedure. Based on overall billings, physicians were classified as billing for both technical (practice/equipment) and professional (supervision/ interpretation) fees, professional fees only, or not billing for either. Logistic regression models were used to evaluate the association between physician billing and use of stress testing, after adjusting for patient and other physician factors.

Main Outcome Measures.—Incidence of nuclear and echocardiographic stress tests within 30 days of an index cardiac-related outpatient visit.

Results.—The overall cumulative incidence of nuclear or echocardiography stress testing within 30 days of the index cardiac-related outpatient visit following revascularization was 12.2% (95% CI, 11.8%-12.7%). The cumulative incidence of nuclear stress testing was 12.6% (95% CI, 12.0%-13.2%), 8.8% (95% CI, 7.5%-10.2%), and 5.0% (95% CI, 4.4%-5.7%) among physicians who billed for technical and professional fees, professional fees only, or neither, respectively. For stress echocardiography, the cumulative incidence of testing was 2.8% (95% CI, 2.5%-3.2%), 1.4% (95% CI, 1.0%-1.9%), and 0.4% (95% CI, 0.3%-0.6%) among physicians who billed for the technical and professional fees, professional fees only, or neither, respectively. Adjusted odds ratios (ORs) of nuclear stress testing among patients treated by physicians who billed for technical and professional fees and professional fees only were 2.3% (95% CI, 1.8%-2.9%) and 1.6% (95% CI, 1.2%-2.1%), respectively, compared with those patients treated by physicians who did not bill for testing ($P < .001$). The adjusted OR of stress echocardiography testing among patients treated by physicians billing for both or professional fees only were 12.8% (95% CI, 7.6%-21.6%) and 7.1% (95% CI, 4.0%-12.9%), respectively, compared with patients treated by physicians who did not bill for testing ($P < .001$).

Conclusion.—Nuclear stress testing and stress echocardiography testing following revascularization were more frequent among patients treated by physicians who billed for technical fees, professional fees, or both compared with those treated by physicians who did not bill for these services.

▶ What this article shows is that incentives work. That is, when you allow physicians to charge for procedures performed in their office and earn money from it, you increase the number of procedures done in their offices.

Is this an appropriate efficiency from 1-stop care or overutilization? We don't know from this article, but understanding the broader implication of these levers warrants careful consideration to avoid unintended consequences. The worst unintended consequence could be that changing it may ultimately make patient care less or more efficient and less or more costly. Make no mistake, this debate is about money. Who bills for what and how that billing pattern influences utilization. I believe the focus should be less about eliminating incentives and more about getting patients the best, most efficient care, maybe even using incentives to prevent them getting sick in the first place. For example, if we pay primary care physicians for normalizing blood pressure, low-density lipid cholesterol, C-reactive protein, hemoglobin A1C, and weight for height, and for tobacco cessation, could we decrease utilization to such a great rate that we would save the system? I think so, but that rests on another large study.

M. F. Roizen, MD

Automated Identification of Postoperative Complications Within an Electronic Medical Record Using Natural Language Processing

Murff HJ, FitzHenry F, Matheny ME, et al (Veterans Affairs Med Ctr, Nashville, TN; et al)
JAMA 306:848-855, 2011

Context.—Currently most automated methods to identify patient safety occurrences rely on administrative data codes; however, free-text searches of electronic medical records could represent an additional surveillance approach.

Objective.—To evaluate a natural language processing search—approach to identify postoperative surgical complications within a comprehensive electronic medical record.

Design, Setting, and Patients.—Cross-sectional study involving 2974 patients undergoing inpatient surgical procedures at 6 Veterans Health Administration (VHA) medical centers from 1999 to 2006.

Main Outcome Measures.—Postoperative occurrences of acute renal failure requiring dialysis, deep vein thrombosis, pulmonary embolism, sepsis, pneumonia, or myocardial infarction identified through medical record review as part of the VA Surgical Quality Improvement Program. We determined the sensitivity and specificity of the natural language processing approach to identify these complications and compared its performance with patient safety indicators that use discharge coding information.

Results.—The proportion of postoperative events for each sample was 2% (39 of 1924) for acute renal failure requiring dialysis, 0.7% (18 of 2327) for pulmonary embolism, 1% (29 of 2327) for deep vein thrombosis, 7% (61 of 866) for sepsis, 16% (222 of 1405) for pneumonia, and 2% (35 of 1822) for myocardial infarction. Natural language processing correctly identified 82% (95% confidence interval [CI], 67%-91%) of acute renal failure cases compared with 38% (95% CI, 25%-54%) for patient safety indicators. Similar results were obtained for venous thromboembolism (59%, 95% CI, 44%-72% vs 46%, 95% CI, 32%-60%), pneumonia (64%, 95% CI, 58%-70% vs 5%, 95% CI, 3%-9%), sepsis (89%, 95% CI, 78%-94% vs 34%, 95% CI, 24%-47%), and postoperative myocardial infarction (91%, 95% CI, 78%-97%) vs 89%, 95% CI, 74%-96%). Both natural language processing and patient safety indicators were highly specific for these diagnoses.

Conclusion.—Among patients undergoing inpatient surgical procedures at VA medical centers, natural language processing analysis of electronic medical records to identify postoperative complications had higher sensitivity and lower specificity compared with patient safety indicators based on discharge coding.

▶ This is an important study because it shows that this process is much better at identifying complications than is the usual postoperative discharge coding. I would encourage all with an interest in electronic medical records, or even all with an interest in postoperative complications, to read this article and see if you can adopt it. It is wonderful.

M. F. Roizen, MD

Intraoperative Waste in Spine Surgery: Incidence, Cost, and Effectiveness of an Educational Program
Soroceanu A, Canacari E, Brown E, et al (Dalhousie Univ, Halifax, Nova Scotia, Canada; Beth Israel Deaconess Med Ctr, Boston, MA)
Spine 36:E1270-E1273, 2011

Study Design.—Prospective observational study.

Objective.—This study aims to quantify the incidence of intraoperative waste in spine surgery and to examine the efficacy of an educational program directed at surgeons to induce a reduction in the intraoperative waste.

Summary of Background Data.—Spine procedures are associated with high costs. Implants are a main contributor of these costs. Intraoperative waste further exacerbates the high cost of surgery.

Methods.—Data were collected during a 25-month period from one academic medical center (15-month observational period, 10-month post–awareness program). The total number of spine procedures and the incidence of intraoperative waste were recorded prospectively. Other variables recorded included the type of product wasted, cost associated with the product or implant wasted, and reason for the waste.

Results.—Intraoperative waste occurred in 20.2% of the procedures prior to the educational program and in 10.3% of the procedures after the implementation of the program ($P < 0.0001$). Monthly costs associated with surgical waste were, on average, $17680 prior to the awareness intervention and $5876 afterwards ($P = 0.0006$). Prior to the intervention, surgical waste represented 4.3% of total operative spine budget. After the awareness program this proportion decrease to an average of 1.2% ($P = 0.003$).

Conclusion.—Intraoperative waste in spine surgery exacerbates the already costly procedures. Extrapolation of this data to the national level leads to an annual estimate of $126,722,000 attributable to intraoperative spine waste. A simple educational program proved to be and continues to be effective in making surgeons aware of the import of their choices and the costs related to surgical waste.

▶ This study documents the intraoperative waste in spine surgery and a reduction in the amount of waste following an educational program designed to alert clinicians to both the degree and causes of waste. The article did not provide the details of the educational program other than what was considered waste and the costs due to waste on both an institutional and individual level. Information not provided that may have been useful includes the size of the department, the specifics of the educational program, whether individual reports of waste were generated for residents as well as faculty, and whether the reports of individual waste were available for all to review. These details would have been useful to all clinicians as they attempt to rein in costs of medical care without compromising quality.

Although details of the methodology were not provided, the results are not really surprising. No one participates in a surgical procedure intending to increase its cost. An awareness of the factors that needlessly increase cost should decrease their occurrence. It would be interesting if the authors were to publish a follow-up report documenting whether the observed changes in behavior were maintained over time. If they were, the educational program developed by these authors is a success.

C. Lien, MD

NICU Care in the Aftermath of Hurricane Katrina: 5 Years of Changes
Barkemeyer BM (Louisiana State Univ Health Sciences Ctr, New Orleans)
Pediatrics 128:S8-S11, 2011

Background.—Hurricane Katrina caused more than 1800 deaths and over $80 billion in damage along the Gulf Coast in August, 2005. A neonatal physician at University Hospital in downtown New Orleans before, during, and after Hurricane Katrina hit that region recounts how neonatology care was accomplished under trying conditions and how it evolved thereafter. The hospital cared primarily for inner-city indigent families.

The Neonates.—All neonatal intensive care unit (NICU) patients at University Hospital survived both the storm and the evacuation. The two sickest NICU patients were premature infants with progressive chronic lung disease dependent on high-frequency ventilators. With no reliable power and running water the morning after the storm, these infants had to be transported through floodwaters by canoe and fire truck to Children's Hospital, then to a third hospital when Children's closed. One infant was eventually hospitalized in Fort Worth, Texas before being lost to follow-up. The other spent 3 months in Baton Rouge, Louisiana before returning to New Orleans. This infant was briefly hospitalized for a viral respiratory infection in the spring of 2006. One child was born preterm 4 days after Katrina made landfall to a mother hospitalized before the storm with threatened preterm labor. The equipment used to care for her was powered by a portable generator, and no routine services (blood gas determinations, laboratory studies, and radiographs) were offered. After 8 hours, she was transported along with 30 other NICU and well infants to Baton Rouge. Reuniting infants and families was challenging because of the city's evacuation and relocations to areas other than New Orleans.

The Hospital.—Both University and nearby Charity Hospital closed because of flood damage, so temporary emergency medical care was provided at other sites. Only after several months of repairs was full-service health care resumed. The first newborn infant after Katrina was delivered at University Hospital in February 2007. As patient volume grew, neonatal care was upgraded stepwise from level 2 to level 3. Over the next 3 years, delivery numbers plateaued at one fourth the volume pre-Katrina. In July 2010 the hospital closed obstetric and neonatal care services because of lack of patient volume and state budget cuts. In addition, many indigent residents did not return to the city and other area hospitals were preferred sites for obstetrics when University Hospital closed.

Evolution of NICU Care.—All three major tertiary care NICUs reopened and reestablished roles fairly quickly after Katrina. Of the nine hospital NICUs present before Katrina, one closed, one reopened without obstetric and neonatal services, two were sold, and one reopened but subsequently closed, so the network of care is four hospitals and the neonatology division is 8 staff members rather than 12.

New patterns in NICU patients developed post-Katrina. Hispanic workers flooded into the area, with a significant increase among NICU patients. Cultural and language barriers caused communication problems. In addition, more infants suffered symptoms of withdrawal from opiates, reflecting an increase in the illicit use of prescription narcotics.

Resident house staff served as key personnel in the prompt and safe evacuation of patients and in triage centers outside New Orleans. However, losing patient populations and training sites reduced educational opportunities. Most residents continued training through the creativity of residency program directors, the hospitality of medical education leaders across the South, and new patient care opportunities related to migrating Katrina evacuees. Training programs returned as New Orleans became repopulated. Graduating medical students often committed to urban residency training programs, but shifts in medical facilities made it difficult to match trainees and patient care sites. New outpatient opportunities have arisen with the development of decentralized outpatient clinics.

Assessment.—Efforts to improve flood-protection systems continue in southern Louisiana, recognizing the continuing threat of hurricanes and other natural disasters. Hospitals have developed mechanisms to allow the safe care or transport of critically ill patients. Depending on risks associated with hospital location and physical plant, some hospitals chose to prepare for patient evaluation and others planned for shelter in place. Hospitals that will evacuate NICU patients plan to use local, regional, and potentially national resources. Those that chose to shelter in place have preferred flood-zone status and enhanced physical plant preparations. Layers of safeguards are in place should local utilities fail, including raised generators to allow extended periods of electric power fueled by underground tanks, on-site wells to provide nonpotable water to cool chillers and dispose of human waste, and stockpiling of food, potable water, and hospital supplies. An elevated heliport allows for transport when typical ground routes are closed.

Efforts were tested in August 2008 when Hurricane Gustav threatened the Gulf Coast. Three million people sought shelter, area hospitals activated their plans, and neonatal patients were managed effectively, fine-tuning the hurricane preparations of New Orleans. Hurricane protection and preparedness in New Orleans are significantly better than pre-Katrina status. Preparation and resiliency and resourcefulness of communities and individuals to meet these challenges are key.

▶ This article reviews the impact of Hurricane Katrina on neonatal intensive care and the responses of the health care system at the time of the disaster and subsequently. Fortunately, in the United States, disasters, natural or man-made, rarely dramatically impact our ability to care for our patients. Nonetheless, it is important that physicians take leadership roles in preparing for those events. As outlined in this article, hospital and community leaders must evaluate each hospital's ability to function safely so that plans can be made to either shelter or evacuate patients. In addition, as the author illustrates, the impact of these events on health care workers is significant, and in the aftermath of a disaster, these issues must be addressed. In recent months, severe storms have impacted our patients and health care systems in several Southern and

Midwestern states. These events should remind us all that each community must be effectively prepared.

S. Black, MD

Paid Malpractice Claims for Adverse Events in Inpatient and Outpatient Settings
Bishop TF, Ryan AM, Casalino LP (Weill Cornell Med College, NY)
JAMA 305:2427-2431, 2011

Context.—An analysis of paid malpractice claims may provide insight into the prevalence and seriousness of adverse medical events in the outpatient setting.

Objective.—To report and compare the number, magnitude, and type of paid malpractice claims for events in inpatient and outpatient settings.

Design and Setting.—Retrospective analysis of malpractice claims paid on behalf of physicians in outpatient and inpatient settings using data from the National Practitioner Data Bank from 2005 through 2009. We evaluated trends in claims paid by setting, characteristics of paid claims, and factors associated with payment amount.

Main Outcome Measures.—Number of paid claims, mean and median payment amounts, types of errors, and outcomes of errors.

Results.—In 2009, there were 10 739 malpractice claims paid on behalf of physicians. Of these paid claims, 4910 (47.6%; 95% confidence interval [CI], 46.6%-48.5%) were for events in the inpatient setting, 4448 (43.1%; 95% CI, 42.1%-44.0%) were for events in the outpatient setting, and 966 (9.4%; 95% CI, 8.8%-9.9%) involved events in both settings. The proportion of payments for events in the outpatient setting increased by a small but statistically significant amount, from 41.7% (95% CI, 40.9%- 42.6%) in 2005 to 43.1% (95% CI, 42.1%-44.0%) in 2009 ($P<.001$ for trend across years). In the outpatient setting, the most common reason for a paid claim was diagnostic (45.9%; 95% CI, 44.4%-47.4%), whereas in the inpatient setting the most common reason was surgical (34.1%; 95% CI, 32.8%-35.4%). Major injury and death were the 2 most common outcomes in both settings. Mean payment amount for events in the inpatient setting was significantly higher than in the outpatient setting ($362 965; 95% CI, $348 192-$377 738 vs $290 111; 95% CI, $278 289-$301 934; $P<.001$).

Conclusion.—In 2009, the number of paid malpractice claims reported to the National Practitioner Data Bank for events in the outpatient setting was similar to the number in the inpatient setting.

▶ Outpatient settings where surgery has migrated face considerable risk of malpractice claims. What is unusual is how low the payout numbers are for anesthesia providers compared with everything else. Clearly, we should take pride in the Anesthesia Patient Safety Foundation (APSF) and in the leadership anesthesia as a specialty has shown. The APSF has made the perioperative period safer and made us less the targets of malpractice claims because we are better able to justify what we do.

M. F. Roizen, MD

Article Index

Chapter 1: Studies of Outcomes, Risks, Costs, and Benefits

Chapter 4: Cardiothoracic and Vascular Anesthesia

Chapter 5: Pediatric Anesthesia

Chapter 6: Head Injury and Neuroanesthesia

Chapter 7: Critical Care Medicine

Chapter 8: Other Perioperative Patient Care Issues

Chapter 9: Patient Safety, Complications, and Mishaps in Anesthesia

Chapter 10: Obstetric Anesthesia

Chapter 11: Pain Management

Author Index

Printed and bound by CPI Group (UK) Ltd, Croydon, CR0 4YY

08/05/2025

01864678-0015